CULVER PUBLIC LIBRARY

SE 05 07

15.00

8/07

Baby Bites

Bridget Swinney, MS, RD

Meadowbrook Press
Distributed by Simon & Schuster
New York

D1376859

Library of Congress Cataloging-in-Publication Data

Swinney, Bridget, 1960-
  Baby bites : homemade food for healthy babies from birth to two / by Bridget Swinney.
     p. cm.
  ISBN-10: 0-88166-495-2, ISBN-13: 978-0-88166-495-9 (Meadowbrook Press); ISBN-10: 0-684-04003-4,
  ISBN-13: 978-0-684-04003-5 (Simon & Schuster)
  1. Infants—Nutrition. 2. Cookery. I. Title.
  RJ216.S924 2007
  641.5'6222—dc22

                                        2006015537

Editors: Christine Zuchora-Walske, Angela Wiechmann
Proofreader: Alicia Ester
Production Manager: Paul Woods
Graphic Design Manager: Tamara Peterson
Desktop Publisher: Danielle White
Cover Photos: © Ariel Skelley/CORBIS, © Norbert Schaefer/CORBIS
Interior Photos: Val Escher
Food Styling: Mike Menner
Index: Beverlee Day

Text © 2007 by Bridget Swinney

All rights reserved. No part of this book may be reproduced or transmitted in any form or by
any means, electronic or mechanical, including photocopying, recording, or using any information
storage and retrieval system, without written permission from the publisher, except in the case of
brief quotations embodied in critical articles and reviews.

"Positioning," "Latch," and "Frequency" stories on pages 44–45 reprinted with permission:
Karen Peters, MBA, RD, IBCLC. Lactation Case Studies. WHRN Report, Winter 2005, page 5.
American Dietetic Association.

"New England Fish Chowder" recipe on page 281, "Quick and Healthy Tortilla Soup" on page 316
are modified from *Quick and Healthy: Low-Fat, Carb-Conscious Cooking* by Brenda Ponichtera, used
with permission.

The contents of this book have been reviewed and checked for accuracy and appropriateness by
professionals in the field of nutrition. However, the author, editors, reviewers, and publisher disclaim
all responsibility arising from any adverse effects or results that occur or might occur as a result of the
inappropriate application of any of the information contained in this book. If you have a question or
concern about any of the information in this book, consult your healthcare professional.

Published by Meadowbrook Press, 5451 Smetana Drive, Minnetonka, MN 55343

www.meadowbrookpress.com

BOOK TRADE DISTRIBUTION by Simon and Schuster, a division of Simon and Schuster, Inc.,
1230 Avenue of the Americas, New York, NY 10020

12 11 10 09 08 07   10 9 8 7 6 5 4 3 2 1

Printed in the United States of America

Dedication

For all babies and those who care for them.
And especially for the new babies in our family:
Addie, Aidan, Emily, Josh, Ethan, and Elaine

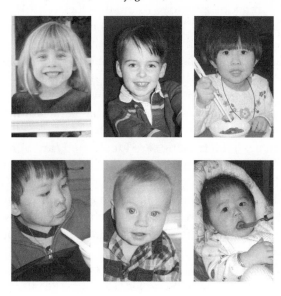

And for our "babies," Nicolas and Robert,
who taught us so much about feeding kids!

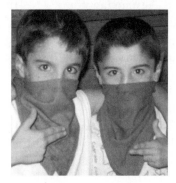

Acknowledgments

Birthing this book has been a labor of love, but it's been a very long labor of love with many complications! Life got in the way more than a few times. Death, birth, illness, jobs, kids, traveling, remodeling disasters—you name it, it happened to the people involved in this book (mostly to me)! We sometimes wondered if this book would ever be born. Luckily for our readers we all stuck with it, through many late nights and weekends (with the help of copious caffeine and chocolate). So I have a lot of people to thank!

First I have to thank my sweet husband, Frank. He has cooked, cleaned, done the laundry, chauffeured kids, provided round-the-clock technical support, and otherwise picked up the pieces of my life while I was researching, writing, cooking for, and revising *Baby Bites*. I couldn't have done it without him!

Next I must thank my sons, Nicolas and Robert. They pitched in when they could, gave advice ("Just finish it!"), offered lots of hugs, and were patient when I couldn't do everything for them that I or they wanted. They even tasted some of the recipes! Most importantly, they provided the hands-on infant feeding and parenting experience that made this book possible.

To my sisters, Colleen (for making sure I took good care of myself) and Judy (my cheerleader): Thank you both for always being there. My father would have been very proud to see another book under my belt, but he passed on before I finished this one. I thank him, too, for his lifelong encouragement and for the positive phrases that still pop into my mind during tough times.

Merci beaucoup to my French family, Nicole and Jean-Yves, for taking care of our household during their visits and for their many encouraging words.

Thank you to John York, MD, FACAAI, our family's board-certified allergist, for his insights on allergy prevention and for reviewing the allergy info in this book. Thanks also to our friends Pat Mitchell, DDS, and Gary Bourgeois, DDS, for reviewing the dental sections of the book. *Merci* to Christina Blais, MSc, DtP, from the University of Montreal for her help with metric conversions. Thanks to Laura Jana, MD, FAAP; Jennifer Shu, MD, FAAP (authors of *Heading Home with Your Newborn*); and Tanya Remers Altman (author of *The Wonder Years*) for their assistance. Thanks to Karen Peters, IBCLC, for her informative breastfeeding case studies. Thanks to my long-time author/dietitian friends, Connie Evers (author of *How to Teach Nutrition to Kids*) and Brenda Ponichtera (author of the Quick and Healthy cookbook series), for their continued support and to Brenda for use of recipes from her book.

Thanks to my friends and family: John and Alicia, Annette and Robert, Debbie, Peggy and Mark, "the TLC" group, and Beatriz. Thanks to my nieces and nephews, Addie, Aidan, Ethan, Emily, Joshua, and Elaine, and to their parents for sharing their feeding stories. Special thanks to the Do family, the Jamison family, and the Holland family for taste-testing. And thanks to all the moms and one granddad who shared their stories with me and you.

Last but definitely not least, I offer my gratitude to my publisher, Bruce Lansky, and my editors, Christine Zuchora-Walske and Angie Wiechmann. (I'm very lucky to have picked a publisher who hires only smart, beautiful, compassionate people who have a sense of humor. Of course, they do live in the land of Lake Wobegon....) Bruce, thanks for setting *Baby Bites* back on course and hopefully sending it on to be a bestseller. Angie, thanks for pinch-hitting and offering an objective eye as the only person on this project without kids. Christine, we didn't always see eye-to-eye, but in the end we created an awesome book (even if we did have to eat a little extra chocolate to get through it). I thank you for your thoroughness and dedication, and I hope the chocolate you ate was especially high in antioxidants.

Special thanks to Christine's family: her husband, Ron, for being super-supportive, and her kids, Tony (four years) and Maria (one year), who provided considerable insight and personal food recommendations. They also had to sacrifice some quality time with mom so this book could go to press. I'm especially grateful for that.

Finally, thanks to all the people who made this book look great: Tami, Val, Mike, Dani, and Paul. And thanks to those whose work is just beginning: Jennifer and Michael.

Contents

Foreword

What can you as a parent or caregiver do to get your little one on track for a healthy food future? Plenty. By reading this book, you're arming yourself with nutrition information and practical advice for each step of your upcoming journey through breast milk or formula, cereals, and solids.

As a pediatrician, every day I see supersize children living on fast-food nutrition and couch potato fitness. And these overweight children not only suffer from adult diseases such as diabetes, high cholesterol, and heart disease, but they also have much higher rates of depression, school failure, and lower self-esteem.

Baby Bites is an excellent all-in-one guide on how to provide the best nutrition possible for your newborn, toddler, and preschooler and how to ensure that he or she continues to enjoy a life of healthy food habits for years to come.

With the tips for success in *Baby Bites*, you can get your child's nutrition off to the right start by breastfeeding, if possible. Breastfeeding provides your infant with the best possible first food for growth and development. In addition, breastfed babies have lower rates of illness, allergies, and childhood obesity than formula-fed babies. When it's time to start solids, think healthy and colorful. Infants will usually eat whatever you give them (although it may take several attempts), so why not get them used to eating a variety of pretty-colored veggies and whole grains as well as drinking water instead of juice and soda? Keep meals and snacks at the table with the family as much as possible, not in front of the television or in the bedroom.

Most of parenthood can be fun and fabulous, but it's rarely a smooth ride. When it comes to nutrition, you're definitely in for some bottle battles and food fights along the way. This book will walk you through which ones are worth fighting, such as not letting your toddler eat only animal crackers three meals a day, and which ones you can let slide, such as giving your toddler orange veggies and hiding those green ones creatively wherever you can.

When it comes to nutrition, the list of delicious, kid-approved recipes in *Baby Bites* is a great place to start. After all, proper nutrition is the building block for your infant's growth and development. And the first few years are crucial for brain, body, and immune system development. It's really amazing to watch your dependent newborn evolve into an individual who can walk, talk, and make his or her own decisions—hopefully healthy ones.

As a parent or caregiver, you are the best role model for your kids. Healthy habits start young, so encourage age-appropriate portions of naturally healthy food. Although it may not always seem so, kids aim to please their parents and like to do as their parents do. By following *Baby Bites*, you can set a healthy example they will want to emulate for life.

Tanya Remer Altmann, MD, FAAP

Pediatrician and Mom

Editor-in-Chief of *The Wonder Years: Helping Your Baby and Young Child*
Successfully Negotiate the Major Developmental Milestones

Executive Board Member, American Academy of Pediatrics Section on Media

Introduction

Good Health Starts with Good Nutrition

Congratulations on taking the first step toward good nutrition for your child!

Why is infant and toddler nutrition so important? Your baby grows by leaps and bounds in the first year, doubling in length and tripling in weight. Brain, vision, and immune system development continue into the second year. Good nutrition provides the building materials for all this growth and development. Good nutrition also sets the stage for a lifetime of healthy eating, which can prevent childhood obesity and a host of other health problems.

The Learning Curve

I speak with hundreds of new parents every year, and they're all hungry for trust-worthy, practical advice about feeding their babies. I was the same way as a new mom. I've never felt more helpless than I did when we first brought Nicolas home from the hospital. There I was with a crying baby and *no instruction book*! You may be lucky enough to have extended family close by, but I didn't—that makes the going a little rougher. I thought feeding my baby would come naturally, but I found there was more to it than intuition and common sense. Even being a dietitian didn't help me much. I needed a few seasoned pros to show me the way.

Now I'm the seasoned pro. Not only did Nicolas and I survive those tough early days, I went back for another round with my second son, Robert. (He survived, too.) I've learned—and continue to learn—new tricks along the way from my boys, my professional research, and the parent network. The parent network is an ever-changing, invaluable tool to help you find a good doctor, learn where diapers are on sale, and get hints on how to sneak veggies into your kid's diet.

Since my boys were little, the parent network has expanded from everyday acquaintances made at work, school, playgroup, or the gym to include those made on the Internet. The Internet is a great source of parenting information and support—but it can also be a source of confusion. If you've ever visited a forum on infant feeding, you know what I mean. Sometimes it's hard to tell fact from fiction....

How Baby Bites *Can Help You*

...And that's where *Baby Bites* comes in. It's the only book that has everything you need to know about feeding your baby from birth to preschool. Some books just discuss one aspect of infant feeding—such as breastfeeding or making baby food. This book has it all!

Evidence-based and real-world–tested, *Baby Bites* is easy to read, sprinkled with humor, and packed with advice from experts—both professional and parental. Here's what you'll find in its fact-filled, friendly pages:

- Key info to consider before your baby's born, to help you make sound decisions and get prepared

- Feeding advice for the entire first two years and beyond, including breastfeeding, formula-feeding, starting solids, transitioning to table foods, dealing with toddler quirks, and everything in-between

- "Tales from the Trenches"—examples and ideas from parents in the thick of it

- How to eat well and lose weight—easily and safely—while breastfeeding (or not)

- The full scoop on your child's digestive system, including all the dirty details you need to deal with poop, spit-up, gas, colic, intolerances, and more

- A chapter explaining the basics of nutrition, how diet affects your child's health, and how to provide balanced nutrition for kids with special dietary needs such as allergies or veganism

- A step-by-step guide to making quick, tasty, healthy meals for babies and toddlers, including dozens of menus and recipes complete with nutrient information

- Insights on developing healthy eating habits and preventing childhood obesity

I hope the knowledge you gain from *Baby Bites* brings you confidence, peace of mind, and a happy, healthy family! I'd love to hear from you personally; you can email me at: bridget@healthyfoodzone.com.

Part 1

The
Liquid Diet

Chapter 1

Getting Ready for Your New Arrival

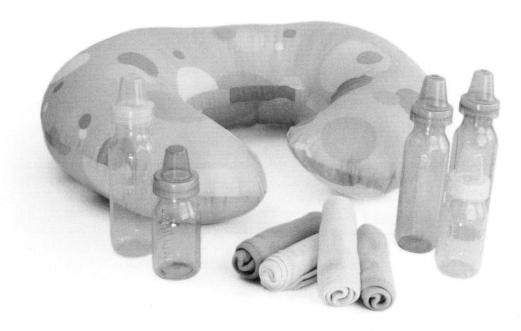

A baby will make love stronger, days shorter, nights longer, bankroll smaller, home happier, clothes shabbier, the past forgotten, and the future worth living for.

—Anonymous

Why Nutrition Is Job One

Chances are, you're an expectant or new parent (or possibly a grandparent) looking for advice on feeding your baby (or grandbaby). Congratulations and welcome to parenthood!

You probably already know that nutrition plays an important role in shaping your baby's future. Here are just a few examples that show nutrition's profound effect on health:

- Breastfeeding can postpone, minimize, or prevent a multitude of health problems in babies, including allergies, asthma, diabetes, and Crohn's disease. In fact, breastfeeding can be a matter of life and death: In the United States, infants who aren't breastfed have a death rate 21 percent higher than that of breastfed infants. Breastfeeding may also be associated with lower blood pressure in children and adults.[1]

- Breastfeeding reduces maternal risk of osteoporosis and some cancers.

- Breastfeeding while eating a diet rich in omega-3 fatty acids provides the nutrients needed for baby's optimum brain development.

- Timing of starting solid foods is important. Introducing them before fifteen weeks increases childhood respiratory illness as well as body fat and weight in childhood.[2]

- Good nutrition prevents iron deficiency. Severe iron deficiency anemia during the first year can cause cognitive problems up to ten years later.

- Following a baby's feeding cues lays the groundwork for a healthy body image and a healthy relationship with food later in life.

- Research shows that negative parental attitudes about feeding—especially being overly concerned about weight and restrictive with food—can lead to obesity in childhood.[3, 4]

- One in every seventeen children under three years has a food allergy. How a child is fed from day one can prevent or postpone allergy development.

The habits you start now can prevent your child from being overweight later. Normally this wouldn't be a topic for a baby book, but childhood obesity is now our number-one health crisis. And kids' eating habits are degrading earlier and earlier. (The most often eaten vegetable of two-year-olds is French fries!)

If you offer your child a consistently healthy diet and also model good choices, chances are very good that you'll have a child with lifelong good eating habits—and a lifetime of good health to go with it.

Your First Big Decision: Infant Feeding

While there's no question that breastfeeding is the best food for babies, North America has been mainly a formula-feeding culture for almost a century. As a result, infant feeding is an emotionally charged topic in these parts.

Will you breastfeed or formula-feed—or both? If, like most parents, you want to breastfeed, take heart: Breastfeeding rates are rebounding—not only in North America, but also around the world:[5]

Breastfeeding Rates Worldwide

Country	Breastfeeding at Birth	Breastfeeding at 4 or 6 Months[6, 7]
United States	70%	33%
Canada	72%	31%
United Kingdom	69%	21%
Sweden	98%	73%
India	95%	43%
Australia	87%	48%
New Zealand	94%	56%

*Rates are for either exclusively or partially breastfeeding at either 4 or 6 months, depending on how data is collected.

Even if you've chosen not to breastfeed, I recommend you read this section before you make your final decision. Why? Because I want to make sure you've had a chance to evaluate all the facts. Perhaps you heard about a friend's breastfeeding difficulties and chose formula then and there. Maybe you can't figure out how to fit breastfeeding into the logistics of your life.

I respect the need for parents to determine what's best for their families. But I also think many parents don't realize that successful breastfeeding is possible for the vast majority of mothers and babies, and that there are very few situations completely incompatible with breastfeeding. Breastfeeding is so important to your baby's and your health that even if you can do it for only a month or can nurse only part-time, it's well worth the effort.

Important Facts about Breastfeeding

I'll discuss the importance of breastfeeding in detail in Chapter 2. Here I'd like to share with you its most impressive health effects.

Why Breastfeeding Is the Best Way to Feed Babies[8]

- Breastfeeding protects your baby in the short term from sudden infant death syndrome (SIDS) and illnesses like ear infections, respiratory infections, urinary tract infections, diarrhea, bacterial meningitis, and gastrointestinal infections.

- Breastfeeding protects your baby in the long term from conditions like type 1 and type 2 diabetes, Crohn's disease, lymphoma, leukemia, high cholesterol, high blood pressure,[9] asthma, and obesity.

- Breast milk naturally contains a vital brain-building nutrient called docosahexaenoic acid (DHA). Some researchers conclude that this is why breastfed children tend to have higher IQs. (For more information on DHA in breast milk, see page 62.)

- Breastfeeding during a painful procedure like a vaccination or heel prick actually provides some pain relief.
- Breastfeeding appears to provide protection against high blood pressure in childhood. In fact, exclusive breastfeeding in infancy is as effective as a low-salt diet and physical activity in controlling hypertension in adulthood.[10]
- The nutrient makeup of breast milk varies according to the changing needs of each unique baby, and is even more beneficial for low birth weight and very low birth weight infants.

Breastfeeding Is Important for Moms, Too

Health[11]

- Breastfeeding releases oxytocin, which helps a mom's uterus contract to its normal size promptly, which in turn controls postpartum bleeding and helps prevent anemia.
- Exclusive, on-demand breastfeeding usually suppresses ovulation and provides natural birth control.
- Breastfeeding lowers a woman's risk of ovarian and breast cancers.
- Breastfeeding may lower a woman's risk of hip fractures and osteoporosis.
- Breastfeeding burns calories, which helps moms lose their pregnancy weight while eating very well.
- Breastfeeding longer than four months lowers a woman's risk of developing rheumatoid arthritis. Breastfeeding a total of twenty-four months cuts a woman's risk by 50 percent.[12]
- Thanks to oxytocin and prolactin, breastfeeding women may have a better mental outlook—lower perceived stress, anger, and depression—than formula-feeding moms.[13]

Cost

- Breastfeeding is free! (Formula, on the other hand, can be expensive.)
- Breastfeeding gives babies their best chance at good health. (Formula-fed babies tend to get sick more often than breastfed babies.) By breastfeeding, moms can minimize their healthcare costs and time away from work.
- Breastfeeding is ecologically sound. Formula manufacturing, packaging, distribution, and disposal take a toll on the environment. Breastfeeding moms avoid contributing to this problem.
- At least 3.6 billion dollars would be saved in the United States alone if its breastfeeding rate increased from 2001 levels (64 percent at birth, 29 percent at six months) to those recommended by the U.S. Surgeon General (75 percent at birth, 50 percent at six months). This figure represents cost savings from the treatment of only three childhood illnesses: otitis media (ear infection), gastroenteritis, and necrotizing enterocolitis.[14]

Convenience

- Breast milk is always fresh, warm, and ready to serve. No shopping, toting, or preparation is ever necessary.

Breastfeeding Challenges

If any of the following situations affect you, breastfeeding your baby could be challenging. The more time you have to educate yourself and prepare, the better. Remember that even in these situations, you most likely will be able to breastfeed exclusively. In fact, if your child has health problems, breastfeeding will be vital to his or her healing, growth, and development.

- **Multiples (twins, triplets, or more)**: If you're expecting multiple babies, breastfeeding them may well be easier than you think. Tandem feeding, a twin nursing pillow, and a bit of experienced advice will get you a long way. If your babies are born prematurely, you may face some additional challenges—but not insurmountable ones. (See page 55 for more on nursing preemies. For information on nursing multiples, visit http://www.lalecheleague.org/NB/NBmultiples.html.)

- **Congenital disorders**: If your baby has Down syndrome, cleft lip and/or palate, phenylketonuria (PKU), autism, or another congenital disorder, breastfeeding may be difficult. But it's almost always in your baby's best interest, and it's almost always possible. Depending on your baby's condition, pumping and bottle-feeding, using a supplemental nursing system (SNS), or supplementing with a special formula may be in order. Enlist support from your child's doctor and a lactation consultant experienced with special needs. You might find it helpful to read La Leche League's information on breastfeeding babies with disabilities at www.lalecheleague.org/NB/NBdisabled.html.

- **Prematurity**: If your baby is born prematurely, you'll make milk suited perfectly to his or her needs. Your milk will be extremely important to help your baby survive and thrive. It'll help prevent infection, reduce the risk and severity of necrotizing enterocolitis and retinopathy of prematurity, and promote optimum cognitive development.[15] Your baby's gestational age, strength of suck, and other health issues may necessitate pumping your milk for a while, but chances are good that your baby will eventually transition to the breast. (See pages 55–56 for more on nursing preemies.)

- **Cesarean section**: C-sections can interfere with breastfeeding initiation for many reasons: incision pain, positioning problems, medication, separation of mother and baby, absence of some hormonal cues from labor, and so on. Nonetheless, plenty of C-section veterans successfully nurse their babies—sometimes two or three of them! It pays to think through the possibility of C-section ahead of time so you can add your success story to the list. If you do end up with a C-section, you'll know how important it is to keep your baby close and to nurse as soon and as often as possible. You'll also know some nursing positions that keep the pressure off your incision. (For more information on positions, see page 39. For a thorough discussion of breastfeeding after cesarean, visit http://www.plus-size-pregnancy.org/CSANDVBAC/bfaftercesarean.htm.)

- **Breast surgery**: Breast surgery may or may not affect your ability to breastfeed. Generally speaking, you can breastfeed if your nipples have not been moved and your ducts have not been cut. If you've had breast reduction, augmentation, lumpectomy, or other surgery on your breasts, your surgeon will know best how much your milk ducts are affected. Discuss with your surgeon your desire to breastfeed. Also, make sure your child's doctor knows about your breast surgery so he or she can monitor your baby's growth closely. (For more information about breastfeeding after surgery, see http://www.lalecheleague.org/NB/NBsurgery.html and http://www.bfar.org.)

- **Maternal illness or chronic health condition**: Virtually all conditions are compatible with breastfeeding, including those in the following list.[16] If you need medication, request a drug that's compatible with breastfeeding. Most medications are—and for those that aren't, there's almost always a safe alternative. As always, if you have concerns, discuss them with your doctor.
  - Common illnesses like cold, sore throat, flu, stomach virus, fever, and mastitis
  - Food poisoning (If it has progressed to septicemia, breastfeeding may continue—possibly after a temporary suspension—along with antibiotic therapy.)
  - Diabetes
  - Lyme disease
  - West Nile virus
  - Hepatitis B surface antigen–positive and hepatitis C
  - Exposure to low-level environmental chemical agents
  - Seropositive carrier of cytomegalovirus (CMV) (If your baby is low birth weight, discuss breastfeeding with your baby's doctor.)
  - Polycystic ovarian syndrome (PCOS)
  - Hypothyroidism and hyperthyroidism

According to the American Academy of Pediatrics (AAP), breastfeeding may not be in your baby's best interest if any of the following rare conditions is present.[17] Discuss breastfeeding with your baby's doctor.

- Untreated tuberculosis
- Human T-cell lymphotropic virus type 1 or 2 (HTLV-1 or HTLV-2)
- Exposure to diagnostic or therapeutic radioactive isotopes or other radioactive materials (for as long as there is radioactivity in breast milk)
- Receiving antimetabolites or chemotherapeutic agents
- Drug abuse
- Herpes simplex with breast lesions (Breastfeeding on the breast without lesions is safe.)
- Human immunodeficiency virus (HIV)

Important Facts about Formula-Feeding

Chapter 4 discusses the details of formula-feeding. Here I'll share with you the key facts you should know about formula:

- Infant formula is the only safe substitute for breast milk.

- Although formula manufacturers try to imitate breast milk, and today's formulas are better than ever, formula will *never* match breast milk. Breast milk contains components that are impossible to reproduce in a lab, and breast milk is a living fluid that changes according to the needs of your baby.

- Because formula is harder to digest than breast milk, your baby will take longer to digest it and will have stinkier poop.

- Depending on the brand and type, formula can cost $2.61 to $7.83 per day (as of October 2006). Exclusively formula-feeding a baby for one year can cost $700 to $3,100 for formula alone.

- If you give birth in a hospital, you may receive formula samples there. Your caregiver or your baby's caregiver may also provide samples or use products that promote formula. This doesn't mean that you should formula-feed, or that the hospital or caregiver recommends a particular brand of formula.

- Around the world, formula is regulated by the Codex Alimentarius (food code), which was developed by the Food and Agriculture Organization of the United Nations (FAO) and the World Health Organization (WHO). The Codex establishes minimal amounts of nutrients that formula must contain. In the U.S., the Food and Drug Administration (FDA) regulates formula ingredients, manufacturing, and packaging by enforcing the Infant Formula Act, a U.S. law that follows the Codex. The regulations give formula companies a lot of flexibility in choosing ingredients, vitamin formulations, and so on. This is how formula ads can tout their differences even though formula is heavily regulated.

- There are three basic types of formula: cow's milk–based, soy-based, and hypoallergenic. (In hypoallergenic formulas, the protein molecules are broken into smaller, more digestible parts.) Among these three basic types, there are also lactose-free formulas and formulas tweaked for other problems your baby might have.

- Formula comes in three forms: ready-to-feed, concentrated, and powdered. Ready-to-feed is the most expensive, and powdered is the cheapest. Although the ingredients are exactly the same (with varying amounts of water), these formulas, when prepared, look slightly different from each other.

Getting Organized

If these two words strike fear in your heart, don't worry. I've been there, and I know how you feel.

When I was expecting my first son, my oldest sister, already the mother of grown boys, said, "You need to get organized." I'm sure the blank look on my face puzzled her. You see, I'm not a natural organizer. (I blame it on my creative-thinking skills.) But my sister was right: It really did help to get organized before Nicolas was born.

Now I'll play "big sister" for you. Having two kids, writing three books, and assuming the role of planner and organizer for a preteen, a teenager, and a husband have taught me a lot about getting my ducks in a row. Ready? Here we go.

The Two Most Important Places in Your Home

People have written entire books about getting organized for a new baby. There certainly is a lot that can be said about preparing for a helpless new addition to your family. But instead of trying to say it all here, I'll focus on the areas where parents of newborns spend most of their time. Daily life in your home will soon revolve around feeding—and its inevitable result, changing.

A Feeding Place

Since you'll be spending a lot of time feeding, it makes sense to set up a feeding place for maximum comfort and convenience. Here are some items you may want in your feeding place:

- **Chair**: Choose a chair that supports your entire body (head, shoulders, back, arms, and bottom) comfortably. Babies—especially newborns—eat often, and they can be really poky! Getting a sore rear or a stiff back from feeding would be a bummer. I recommend a cushioned rocking chair, a glider, an overstuffed easy chair, or a recliner. It's not unusual for nursing moms to fall asleep while feeding, so choose a chair you won't topple out of.

- **Pillows**: A pillow on your lap in the feeding chair provides a resting place for your arms and brings your baby to the correct height for feeding. (A C-shaped nursing pillow is especially handy, but any pillow will do.) Using a pillow for feedings can prevent bad positioning and muscle aches and help you relax while feeding. You may also find pillows helpful for positioning you and your baby during night feedings in bed.

- **Footstool**: Feeding sessions may be the only times you get to sit down. Make the most of them by putting your feet up! When you're nursing, a footstool also helps bring your lap to the proper height for feeding.

- **Side table**: A small table next to your feeding chair is handy for holding things you might want while feeding: a glass of water, a snack, a notepad, a book, the phone, and so on.

- **Kid-size chair**: A kid-size chair can help you include an older child in the feeding process and ease his or her adjustment to the new baby. For example, some moms find feedings a good time to talk or read with their older kids.

A Changing Place

Because feeding will usually inspire your baby to poop and/or pee, you'll be changing diapers almost as often as you feed. Having a handy changing place will make your life a lot easier.

If your place is small, one changing station should do the trick. If your home is big and you tend to roam all over it, you might want more. For example, you might set up one station in the room where your baby sleeps and one in the room where you spend most of your time. In our house, the baby's room was always upstairs—a long way to go to change a diaper—so I made a small changing station in the family room.

Here are some items you may want at your changing place(s):

- **Changing table, changing pad, or blanket**: I never owned a changing table. At the time, it seemed like an unnecessary expense. We made do with a blanket on the couch when our boys were newborns, followed by a blanket on the floor. (One advantage of using a towel or blanket on the floor is that you don't have to worry about your baby rolling off and getting hurt.) Use whatever works best for you.
- **Diapering supplies**: Keep a stash of diapers, wipes, and diaper cream within reach at your changing place(s).
- **Clean outfit**: Even the best diapers leak sometimes, and it's nice to have a clean onesie or sleeper at hand when you're changing a blowout.
- **Gizmos and gadgets**: If you're into gadgets, there certainly are a lot of diapering gizmos you can buy: a wipe warmer, a Diaper Genie, a Wee Block (for boys), and so on. Your baby will be just fine without these things, but they may make life more comfortable for you.

Setting Priorities

When you have a newborn, your old priorities go out the window. Obviously, caring for your baby will take top priority now because your baby is helpless without you. But don't forget to take care of yourself, too. If you don't recharge your own batteries occasionally, you'll be of no use to that baby!

Before having your baby, you were probably used to controlling your own schedule. It's disorienting to suddenly lose that control when you become a parent. Now your day is dictated by your baby's relentless, ever-changing needs. Don't worry, you'll get used to it! Just remember that you really do need to follow your baby's lead. Your baby learns to trust you when you meet his or her needs promptly, and this secure attachment to you is vital for normal development.

When you do have time of your own, which may be rare the first weeks, you'll need to use it wisely. Your top three personal priorities should be sleep and rest, staying healthy and hydrated, and enjoying your baby. Everything else is just icing on the cake! Here's how your first month might look:

First Week

- Sleep when your baby sleeps.
- Housework? Ha!
- Don't feel bad if you never manage to shower some days.
- Unless you're expecting someone besides friends or family, it's okay to stay in your pajamas!
- Let someone else shop for you or postpone shopping until next week.

Second Week

- Refresh your memory by reading baby-care books.
- You might want to think about picking up the house a bit—then again, you might not.
- Let your partner or a friend stay with your baby during naptime while you:
    - Take a walk.
    - Take a shower.
    - Go to the grocery store.
    - Just get out of the house.

Third Week

By the third week, you and your baby should be getting into a rhythm. You might feel comfortable venturing out together now. (Or you might not, which is also okay.) Avoid taking your baby to crowded places for a couple more weeks, though; your baby's immature immune system makes him or her susceptible to airborne illnesses.

If this is your first baby, you may find that just getting out the door is an adventure. Depending on where you're going and what the weather's like, you may find yourself lugging a car seat, a diaper bag, and a stroller or baby carrier. And don't forget your appropriately-dressed baby! Whew—it's a lot to think about. But don't worry: It'll get easier as you get used to preparing for excursions.

Here's what might make sense the third week of your baby's life:

- Take a long, long, shower.
- List things you really need to do or buy. Forget about the nonessentials.
- Pick one task on your list for each day. (For example, you might have laundry day, bill-paying day, and so on.) When my boys were little, this system made my responsibilities more manageable and helped me feel I was actually accomplishing something. Without it, I found myself doing each task constantly, which was exhausting and demoralizing.

Fourth Week

By this time, you'll probably feel comfortable taking your baby out. If venturing out of the house with your baby still seems daunting, try to nudge the edges of your comfort zone. A change of scenery is good for both you and your baby.

You should be well on your way to full recovery from birth, unless you had a C-section. You should also be turning the corner on any breastfeeding discomfort.

If you'll be going back to work full-time, consider introducing expressed breast milk by bottle or cup this week. This is also a good time to start stocking your freezer with breast milk. (See Chapter 5 for more tips on preparing for your return to work.)

If you'll return to work only part-time, you may or may not need to express milk for your baby while you're away. If your baby wants to feed while you're gone, he or she will need to learn to drink from a bottle or cup. Some babies, however, decide to just wait for their moms (often sleeping through the separation) and tank up when they're together. Only time will tell which type of baby yours will be, so be prepared for either.

Chapter 2

Breastfeeding

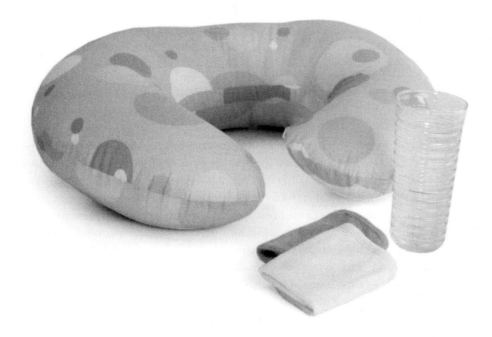

I just pulled up my shirt, stood off to the side, and did it.
Everyone was pretty mature about it.

—Joy Fawcett, Olympic soccer champion

Breast milk truly is liquid gold. No other food approaches its amazing properties or is anywhere near as important to humans. It's a living fluid, containing antibodies to protect babies from illness; healthy bacteria that prevent the growth of harmful bacteria; macrophages that kill harmful bacteria, fungi, and viruses; nucleotides to help babies' developing immune systems; and other immunological compounds such as interferon and complement, T and B lymphocytes, and many types of hormones. Breast milk constantly changes to meet babies' immune and growth needs. Babies are never allergic to their mothers' milk (though they're occasionally allergic to foods their mothers eat). Suckling at the breast promotes good jaw development and straight, healthy teeth. And that's just the beginning: Breastfeeding also provides countless developmental, psychological, social, and environmental benefits necessary for healthy children and a healthy world.

The Amazing Traits of Breast Milk

What makes breast milk so powerful? It contains more than two hundred amazing, ever-changing ingredients—so many and so complex that there are whole textbooks on the subject! On the following pages I'll summarize breast milk's most important traits.

Tailored to Your Baby's Needs

Before I explain the components of mom's milk, I need to point out one important feature of these ingredients: They're always changing to meet the physiological needs of *your* baby.

First of all, your milk changes as your baby ages:

- **Colostrum**: For the first few days after your baby's birth, your breasts produce small amounts of colostrum—perfect for your newborn's marble-size stomach. Colostrum is very digestible and has a laxative effect, which encourages your baby to pass meconium (first poop). This, in turn, encourages your baby to feed more, which encourages more pooping (and so on), which prevents or alleviates jaundice. Colostrum is rich in antibodies tailored to your surroundings. It's also rich in sodium, potassium, chloride, and cholesterol to encourage optimal heart, brain, and nervous system development. Its high protein content defends your baby against infection, helps your baby's body grow and develop, and stabilizes your baby's blood sugar. Its yellowish color comes from beta carotene, an antioxidant the liver converts to vitamin A.

- **Transitional milk**: From a few days postpartum until about two weeks postpartum, your milk changes from colostrum to mature milk. During this period it's called transitional milk. Its texture gets thinner, and its color becomes creamier. Its protein and immunoglobulins decrease while its lactose, fat, calories, and quantity increase to meet your baby's accelerating growth needs.

- **Mature milk**: The transition to mature milk is usually complete two weeks after your baby's birth. Mature milk is about 90 percent water to keep your baby hydrated. The other 10 percent is carbohydrates, proteins, and fats in quantities tailored to your baby's growth and energy needs. Mature milk contains fewer antibodies than do colostrum and transitional milk, but it contains dramatically more macrophages (white blood cells that gobble up bacteria and other foreign bodies). Your breasts continue to produce mature milk as long as you continue to breastfeed. After the first year, as your baby becomes a toddler and begins to nurse less and eat more solid foods, both the fat content and the levels of certain antibodies increase to give your active (and probably picky) child extra energy and extra protection from illness.

Here's another way your milk changes to meet your baby's needs: Its fat content is in almost constant flux. It increases as a feeding progresses: The low-fat milk at the beginning of a feeding encourages your baby to get all of the fluid, protein, and vitamins he or she needs. At the end of the feeding, the higher-fat milk makes your baby feel satisfied. Your milk's fat content also increases when your baby eats more—when feedings are closer together (such as during a growth spurt or a spell of cluster-feeding when your baby is very hungry).

> **Preemie Colostrum**
>
> If your baby is premature, your milk will contain more nitrogen, calories, vitamin A, zinc, and sodium than the milk of a mom with a full-term baby. These extra nutrients help your baby catch up in growth and development. Your colostrum will also be higher in anti-infective properties like immunoglobulin A (IgA), lysozyme, and lactoferrin to protect your preemie from bacterial or viral infection. You'll experience a slower transition to mature milk so your preemie can have more nutrient-rich colostrum.

Finally, your milk changes to protect your baby from the ever-changing germs in your environment. Breast milk contains high amounts of secretory IgA, an immunoglobulin that protects the ears, nose, throat, and digestive tract. Your milk levels of IgA targeted against specific viruses and bacteria increase when you're exposed to these organisms. In other words: Your milk protects your baby from the exact germs he or she is likely to be exposed to.

What's in Breast Milk?

Fat

One of the best things about breast milk is its rich, brain-building fat. Fat provides about 50 percent of the calories in breast milk. The amount of fat in your milk stays pretty constant even when the amount of fat in your diet changes. (However, the type of fat you eat does change the type of fat in your milk.) The fat in breast milk naturally contains the long-chain polyunsaturated fatty acids docosahexaenoic acid (DHA) and arachidonic acid (ARA) that are critical for brain and eye development. The fat in breast milk is easily digestible because it contains lipase, the enzyme required for breakdown into useful fatty acids. This allows maximum absorption by your baby's body.

Cholesterol

Cholesterol in the adult diet has a bad reputation, but it's well-known as a "good guy" in the infant diet. Breast milk has a fairly high cholesterol content, which is critical for the growth and maintenance of cell membranes. The higher cholesterol levels in breastfed infants may protect them against high blood cholesterol later in life. If you have a family history of heart disease or high cholesterol, breastfeeding could change your baby's heart disease risk as an adult—another great reason to breastfeed!

Proteins and Protein Components

Breast milk contains many proteins as well as the building blocks of protein. Many of them are biologically active and can never be reproduced in formula. The smaller protein components are easily absorbed and utilized by your baby's body. Just a few of these proteins and protein components are noted on the following pages.

- **White blood cells**:
    - *Antibodies*: Antibodies (also called immunoglobulins) are proteins that offer immune protection. IgA and immunoglobulin G (IgG) are the most plentiful in breast milk. IgA is particularly resistant to enzyme destruction and coats the lining of the intestine, creating a barrier against viruses and bacteria. As you're exposed to various germs in your environment, your body makes antibodies against them, and you pass these on to your baby in your breast milk.
    - *Lymphocytes*: There are two types of lymphocytes: B lymphocytes and T lymphocytes (also called B cells and T cells). Both are important to your baby's immune system because they make the IgA antibody.
    - *Macrophages*: This cell's job is to devour germs and cellular "garbage." The word *macrophage*, translated literally, means "big eater."
- **Glycoproteins**: Many proteins in breast milk are actually glycoproteins. A glycoprotein is a molecule that contains both protein and carbohydrate. This combination packs a powerful punch in the immune system; some glycoproteins like IgA protect against bacteria and viruses, while others improve absorption of minerals like iron and copper. Lactalbumin has been shown to fight against the bacteria that causes pneumonia, while lactoferrin keeps both bacteria and viruses from growing.
- **Enzymes**: Breast milk contains more than twenty active enzymes that perform various important functions. Digestive enzymes like amylase and lipase help break down carbohydrates and fats. Some enzymes act as mineral carriers, while others protect immunoglobulins. Others, like lysozyme and peroxidase, are antibacterial.
- **Hormones and hormone-like proteins**: Hormones and related proteins are chemical messengers. There are many different types: Some stimulate growth; some activate the immune system; and others regulate metabolism, reproduction,

and breast milk production. Breast milk contains many hormones and hormone-like proteins, and they all influence your baby's growth and development. For example, insulin regulates your baby's metabolism; thyroxine regulates both metabolism and growth; nerve growth factor helps nerves form and function; epidermal growth factor stimulates the skin and cell lining growth; and prostaglandins can have powerful effects over body processes like blood pressure and inflammation.

- **Amino acids**: Amino acids are special molecules that link to form proteins. Breast milk is rich in highly bioavailable forms of the important amino acids taurine and carnitine. Taurine is important for brain and eye development. Carnitine plays a big role in fat metabolism. It's especially important for newborns, who use fat as the preferred energy source for the heart, brain, and other organs with high energy needs.

- **Nucleotides**: Nucleotides are the building blocks of deoxyribonucleic acid (DNA) and ribonucleic acid (RNA), which carry the genetic information in cells. Nucleotides help your baby's cardiovascular and neurological systems and also aid the metabolism of carbohydrates, fats, and proteins. They're well-known for their part in defending against bacteria, viruses, parasites, and some cancers.[1]

> **Bioavailability**
>
> Bioavailability refers to how much of a nutrient is actually absorbed and available at the place in the body where it's needed. You may see the term *bioavailable* a lot when reading about breast milk because its nutrients are better absorbed and used by a baby's body than are the same nutrients in formula.

Carbohydrates

The main carbohydrate in breast milk is lactose. Lactose enhances calcium absorption and provides a source of galactose, another carbohydrate. Galactose is the base of a nutrient your baby needs for central nervous system development. The lactose content of breast milk stays constant throughout the day, providing a steady source of carbohydrates.

Breast milk also contains oligosccharides, yet another type of carbohydrate. Oligosaccharides are small chains of sugar molecules that your baby only partially digests. The undigested portions feed the friendly bacteria (bifidobacteria and lactobacillus) that populate your baby's digestive tract. (Oligosaccharides are also known as probiotics.) Oligosaccharides combine with proteins to form glycoproteins, which protect your baby against certain germs. (For more on glycoproteins, see page 18.)

Vitamins and Minerals

Breast milk contains all the vitamins and minerals your baby needs, in exactly the right amounts and in highly bioavailable forms. Formula manufacturers try to match the nutrient profile of breast milk, but the vitamins and minerals in formula tend to be far less bioavailable than those in breast milk. (For example, the iron in breast milk is 50 to 70 percent absorbed, whereas the iron in iron-fortified cow's milk formula is 3 to 12 percent absorbed.) This means formula must contain much greater amounts of these nutrients, which makes it harder for babies to digest.

Why Breastfeeding Is Important

For Your Baby

Human babies are designed to drink human milk; it's uniquely and perfectly suited to their needs. Because breast milk is babies' normal, natural food, it gives them their best shot at reaching their health, growth, and development potential.

There's strong evidence that breastfed babies experience fewer and less sever incidences of the following conditions than formula-fed babies.[2]

- Diarrhea
- Respiratory infection
- Middle ear infection
- Bacterial infection in the bloodstream
- Bacterial meningitis
- Botulism
- Urinary tract infection
- Necrotizing enterocolitis

Some studies suggest that breastfeeding protects children from the following diseases and conditions (sometimes in later life).[3]

- Sudden infant death syndrome (SIDS)
- Type 1 and type 2 diabetes
- Lymphoma
- Leukemia
- Hodgkin's disease
- Overweight and obesity
- High cholesterol
- Asthma

Breastfeeding also fosters optimum cognitive, social, and emotional development. A newborn can see clearly only eight to fifteen inches, the distance between the faces of a nursing baby and mother. Nursing, therefore, provides a vehicle for strong, early attachment between a mother and her baby. It allows not only regular eye contact, but also regular skin-to-skin contact. Psychologists believe nursing babies reap a special sense of security from the warm, close presence of their mothers. Babies require this secure attachment in order to venture forth normally in all areas of mental development.

Did You Know?

As early as one week after birth, babies can distinguish the smell of their own mothers' milk from the milk of other mothers.

For You

Breastfeeding Helps You Physically...

Just as your baby is designed to drink your milk, your body is designed to feed your baby. Breastfeeding gives you, too, your best shot at good health.

- Breastfeeding causes your pituitary gland to release oxytocin regularly, which makes your uterus contract. This prevents postpartum hemmorhage and promotes speedy return of your uterus to its normal size.

- Exclusive breastfeeding delays ovulation and menstruation, thereby preventing both pregnancy and iron-deficiency anemia. (However, you may still want to discuss birth control options with your doctor.)

- Milk production burns two to five hundred calories per day, which helps you lose pregnancy weight and keep it off.

- Breastfeeding helps control blood sugar, which lowers your risk of developing diabetes. In fact, one study found that women with gestational diabetes who didn't breastfeed were twice as likely to develop type 2 diabetes as women who did.[4]

- Breastfeeding improves cholesterol and triglyceride levels, which rise during pregnancy.[5] Taking into account the weight loss, cholesterol, and blood glucose improvements of breastfeeding, it could lower your risk of heart disease and metabolic syndrome.[6]

- After weaning, your bone density returns to prepregnancy or higher levels, which reduces your risk of osteoporosis and postmenopausal hip fractures.

- Breastfeeding protects you against some reproductive cancers. Ovarian and uterine cancers are more common in women who don't breastfeed. Breastfeeding for a total of from six to twenty-four months in your lifetime reduces your risk of breast cancer by 11 to 25 percent.

...And Mentally...

- When you breastfeed, you know you're giving your baby the best possible chance at good health, and this brings tremendous peace of mind.

- Formula-fed babies tend to get sick more often than breastfed babies, and caring for a sick baby can be very stressful. When you breastfeed, you minimize this source of stress in your life.

- Breastfeeding provides interaction and closeness between you and your child that's unlike any other relationship.

Sleep Secrets

Because newborns spend so much time at the breast, nursing sessions are great times to catch a few winks. Just make sure you're nursing in a comfy chair with a pillow supporting your arms, or in bed side-lying with your baby. (Be aware that sleeping the night in the same bed with your baby isn't recommended by the American Academy of Pediatrics, while other researchers and public health organizations support it.) Sweet dreams!

- Breastfeeding triggers your body to release prolactin, a hormone that not only helps your body make milk, but also keeps you calm. Breastfeeding mothers have been shown to have a less intense response to adrenaline than other women.

- Breastfeeding gives you a bottomless supply of warm, fresh, ready-to-serve food for your baby at all times. You never have to worry about preparation, toting, cleaning, or contamination.

- It's easy to multitask while breastfeeding. Once your baby's latched on, you need only one arm—or zero if you're using a nursing pillow or a sling—to support him or her. You can read, tend to another child, make a sandwich, or do whatever you need to keep your day running smoothly.

- You can sleep while breastfeeding your baby, which helps you get much-needed rest. Adequate rest not only makes your body healthier, it also makes your days brighter.

...And Financially

- Because breastfeeding is free, it puts no strain on your finances.
- Its infant health effects save you money on:
  - Doctor visits
  - Leave from work to care for a sick baby
  - Prescription and over-the-counter medication for your baby
- The maternal health effects of breastfeeding save you money on your own health care, including
  - Osteporosis care
  - Cancer treatment
  - Diabetes care
  - Weight control therapy
- In October 2006, formula costs $2.61 to $7.83 per day. Doesn't sound like too much...until you do the math for a year! (And if your baby has a cow's milk protein allergy, you'd pay much more.)

For Everyone

When you're knee-deep in diapers, it's tough to see the big picture. Breastfeeding not only has an economic and environmental impact in your own backyard—the effect is also global![7]

Economic Impact

For a country's economy, the loss of work days, drop in productivity, and cost of insurance claims take its toll. The cost of insurance claims alone adds up to over three billion dollars a year in the U.S. for illnesses that could be prevented if breast-feeding levels were increased.[8] Necrotizing enterocolitis, a condition that tends to

Ideas for the Cash You Don't Spend on Formula

Time Frame	Money Saved	Spending Ideas
One day	$5.22	Rent a movie or buy one book or two magazines
One week	$36.00	Pizza and salad delivery plus two movies on demand; Boppy breastfeeding pillow; or one-month fitness membership
One month	$156.00	Haircut, manicure, and pedicure; baby gym, musical mobile, and baby outfit; cleaning service; two tickets to see a concert; or electric breast pump
Two months	$302.00	Four-in-one convertible crib plus sheets; round-trip plane ticket to visit grandma; digital camcorder; or six sessions with a registered dietitian or personal trainer
Three months	$468.00	One-year fitness membership plus new workout clothes or savings bond for baby's college
Four months	$624.00	Weekend ski getaway for mom, dad, and baby; annual family fitness membership; or two new bicycles plus a baby carrier
Five months	$780.00	New computer; new leather sofa; 32-inch flat-screen TV; or new king-size front-loading washing machine
Six months	$936.00	Very nice new wardrobe for mom; new dining room set; or furniture for new home office
Nine months	$1,404.00	Monthly house cleaning or yard service for one year; biweekly dinner and a movie out for one year; or a home gym
Twelve months	$1,872.00	Round trip tickets, hotel, and car rental for one week in Hawaii; side-by-side refrigerator-freezer; five-piece queen bedroom set; or one year of monthly car payments

How costs were calculated: Prices were gathered from http://www.walgreens.com, http://www.drugstore.com, and http://www.similac.com. An average price per ounce was calculated from the least expensive powdered formula (nine cents per ounce prepared) to the most expensive ready-to-feed formula (twenty-seven cents per ounce). The amount of twenty-nine ounces per day of formula was used as an average amount of formula a baby might drink between two and twelve months.

strike premature infants, occurs ten times more often in formula-fed infants. Each case of necrotizing enterocolitis can cost up to $200,000! Close to $600 million of federal funds is spent each year on formula for the Women, Infants, and Children (WIC) program, a supplemental food program for low-income women, babies, and children.

In 2005, total U.S. spending on healthcare was $1.9 trillion dollars or 16% of the gross domestic product (GDP). It's expected to rise to $2.9 trillion in 2009. The U.S. spends more on healthcare than any industrialized nation.[9] Increasing breastfeeding rates and offering more support to breastfeeding women are ways our skyrocketing healthcare costs could be reduced.

Environmental Impact

Breast milk is delivered on demand to an infant without manufacturing, transportation, or packaging. The impact on the environment from not breastfeeding can be huge. It has been reported that for every 80,000 mothers who breastfeed, 17,200 tons of tin that would have been used for formula cans (that most likely end up in landfills) are saved.[10] Current estimates say that 550 million formula cans (including 86,000 tons of metal and 800,000 pounds of paper packaging) end up in U.S. landfills. Then there's the environmental cost of getting formula from the factory to the stores. Don't forget last-minute runs to the store for formula; extra driving contributes to global warming.

Challenges That Affect Breastfeeding

Most women and babies can breastfeed, even if they have health problems. Some conditions make nursing difficult, but very few make it impossible. Where there's a will, there's a way—and pity the person who gets in the way of a woman's will!

Your Baby's Health and Birth Experience

If your baby is born prematurely or has other health problems, you might assume that he or she won't be able to breastfeed. However, most babies—including those with the conditions listed below—can breastfeed or at least receive pumped breast milk. You and your baby may simply need advice from a lactation consultant, help with positioning, more frequent nursing sessions, or special equipment to make breastfeeding work for you.[11]

- Birth injury
- Premature birth
- Hyperbilirubinemia (jaundice)
- Hypoglycemia
- Small for gestational age (SGA)
- Large for gestational age (LGA)
- Intrauterine growth restriction (IUGR)
- Tongue-tie (ankyloglossia)
- Down syndrome
- Cleft lip or palate

Even if your baby can't suckle right away (or ever) due to these or other special needs, you can pump your milk and feed it another way. In fact, you may find (as many women in this situation do) that pumping milk for your baby is very healing. When babies are ill, their parents often feel stressed out and helpless. Pumping milk is one very valuable way you can be present for your child and improve his or her health outlook. Remember that breastfeeding your baby for as long as possible—however long that may be, and regardless of your baby's condition—can help your child immensely.

If your baby is hospitalized and you want to provide breast milk for him or her, make sure to mention it to your doctors. You should start pumping as soon as possible after your baby's birth. The hospital will probably have a pump you can use while you're there and may also rent pumps for home use. At first, if your baby's sucking isn't strong enough, your milk may have to be fed via tube, supplemental nursing system (SNS), cup, or eyedropper.

Your Health and Birth Experience

If you have health issues of your own, or if your birth experience is particularly challenging, you may be overwhelmed by the prospect of breastfeeding. That's normal—and here's the good news: breastfeeding in these situations is normal, too. It may be challenging, but the challenges are surmountable. And you'll feel great about overcoming them! Here are some common maternal challenges that may affect breastfeeding, along with a few tips and tidbits to get you off to a good start.

Cesarean Section

- Most medications given during a C-section will not seriously affect your baby. However, they may make your baby sleepy or unenthusiastic about breastfeeding at first. Ask your caregiver for pointers on encouraging your baby to nurse and keeping him or her awake during feedings. Early and frequent nursing will make up for some of the hormonal signals your body may have missed due to anesthesia and/or a shortened labor.

- Pain medication given after a C-section may make your baby a little sleepy, but it's important for initiating breastfeeding. Pain interferes with your body's release of oxytocin, a key breastfeeding hormone. Don't be afraid to control post-surgical pain; it'll not only help you feel more comfortable and get more rest, it'll also help your body feed your baby.

Why Preemies Need Breast Milk

- Preemies are at greater risk for infection and illness than full-term babies. Their immune systems are even less mature, and they're exposed to more germs while they're hospitalized.
- Necrotizing entercolitis (NEC), a condition in which part of the tissue of the intestine is destroyed, is most common in premature and underweight babies, but happens ten times more often in formula-fed babies than breastfed babies. Breastfeeding is so successful in the prevention of NEC that some hospitals are using banked human milk for feeding premature infants.[12]
- Breast milk contains enzymes that help a preemie's immature digestive system develop.
- Preemie breast milk contains more antibodies and anti-inflammatory substances, which help protect the premature baby's fragile bowels.
- Preemie breast milk contains higher levels of protein, nitrogen, calories, calcium, phosphorous, zinc, and sodium to better meet a preemie's nutrient needs.
- Although preemies fed fortified human milk grow more slowly than formula-fed preemies, they're healthier. One study shows that they're discharged from the hospital two weeks earlier than formula-fed preemies.[13]
- Premature babies absorb fat more efficiently from breast milk than from formula. Fat is important for preemies because it's calorie-dense, packing a nutritional punch for babies with tiny stomachs. The essential fatty acids in breast milk are also important for brain and eye development, which lags in preemies.

- Positioning can help you minimize incision pain while breastfeeding. Side-lying and the football hold will keep your baby completely off your incision. If you prefer the cradle hold, prop your baby on one or more soft pillows to protect your incision.

Multiples

- In most cases, moms of multiples—even triplets and quadruplets—can exclusively breastfeed their babies. (Breast milk production is a supply and demand process, so if much is demanded, much is made.) Remember that because your babies are at higher risk for prematurity, low birth weight, and other health problems than singletons are, breastfeeding is especially important for them.

- Naturally, breastfeeding multiples requires extra work and help—but every aspect of parenting multiples requires extra work and help. The best strategy for success is to arm yourself with knowledge and line up support before your babies are born. Find a lactation consultant who has experience with multiples. Network with your local La Leche League. Arrange for postpartum help at home. Visit the following websites, which contain lots of useful information, links, and tandem feeding photos:
  - http://www.karengromada.com
  - http://www.mostonline.org/faq_bf.htm
  - http://www.kellymom.com/bf/start/basics/bf-links-multiples.html

- When you're nursing multiples, it'll be even more important for you to eat right and get plenty of rest. This is another good reason to plan ahead for postpartum help at home.

> ### Tales from the Trenches: Nursing Twins
>
> Kelly, from Santee, California, has this to say about nursing twins: "You can do it!" Kelly is exclusively breastfeeding her twins, Anna and Isabelle. She usually feeds them one at a time; she sees feedings as her special one-on-one time with each baby. Even though she doesn't tandem-feed, Kelly doesn't find nursing time-consuming. Her babies have become very efficient feeders; they can empty one breast in five to seven minutes. She says, "Nursing is easier than bottles for me. I'd rather spend time nursing than preparing all that formula. And when I add up all the health benefits—for them and for me—it's obviously time well spent." Another benefit: Kelly notes that she lost all thirty-eight pounds of her pregnancy weight by six weeks postpartum!

Chronic Illness

- **Thyroid problems**: About one in twenty women don't produce adequate thyroid hormones; this is called hypothyroidism. Breastfeeding is recommended for all mothers with thyroid problems. Medications commonly prescribed for both overactive and underactive thyroid, such as levothyroxine and methimazole, are approved by the American Academy of Pediatrics (AAP) for use during breastfeeding. Be aware that untreated hypothyroidism may result in a decreased milk supply.

- **Polycystic ovarian syndrome (PCOS)**: PCOS is said to affect about 5 percent of women and can cause symptoms such as irregular periods, acne, elevated insulin levels, excess hair on the face and body, and overweight. PCOS is one of the leading causes of infertility in women. It's caused by an imbalance of insulin, estrogen, and progesterone, all important hormones for successful breastfeeding.

  Some women with PCOS have no problems breastfeeding, while others have an undersupply or oversupply of milk. A medication called metformin appears to be the best treatment of choice—both during pregnancy and lactation. Thomas Hale, a well-known expert on the use of medications in nursing mothers, along with his colleagues in Western Australia, have concluded that the use of metformin by breastfeeding moms is safe.[14] Because 80 percent of women with PCOS are overweight, lifestyle changes are also vital for treatment. A diet that promotes weight loss or maintenance and includes high-fiber foods, limited sugar, and healthy fats and regular exercise are keystones of treatment.

- **Diabetes**: A lot of attention is given to women with diabetes during pregnancy, with good reason. However, the topic of breastfeeding for the diabetic mom often gets overlooked. Whether you have type 1 or type 2 or had gestational diabetes during pregnancy, breastfeeding may decrease your baby's chances of being diabetic—and it will help control your blood sugar. Some things you should be aware of:[15, 16]

  - It's important to keep in touch with your healthcare team while breastfeeding because insulin levels may need adjustment, and your dietitian may need to change your meal plan.

  - Breastfeeding tends to lower blood glucose, so you may need to adjust your insulin and/or have a snack before or after breastfeeding. Testing your blood glucose before and after nursing can help you see the effect.

  - When your baby has a growth spurt, you may also need to increase your energy intake or adjust insulin.

  - If you have type 2 diabetes, you will probably need to stay on insulin for a while after delivery.

  - Your hospital may have a policy to keep babies of diabetic moms in the nursery the first twenty-four hours. If so, make it clear that you want to breastfeed and avoid any formula.

  - Ask for help from a lactation consultant at the hospital to make sure breastfeeding gets off to a good start.

  - If you can't breastfeed your baby right away, ask for an electric pump and begin pumping to establish your milk supply.

  - Prevent infection by learning how to prevent plugged ducts and cracked nipples.

- **Depression**: As many as 80 percent of new moms briefly get the baby blues, but one in seven has a more serious problem: postpartum depression. Postpartum depression is nothing to be ashamed of—it's simply a complication of pregnancy and childbirth. If you feel like you have more than a touch of blues, don't hesitate to get help fast. Why? Depression can affect your ability to take care of your baby. It can also hinder your baby's physical and psychological development.

  - *How depression affects breastfeeding*: Depressed moms are less likely to breastfeed, and if they do breastfeed, they do it for shorter periods of time. One theory is that depressed moms perceive negative reactions in their babies differently and this causes early weaning.[17]

  - *How breastfeeding affects depression*: The psychological and physical benefits of breastfeeding mitigate some of the negative physical effects of depression on the infant such as reduced brain activity and negative responsiveness. Breastfeeding moms and babies also respond better to each other than they would if not breastfeeding.

  - *Antidepressant use and breastfeeding*: Many women with postpartum depression remain untreated due to misinformation about using antidepressants while nursing. Of the more frequently studied antidepressants, Zoloft (sertraline), Paxil (paroxetine), and Pamelor (nortriptyline) have been to shown to have no adverse affects on infants.[18] Zoloft is reported to be the best drug choice so far for breastfeeding moms according to Hale.[19] What about herbal products? Saint John's Wort is weaker than the medications mentioned above and may decrease the action of other drugs. There can also be contaminant and standardization issues in using an herbal product.

If you need to take medication for any chronic illness, talk with your doctor about your plan to breastfeed, and inquire about breastfeeding-safe options. According to the AAP, most drugs likely to be prescribed to a nursing mother won't affect her milk supply or her baby's well-being.[20] Make sure your caregiver consults the latest edition of Thomas Hale's *Medications and Mothers' Milk* when advising you; this reference book is the gold standard for answers on pharmacology and breastfeeding.

Breast Conditions

- **Breast surgery**: Breast surgery may or may not affect your ability to breastfeed. Generally speaking, you can breastfeed if your nipples have not been moved and your ducts have not been cut. If you've had breast reduction, augmentation, lumpectomy, or other surgery on your breasts, your surgeon will know best how much your milk ducts are affected. Discuss with your surgeon your desire to breastfeed. Also, make sure your child's caregiver knows about your breast surgery so he or she can monitor your baby's growth closely. (For more information about breastfeeding after surgery, see http://www.lalecheleague. org/NB/NBsurgery.html.) Breast reduction tends to affect breastfeeding more than other breast surgeries. However, many women have breastfed successfully after reduction. (For detailed information and support on breastfeeding after reduction, see http://www.bfar.org.) Breastfeeding with silicone implants appears to be safe, according to the AAP.[21] However, some argue that the effect of silicone on infants has not been studied enough. Ask your doctor for the most up-to-date opinion.

- **Breast or nipple abnormality**: Flat nipples do not protrude or become erect when stimulated; inverted nipples retract rather than protrude when the areola is pressed. There are varying degrees of flat and inverted nipples; in some cases these conditions may affect a baby's ability to latch on. If you discover you have flat or inverted nipples while you're pregnant, some lactation consultants recommend that you try to draw out your nipples using your fingers. Others recommend using breast shells during pregnancy to help the nipples protrude more. Don't worry if you don't discover the shape of your nipples until after your baby arrives. Using a breast pump immediately before nursing can help draw out the nipple for easier latch. Getting a good latch is critical—seek the advice of a lactation consultant if needed.

- **No prenatal breast changes**: This may affect your ability to breastfeed if you have insufficient glandular tissue (a rare condition) or if you have a condition (like PCOS) that affects your hormone balance. However, lack of breast changes in pregnancy may also mean nothing at all—so don't get discouraged. Speak with your caregiver and a lactation consultant to set your mind at ease and, if necessary, to lay out a plan for successful breastfeeding.

Getting Ready for Breastfeeding

Gearing Up

Hasn't nature provided all the equipment you need to breastfeed? Yes. But there are a few additional items you may find useful:

- **Nursing bra**: Though any bra with cups that can be pulled up or down to expose your breasts will do, a lot of moms prefer the easy access nursing bras provide. If you find that you need new bras for your expanding chest while you're pregnant, you might want to skip straight to nursing bras and save some money.

- **Nursing clothes**: Any ordinary two-piece outfit will work for nursing; there's no need to buy an entire closet full of nursing clothes. However, they can come in handy for nursing in public if you're particularly modest or if you're still getting the hang of maneuvering baby, breast, and clothing simultaneously. To see how you like nursing clothes, you might want to buy just a few shirts or dresses. Here are some good online sources for nursingwear:
    - http://www.motherwear.com
    - http://www.expressiva.com
    - http://www.motherhoodnursing.com
    - http://www.onehotmama.com

- **Nursing pads**: Most breastfeeding moms need to use nursing pads for at least the first few weeks. (Some women stop leaking after their supply settles down; others continue to leak until their children wean.) You have three choices:
  - *Disposable pads*: These are very absorbent and discreet; they're a practical choice if you're a super-soaker. Unfortunately, they're also expensive and wasteful. Nursing moms rate Lansinoh disposable pads very highly. (Visit http://www.lansinoh.com for more information.)
  - *Cloth pads*: If you leak only occasionally or moderately, cloth pads may work well for you. They're usually made of cotton; some wool ones are also available. Cloth pads are more economical and environmentally friendly than disposables, but they also tend to be bulkier and less absorbent. Nursing moms give high marks to Medela lace washable nursing pads. (Visit http://www.medela.com for more information.)
  - *Lilypadz*: These reusable pads work well for leakers of all kinds. They combine the advantages of disposables (reliability and discreetness) with those of cloth pads (cost and sustainability). They actually prevent leaks (instead of absorbing milk) by putting constant pressure on your nipples. They're made of soft, flexible, form-fitting silicone that sticks to your skin without adhesive—they can even be worn while swimming! A small, unpublished study at the Medical Center of Central Georgia found that moms using Lilypadz had fewer cases of mastitis, clogged ducts, and thrush than women using traditional pads.[22] One pair is quite expensive (twenty-five to thirty dollars), but this drawback is balanced by the fact that you'll only need one pair. (Visit http://www.lilypadz.com for more information.)
- **Comfortable chair and footstool**: Babies—especially newborns—eat often, and they can be poky. Getting a sore rear or a stiff back from feeding would be a bummer. Check out the chairs in your home and choose one that supports your entire body (head, shoulders, back, arms, and bottom) comfortably. It's also wise to choose a chair you won't topple out of if you doze off while nursing. Add a footstool so you can maximize the rest you get during feedings by putting your feet up. A footstool also helps bring your lap to the proper height for nursing.
- **Pillow**: I got tendonitis in my elbow after a month of nursing from holding my arm up too long without support. Take a lesson from me and use a pillow instead! Even with a comfortable chair and footstool, you'll probably need some sort of pillow on your lap to bring your baby to the right height without straining your arm. An ordinary couch or bed pillow will do, but you may also want to check out these pillows made especially for nursing:
  - *My Brest Friend*: This wraparound pillow supports your back, arms, and elbows as well as your baby. It even has a pocket to store supplies. Because it encircles your body, it won't shift during a feeding and is especially helpful when sitting on the floor. (For more information, visit http://www.mybrestfriend.com.)

- *Boppy*: This C-shaped pillow is very popular and widely available. (For more information, visit http://www.boppy.com.)
- *EZ-2-Nurse Twins*: This pillow is specially designed for tandem nursing multiples. It's bigger than other nursing pillows and holds more weight. Its top slopes toward you so you can properly position your babies without using your arms to prop them. It secures with a strap around your back and also comes with a back pillow. (For more information, visit http://www.doubleblessings.com.)
- *The Nursing Nest*: This pillow was developed by a mom who found it difficult to nurse after a C-section. Designed for side-lying, the pillow creates a barrier between sleepers in the bed. It can also be used for table-top nursing. (For more information, visit http://www.peacefulpea.com.)

- **Notebook**: When you're a sleep-deprived mom of a newborn, the days and nights blend together. It can be hard to keep track of what day it is—much less your baby's intake and output. But tracking this info will tell you that your baby is doing well (or if you should be concerned), and it'll give you confidence in your parenting skills. Do yourself a favor and jot a note about each feeding and diaper change. (Simply note nursing times and wet and poopy diapers. If you like, you can also track your diet to see if it affects your baby.) Take your diary to your first few visits with your baby's caregiver. If you find it a pain to write everything down, how about wearing a bracelet that keeps track of it for you? The Nursing Bracelet, an ingenious, pretty combination of colored and numbered beads and moveable charm(s) on memory wire, can be used in several ways: to track when you last fed your baby, to mark which breast your baby fed from last, to count your baby's feedings per day, and/or to count wet or poopy diapers. (For tips on how to use the bracelet, visit http://www.thenursing-bracelet.com.) A more basic and less expensive product is called Milk Bands nursing bracelets. Made of soft silicone with small holes and two plastic pegs, it can track number of feedings or time and side of last feeding. You can even shower in it. (For more information, visit http://www.milkbands.com.)

To Cover or Not to Cover

The best way to nurse in public is: Just do it! The more you do it, the easier it is, and the less you—and others—give it a second thought. It's amazing how discreetly you can latch your baby on with just a little practice. You'll also be amazed at how seldom people even notice that you're nursing.

Some women choose to cover up with a blanket or other gear when nursing in public. You may want to do this if you're very modest or shy. Be warned, though: Many babies hate nursing under cover. It's hot, stuffy, lonely, and boring. Many moms find cover-ups awkward, too: They make it tricky to latch baby on; they tend to slip around; babies yank on them; and ironically, they call attention to nursing.

If you do want to keep a cover-up handy, a small, light blanket or scarf will do the trick. Or check out the stylish nursing shawl at www.lovedbaby.com.

- **Breast pump**: Regardless of your postpartum plans, it's a good idea to have some sort of breast pump on hand. A pump can come in very handy if you need to be away from your baby or (along with frequent nursing) to help alleviate engorgement or plugged ducts. What kind of pump do you need? It depends on where and how often you'll be pumping. Pumps are powered in a variety of ways; some pumps can be powered in two or three different ways. Check out your options in the following list.

  - *Manual pump*: A manual pump is best for occasional use (no more than once a day). If you find yourself needing to pump at unpredictable times and places, this may be the pump for you, since it requires no electricity or supply of batteries. Some manual pumps require more muscle power than others; if you can, try out a manual pump's action before you buy it to make sure it doesn't strain your hand. Well-reviewed manual pumps include the Avent Isis, the Medela Harmony, and the Ameda One-Hand. In two clinical studies, the Avent Isis had equal or better milk volume and moms found it more comfortable than a mini-electric pump or electric pump.[23, 24] If you have limited use of your hands but still want a manual pump, look for one with a foot pedal, such as the Medela PedalPump.

  - *Battery-operated pump*: Like a manual pump, a battery-operated pump is also recommended for occasional use. It requires less muscle power and *may* extract milk more efficiently, but its batteries must be kept fresh because its suction weakens as the batteries weaken. A battery-operated pump typically uses AA batteries but may also have an AC adapter. This type of pump gets mixed reviews; a couple of options are The First Years Natural Comfort Pump and Gentle Expressions Pump.

  - *Personal electric pump*: This type of pump is best for a mom who needs to pump a few times a day (for example, while working outside the home). Personal electric pumps strive to be comfortable, portable, and very efficient. They usually pump both breasts simultaneously and can be powered in various ways (AC adapter, car adapter, and/or AA batteries). Some well-reviewed models are Medela Pump in Style and Ameda Purely Yours.

  - *Hospital-grade electric pump*: This type of pump is designed to build and maintain milk supply. It's recommended for heavy use (for example, by a mom who's exclusively pumping). It's extremely sturdy and efficient, but also quite expensive and less portable than a personal electric pump. Because it can be used safely by multiple moms with individual accessories,

Pumping Resources

Here's an excellent resource to help you choose the right pump for your needs:
- http://www.leron-line.com/updates/Breast_Pumps.htm

And here are a few more great websites for pumping support and information:
- http://www.breastfeeding.com/pumps&pumping.html
- http://www.pumpingmoms.org
- http://www.kellymom.com/bf/pumping/milkstorage.html
- http://www.kellymom.com/bf/pumping/reusing-expressedmilk.html

this type of pump is typically available for rent from hospitals, lactation consultants, health departments, and medical equipment rental stores. Some well-reviewed models are Medela Symphony, Medela Lactina, Medela Classic, Ameda Elite, Ameda SMB, and Ameda Lact-e.

- **Insulated tote**: If you'll be pumping regularly away from home, you'll need an insulated tote for your milk. Many personal electric pumps have built-in coolers. But if yours doesn't, or if you'll be leaving your pump at work, you'll want a separate cooler. An insulated lunch sack with an ice pack works well.

- **Comfort measures**: To prevent or soothe irritated nipples—especially in the first few weeks—you may want to keep some nipple cream on hand. Experts recommend that you use only 100 percent modified lanolin on your nipples, as other ingredients may be harmful to your baby. (Both Lansinoh and Medela make widely available lanolin creams.) If you're allergic to lanolin or are strictly vegan, ask a lactation consultant to recommend an alternative cream. If you choose anything besides 100 percent lanolin cream, read the label carefully and strictly avoid arachis oil, which is peanut oil. Research shows that using arachis oil on your skin or your baby's can cause a peanut allergy. Another handy item, this one for soothing engorged breasts or alleviating plugged ducts, is a hot/cold pack. Any hot or cold pack—such as a rice sock or a package of frozen peas—will do, or you may want to try a reusable breast-shaped hot/cold pack, such as those made by Lansinoh, Gerber, and Ameda.

Putting Together Your Team

You've probably heard the saying *It takes a village to raise a child*. It also takes teamwork to breastfeed successfully. Here's a list of people and places to recruit for your team.

Your Obstetrician or Midwife

You might not think of your obstetrical caregiver as an important part of your breastfeeding team, but he or she has a very important job: getting you off to a good start. You're probably visiting your caregiver regularly throughout your pregnancy, and these visits can be a valuable source of breastfeeding information and support. Make sure to tell your caregiver that you want to breastfeed exclusively, and work together to create a birth plan that facilitates this.

Your Baby's Doctor

As you ask for recommendations and schedule interviews with potential doctors for your baby, find out if they're knowledgeable and supportive of breastfeeding. Your baby's doctor will be your key postpartum health resource, so it's very important to choose one who not only understands how important breastfeeding is to your baby's health, but also how to help you over the inevitable bumps in the road.

Following are some questions you can ask to gauge a doctor's breastfeeding know-how. Ideally, the doctor will know how to answer them or will be able to refer you directly to a lactation consultant.

- **What percentage of babies in your practice are breastfed?** The higher, the better.
- **How will I know if my baby is getting enough milk?** See page 43.
- **When do you suggest breastfed newborns have a checkup?** The AAP recommends a first checkup at three to five days for extensive evaluation of latch, hydration, weight, and/or breast problems and another checkup at two to three weeks to check weight gain.
- **If I need help with breastfeeding, can you help me or refer me to a lactation consultant?** Ideally, the answer should be *yes* to both. At the very least, the doctor should have a partnership with one or more lactation consultants.
- **Do you recommend rooming-in with my newborn?** That's the best way to get breastfeeding off to a good start.
- **How long should I breastfeed?** The AAP recommends breastfeeding your baby exclusively (no formula, water, solid foods, or anything else besides breast milk) for the first six months, followed by breastfeeding with complementary foods for *at least* the first year of your baby's life.
- **If my baby doesn't nurse right away, what can we do?** You should avoid bottles completely during the first few weeks to prevent nipple confusion. If your baby is losing weight too quickly or showing signs of dehydration, you should feed him or her expressed colostrum or breast milk using an SNS, eyedropper, or small cup.

Ten Steps for a "Baby Friendly" Facility[25]

1. Maintain a written breastfeeding policy that is routinely communicated to all healthcare staff.
2. Train all healthcare staff in skills necessary to implement this policy.
3. Inform all pregnant women about the benefits and management of breastfeeding.
4. Help mothers initiate breastfeeding within one hour of birth.
5. Show mothers how to breastfeed and how to maintain lactation, even if they are separated from their infants.
6. Give infants no food or drink other than breast milk, unless medically indicated.
7. Practice rooming-in: Allow mothers and infants to remain together twenty-four hours a day.
8. Encourage unrestricted breastfeeding.
9. Give no pacifiers or artificial nipples to breastfeeding infants.
10. Foster the establishment of breastfeeding support groups and refer mothers to them on discharge from the hospital or clinic.

Your Birth Site

Depending on your insurance (or lack of insurance), your health status, and where you are, you may or may not have a choice about where you give birth. If you don't have a choice, find out how breastfeeding-friendly your birth site is so you can be prepared to deal with it. If you do have a choice, try to select a place that will help instead of hinder breastfeeding establishment.

Delivering your baby at home or at a birth center usually provides the best conditions for initiating breastfeeding. Some hospitals are very breastfeeding-friendly, too—but be aware that hospital policies can sometimes be obstacles. In the end it often comes down to luck—if the nurse assigned to you has the initiative, time, and knowledge to support your breastfeeding efforts and if there is a lactation consultant available when you need one.

If you'll be birthing at a hospital, find out if it's a Baby-Friendly Hospital. This certification developed by the United Nations Children's Fund (UNICEF) and the World Health Organization (WHO) helps hospitals give mothers the information, confidence, and skills they need to successfully initiate and continue breastfeeding their babies, and it gives special recognition to hospitals that do so.

Even if your hospital isn't officially Baby-Friendly, it may still follow the Baby-Friendly Hospital Initiative's Ten Steps to Successful Breastfeeding. Find out which of these steps are followed at your hospital.

Your Family and Friends

If possible, surround yourself with family and friends who support your breastfeeding efforts. Experienced breastfeeders are the best sources of advice and camaraderie—but anyone who's willing to cheer you on and help you out should be welcomed with open arms! (On the flip side, be prepared to politely ignore naysayers in your social circle.)

If your partner feels out of the loop when you talk about nursing, try to help him feel more comfortable. Tell him how important breastfeeding is for your entire family. Explain that it'll be his job to teach your baby about all the other important and enjoyable things in life, like baths, clean diapers, playtime, hugs, and kisses. Share information you've found on the Internet or in books or magazines and take him to a breastfeeding class. (He won't be the only father there; most breastfeeding classes encourage partners to attend.) Explain how he can be a part of your breastfeeding experience. Here are some things he can do:

- Have a positive and supportive attitude.
- Bring you snacks, water, or whatever else you need while you're nursing.
- Prepare meals and take over household chores.
- Spend one-on-one time with your other child(ren).
- Feed your baby expressed milk after breastfeeding is well-established.
- Feed your baby solid foods when he or she gets older.

Your older child(ren) also can help you in your nursing venture by keeping you company or bringing you things while you nurse.

Your Employee Benefits

While you're checking on your insurance plan's coverage of your prenatal care and birth, also find out if it will cover postpartum services such as a lactation consultant or breast pump rental or purchase. Recruit help from your employee benefits representative if necessary.

Also consult with your benefits representative to see if your employer offers any special assistance for new moms, such as a workplace lactation program or pump rental. Some employers also arrange for discounted lactation consultant fees or free telephone support. For more information about maintaining breastfeeding while working outside the home, see Chapter 5.

La Leche League

If you don't know many—or any—other breastfeeding moms, La Leche League International (LLLI) can help you get connected. LLLI is a mother-to-mother breastfeeding support and education network with local groups all over the world. To find the group nearest you, visit http://www.lalecheleague.org/ WebIndex.html or call one of the following phone numbers.

- For leaders or groups in the United States: 800-LALECHE or 847-519-7730 (The second number leads to an automated system for finding leaders by entering a zip code.)
- For leaders or groups in Canada: 800-665-4324 or 514-LALECHE (The second number is for finding a French-speaking leader.)

Gathering Information While You're Pregnant

Many a new parent has said that babies should come with instruction books. Since they don't—and you won't have time to read after your baby's born anyway!—it's a good idea to educate yourself while you're pregnant. There are several ways to do that.

Take a Class

- Sign up for a breastfeeding class through your doctor's or midwife's office or your local hospital's childbirth education department.
- Attend meetings of your local LLLI group.
- Call local lactation consultants to find out if they offer classes or one-on-one prenatal counseling.

Read a Book

- *Breastfeeding with Confidence* by Sue Cox
- *The Nursing Mother's Companion* by Kathleen Huggins
- *The Ultimate Breastfeeding Book of Answers* by Jack Newman and Teresa Pitman
- *The Breastfeeding Book* by Martha Sears and William Sears
- *American Academy of Pediatrics New Mother's Guide to Breastfeeding* by Joan Younger Meek
- *The Womanly Art of Breastfeeding* by La Leche League International
- *Nursing Mother, Working Mother* by Gale Pryor
- *So* That's *What They're For!* by Janet Tamaro
- *Eat Well, Lose Weight, While Breastfeeding* by Eileen Behan
- *Mothering Multiples* by Karen Kerkhoff Gromada
- *Defining Your Own Success: Breastfeeding after Breast Reduction Surgery* by Diana West
- *Breastfeeding the Adopted Baby* by Debra Stewart Peterson

Subscribe to a Magazine

- *Mothering*
- *New Beginnings*
- *The Compleat Mother*

Surf the Net

- http://www.kellymom.com
- http://www.lalecheleague.org
- http://www.askdrsears.com
- http://www.4woman.gov/breastfeeding
- http://www.breastfeeding.com
- http://www.mothering.com/discussions

The First Two Weeks

The First Few Days

Labor and Birth

After forty weeks of waiting, great growth in girth, and untold hours of contemplation... finally the big moment is almost here! Welcome to childbirth. As you begin labor, breastfeeding may be the last thing on your mind. You're probably either focused on coping with your contractions or contemplating pain management. But even though there's a lot going on, this is the perfect time to make your feeding wishes very clear.

If you're birthing at a hospital or birth center, tell the staff:

> ### What's a Lactation Consultant?
>
> A lactation consultant is a specialist who helps mothers with breastfeeding. She's both a teacher and a troubleshooter. She often helps mothers and babies with latching problems, pain, low milk supply, and/or low weight gain. She also helps women breastfeed through challenges such as premature birth or returning to work. She's familiar with the latest, greatest breastfeeding equipment and supplies.
>
> A lactation consultant may work at a hospital, clinic, doctor's office, or her own private practice. She's typically a health professional like a registered nurse (RN), registered dietitian (RD), or certified nurse-midwife (CNM). Sometimes she's another type of midwife, a social worker, or a speech therapist.
>
> There are many lactation monikers in use, and they can mean different things when used by different people. The best way to ensure that you get knowledgeable, experienced, up-to-date help is to look for an International Board Certified Lactation Consultant (IBCLC). IBCLC is considered the gold standard for certifying lactation consultants. (You may also see the credential Registered Lactation Consultant (RLC), a trademarked name used by some IBCLCs.)
>
> To find an IBCLC near you, visit http://gotwww.net/ilca.

- You want to breastfeed your baby exclusively. You don't want your baby to have anything except breast milk unless it's medically necessary.

- You don't want your baby to have any artificial nipples (bottles or pacifiers). If necessary, you want your baby fed via eyedropper, SNS, or cup.

- You want to room-in with your baby.

- You'd like to meet with a lactation consultant after your baby is born.

If your labor is long, the nursing staff may turn over, and you might have to repeat your wishes. (This is a good task for your partner.)

The First Feeding

Finally, you have the prize: your new baby! The hustle and bustle around you blurs into the background as you focus on this tiny person.

After birth, your baby should be placed skin-to-skin on your belly or chest with warm towels over both of you. This will help your baby stay warmer, breathe easier, and cry less than being placed in a crib or warmer. Early skin-to-skin contact also helps breastfeeding get started. Most babies will instinctively find the breast and begin breastfeeding without help within the first hour, which is the time frame recommended for a successful start to breastfeeding.

Your baby may just lick your nipple or suckle a bit—or may latch on with full force. Every experience is different. And no matter how many times you've lived this moment in your mind, it may not feel like you expected it to. It may, in fact, feel downright strange. Don't worry: All types of emotions are normal at this time!

As you snuggle and get to know each other, you'll both get comfortable with the idea of nursing and will find your way on your own—provided you're not disturbed. It's best to be alone with your baby and partner at this time. If you want expert help handy, your doctor or midwife or a lactation consultant can wait quietly nearby.

If you or your baby has medical complications, breastfeeding within the first hour might not be possible. Breastfeeding may also be delayed if you've had pain medication, which can make your baby too sleepy to nurse. If your first feeding is delayed for any reason, ask to speak to a lactation consultant. The consultant may recommend pumping to get your milk supply going or may have suggestions for encouraging a sleepy baby to nurse.

Nursing as soon as possible after birth is important because it sends your body a message to fire up the milk factory and helps your uterus contract, preventing excessive bleeding. Nursing early and often also gives your baby a good dose of colostrum, the important first milk your breasts make. (For more on the value of colostrum, see page 16.)

Pacifier Use and Bed Sharing: Impact on SIDS

In late 2005, the AAP Task Force on Sudden Infant Death Syndrome (SIDS) published a policy statement that recommended that parents consider using a pacifier at naptime and bedtime but that for breastfeeding infants, pacifier introduction should be delayed one month to ensure that breastfeeding is well established. The policy also suggested a separate but close sleeping environment. Many breastfeeding advocates disagree with the policy.

How can you decide what to do? Read the facts and discuss it with your doctor. For more information, see:
- http://www.bfmed.org/documents/ SIDS-Bedsharing.doc
- http://www.lalecheleague.org/ Release/sids.html
- http://www.drgreene.com/21_2051. html
- http://www.sidsalliance.org/research/ pacifiers_position_paper.pdf

What Is Colostrum?

If colostrum could be bottled and sold, the health claims would look something like this:

- More immunoglobulins and good bacteria than any other breast milk!
- Keeps bacteria and viruses from invading the intestinal wall!
- An immunization your baby can drink!
- Easy to digest!
- Helps your baby pass meconium!
- Prevents jaundice!
- Rich yellow color from natural antioxidant beta carotene!
- Absolutely free!
- Just four ounces is all your baby needs in the first twenty-four hours!

> **Checklist for Early Breastfeeding**
>
> - Relax.
> - Room-in.
> - Request no bottles or pacifiers.
> - Nurse within one hour of birth.
> - Ask for a lactation consultant.
> - Nurse on demand.
> - Enjoy getting to know your baby.

An additional note on that last claim.... Colostrum is so rich in nutrients and everything else your baby needs to jump-start his or her digestive tract and immune system that only very small amounts are necessary. Don't worry about not having enough. If you feed your baby on demand, it will be exactly the right amount.

After the First Feeding: Positioning

After your first nursing encounter, it's time to work on the breastfeeding techniques you've heard so much about.

Position, position, position. Obviously, it can't be said enough: Good positioning of your baby is vital! It helps your baby latch properly and extract milk effectively. It can also prevent sore nipples. Here's a basic guide to proper positioning:

1. **Get comfortable**. Grab your pillow(s), footstool, glass of water, and/or whatever else you need to be comfy and relaxed, and set up shop in a chair or in bed.

2. **Choose a hold**.

   Cradle hold: With this hold, you support your baby with the arm nearest the breast you're feeding from. Your baby's head is in the crook of your elbow, with your forearm supporting baby's back and your hand supporting baby's bottom. This is the most commonly used hold.

   Cross cradle hold: With this hold, you support your baby with the arm opposite the breast you're feeding from. Your hand holds your baby's head, and your forearm supports your baby's back and bottom. This hold is useful if your baby needs help latching because it lets you direct your baby's head.

   Football hold: This hold resembles the way a football player clutches the ball while running to the end zone. As with the cross cradle hold, your hand holds your baby's head, and your forearm supports your baby's back and bottom. But instead of lying across your front, your baby lies at your side. A pillow or two lifts your baby and your arm to the right height. This hold keeps your baby off your incision if you had a C-section. It's also useful for tandem nursing.

Side-lying: With this hold, you and your baby lie on your sides facing each other. Align your baby's mouth with your nipple by adjusting your position or supporting your baby's head with your upper arm. To switch breasts, just put your baby on your chest and roll over so you're lying on your other side.

Combination of holds: Once you become more experienced at breastfeeding, you may discover that a combination of different holds works best for you. For example, if you're left-handed, you might use the football hold on your left breast and the cross cradle hold on your right.

3. **Align your baby**: Good alignment is the key to a good latch. If you're using the cradle, cross cradle, or side-lying hold, you and your baby should be tummy-to-tummy. If you're using the football hold, you and your baby should be side-to-tummy. Your baby's nose should be pointing at your nipple, and your baby's body should be straight— you should be able to draw an imaginary line from ear to shoulder to hip.

4. **Introduce your nipple**: If you're using the cradle, cross cradle, or football hold, cup your breast in a U-hold by placing your thumb on one side of your areola and your fingers on the other. If you're using the side-lying hold, cup your breast in a C-hold by placing your thumb above your areola and your fingers below it. Both the U-hold and the C-hold create a "breast sandwich" that make it easier for your baby to latch onto as much breast as possible. Tickle your baby's mouth with your nipple. When your baby opens his or her mouth wide, quickly but gently guide baby's mouth onto your nipple. Be sure to bring your baby to your breast instead of bringing your breast to your baby. Your baby should extend his or her neck a bit to reach your nipple; this makes it easier for baby to breathe and swallow. If baby's chin is tucked in, breathing and swallowing will be harder. Make sure your baby's mouth covers as much of your areola as possible, and that baby's lips are flanged outward.

5. **Vary your holds**: Once you master one hold, try another. The different positions put pressure on different milk ducts, so rotating positions can help prevent clogged ducts.

On Your Own

If you've given birth in a hospital or birth center, you may be eager to return to the cozy security of home. At the same time, you may feel apprehensive about breastfeeding on your own where there are no nurses or other expert helpers. However you're feeling, trust your baby, your body, and your instincts. Your baby is born to breastfeed. Your body is designed to feed your baby. And your common sense will tell you if something's amiss. All you need to remember are a few basic signs and guidelines.

Basic Guidelines

For continued breastfeeding success, here are some important guidelines to follow during your baby's first two weeks:

- Nurse your baby on demand, *at least* eight to twelve times per twenty-four hours. Don't expect your newborn to eat at regular intervals; instead, simply feed whenever your baby shows signs of hunger. (See below.)

- If your baby sleeps more than four hours straight, wake him or her up for a feeding. This will help prevent dehydration and establish your milk supply.

- Continue giving your baby only breast milk—no water, formula, or anything else.

- Only nurse at the breast; do not express any milk unless you've already been pumping for medical reasons. When your milk first comes in, frequent nursing is your best bet to alleviate engorgement. If your baby can't keep up with your supply, pumping briefly after nursing will help.

- Continue avoiding artificial nipples.

- If you have latching problems or nipple pain, seek help immediately from a lactation consultant. (See page 37 for more on lactation consultants and page 49 for more on nipple pain.)

- Monitor your baby's diapers (see page 43) and watch for signs of dehydration. (See sidebar on the following page.)

- Have your baby's doctor examine him or her two to four days after birth. Among other things, having your baby weighed may resolve any fears you have about having enough milk for your baby. Your baby's doctor can also observe a nursing session and offer tips if necessary.

Signs of Hunger and Fullness

Crying may seem to be your newborn's only mode of communication. You know crying is a sign of discomfort, but what kind of discomfort? Only trial and error will tell. Isn't there a better way to meet your baby's needs?

Yes, there is. If you watch carefully, you'll see that your baby is often trying to tell you something *without* crying. For example, your baby uses many distinct signs to show that he or she is hungry or full. If you heed them, you can minimize the amount of crying in your house—from both you and your baby!

Signs of Hunger

Early Signs

If you nurse your baby promptly when you see these early signs of hunger, you'll prevent the fussing and crying that comes next. You'll also teach your baby that you can be trusted to meet his or her needs.

- Smacking or licking lips
- Opening and closing mouth
- Sucking on lips, tongue, hands, fingers, toes, toys, or clothing

Signs of Dehydration

If you notice these signs, you'll need to take your baby to his or her caregiver or to an urgent care clinic immediately.

- Your baby's eyes are dull.
- Your baby's mouth and lips are dry.
- Your baby's skin feels loose. When you gently pinch it, it doesn't spring right back into shape.
- Your baby's skin and the whites of his eyes are growing yellower.
- Your baby's diapers are damp, not wet, and are stained yellow.
- Your baby is sleepy and doesn't wake to feed often (at least six–eight feeds every twenty-four hours). Or your baby wakes often to feed, but just sucks quickly with only a few swallows before falling asleep again at most or all feeds.
- Your baby doesn't swallow frequently and rhythmically in the first five minutes of each feed.
- Your baby is unsettled (searching for the breast or crying) after a feeding.
- Your baby frowns while sucking at the breast.
- Your baby has tiny amounts of black or brown stool.
- You have no change in breast fullness from the beginning to the end of each feeding.

Active Signs

When you see these signs, it means your baby's getting impatient because you haven't been paying attention!

- Rooting around on the chest of whoever's handy
- Fidgeting or squirming
- Hitting you
- Fussing or breathing fast
- Shaking head quickly from side to side

Late Signs

These are signs of extreme hunger and desperation; your baby's wondering if he or she will ever eat again. Be aware that nursing may be difficult or impossible. You'll have to find a way to calm down your agitated baby first.

- Crying
- Refusing the breast

Signs of Fullness

Just as your baby can show hunger, he or she can also communicate fullness. The signs listed below may also signal a need to pause briefly and burp.

- Detaching from the breast
- Falling asleep

Common Questions

Q: How often should I nurse?

A: Nurse your baby whenever you see signs of hunger. This is called feeding on demand. You should expect to nurse at least eight to twelve times per twenty-four hours. This doesn't mean feedings will be spaced regularly; for example, your baby might feed every hour for several hours, then take a three-hour break, and so on. Don't expect or force your baby to follow a schedule, because his or her needs change throughout the day and from day to day. Remember that cluster feeding is common and isn't a sign of insufficient milk production—and that the more you nurse, the more milk you'll produce. If your baby sleeps more than four hours straight during the first two weeks, you should wake him or her up to nurse.

During growth spurts (which occur at about 2–3 weeks, 6 weeks, and 6 months), your baby may drink more often. When he begins sleeping longer hours in the night, his feedings will be more spread out.

Q: How long should I nurse at each feeding?

A: You should nurse your baby on each breast for as long as your baby wants to feed. The fat content of your milk increases as your baby nurses at each breast, so it's important not to cut it short! Let your baby detach instead of detaching him or her. If your baby's awake after finishing a breast, burp him or her and offer the other breast. Repeat until your baby is no longer interested in feeding.

Q: How do I know if my baby is eating enough?

A: There are two ways to measure this—by output and weight gain.

- *Output*:
    - The first week: During the first three or four days, your baby should have at least one wet diaper and one poopy diaper for each day of life (one on day one, two on day two, and so on). Your baby's poop should turn from thick, tarry, and black to greenish yellow. After day four your baby should have at least five wet diapers and at least three quarter-size poops per day. The poop should be loose, yellow, and curdy. To feel how heavy a sufficiently wet diaper is, pour three tablespoons of water into a clean diaper.
    - Weeks two through four: Your baby should have at least five wet diapers and at least three quarter-size poops per day.
    - After four to six weeks: Some babies begin to poop less often at this time—as infrequently as once every seven to ten days. As long as your baby is gaining well, this is normal. After six weeks, your baby's wet diapers may drop to four per day, but the amount of urine in them will increase to four to six tablespoons as your baby's bladder capacity grows.
- *Weight gain*: It's normal for a newborn to lose up to 7 percent of birth weight in the first few days of life.[26] If your baby was born healthy and at term, he or she

Every Feeding IS an Opportunity

When your baby is asking to nurse a lot, it's easy to get impatient. It might help to look at each feeding as an opportunity to focus on and bond with your baby. Feedings are wonderfully quiet times to reflect on the miracle of life. Alternatively, you can look forward to feedings as chances to rest. Use them to put your feet up and close your eyes for a few minutes!

Which Breast First?

If your baby nurses from both breasts, he or she usually takes more milk from the first one. Begin each feeding on the breast you ended with at the last feeding (or the breast that feels most full). If your baby nursed from only one breast at the last feeding, begin the next feeding with the other breast. By switching back and forth between breasts when you start feedings, you make sure both breasts get the message to make plenty of milk. To remember which breast you want to start the next feeding on, tie a ribbon or slip a small safety pin around the bra strap on that side.

should be back to birth weight within fourteen days. A good time to check your baby's weight is at the end of the first week or the beginning of the second week. After your milk comes in, your baby should gain about 6 ounces (170 grams) per week.

Q: How will I know if my baby is correctly latched?

A: Your baby's mouth should be wide open, lips flanged outward, and nose, cheeks, and chin should be touching or almost touching your breast. Your baby's mouth should cover as much of your areola as possible, not just your nipple. Correct latching will minimize sore nipples and help your baby extract milk efficiently.

Q: How will I know if my baby is actually drinking?

A: If you listen carefully, you'll hear your baby suck and swallow rhythmically, with occasional pauses. After nursing effectively, your baby will have a moist mouth (perhaps a milk mustache, too) and will seem satisfied. Your breast will soften as your baby empties it.

Common Problems and Practical Solutions

The first three stories in this section (about positioning, latch, and frequency) are about three real women who experienced the most common breastfeeding problems. Karen Peters, a lactation consultant and executive director of Breastfeeding Task Force of Greater Los Angeles, helped these women overcome their problems and successfully breastfeed their babies.

Positioning

Mary came to Karen for help at three weeks postpartum. Her baby was gaining plenty of weight, breastfeeding often, and peeing and pooping well—but Mary had sore nipples.

Karen watched Mary nurse and noticed her awkward positioning. Mary lifted her breast high, hiked up her shoulder, and pressed her baby's head forcefully to her breast. Her baby resisted this pressure by pushing back against her hand. The breast distortion and pushing made it impossible for Mary's baby to latch well. With all the tension in both Mary and her baby, breastfeeding felt like a battle.

Karen taught Mary to let her breast rest in its normal position and to cradle her baby with his nose at nipple level. Karen also showed Mary how to support her son's body while giving him control of his head. After Mary changed her positioning, her nipple pain disappeared, and she and her son both began to enjoy breastfeeding.

Latch

Sharon sought Karen's help at five days postpartum, complaining of sore nipples. Her left nipple had an open wound, and she was beginning to resent her son's frequent feeding.

Karen observed a nursing session and saw that Sharon positioned Jason well, on his side with his body completely facing her body. She supported his shoulder blades and the base of his head. She brought his nose to nipple level using the cross cradle hold. When Jason opened his mouth only slightly, she leaned forward to insert her nipple. She cried out in pain, but let him stay latched.

Quickly, Karen instructed Sharon to release the suction with her finger and detach Jason. Her nipple had white crease on it, passing right through the wound on the top. Karen taught Sharon to correct the latch by waiting for Jason to open his mouth wide, then bringing him quickly up and onto her breast. Karen also explained that comfort should be Sharon's guide; if latching hurt, she should detach and relatch Jason with a wider mouth.

Sharon shared in a support group the next week that her nipples were completely healed. Jason was opening his mouth wide to latch. She was now looking forward to each feeding instead of dreading it.

Frequency

Emily's son, Luke, was still below his birth weight at his two-week checkup, and she was referred to Karen's breastfeeding support group. Emily said she'd been instructed to feed Luke every three hours. Sometimes he was deeply asleep and difficult to rouse. He often fell asleep at the breast. Between feedings Emily placed him in the car seat.

Karen explained that Emily and Luke were the victims of bad advice. Because Emily had been told to schedule Luke's feedings, she was watching the clock instead of Luke. She was missing his hunger signs, like putting his hands in his mouth, and was thus missing opportunities when he was alert and eager to eat. The warm, rounded car seat probably contributed to Luke's oversleeping and may also have impeded his breathing.

Karen told Emily that instead of feeding Luke every three hours (or on any schedule), she should feed Luke on demand, a *minimum* of eight times per twenty-four hours. Karen also recommended holding Luke or laying him on his back between feedings and using the car seat only for car rides. Finally, she suggested that Emily continue attending the support group, where she could listen to other mothers share how they read their babies' cues. Emily did all these things and reported that Luke was gaining weight well.

Engorgement

Your milk will "come in" anywhere from two to five days after you give birth. Most women will feel at least some engorgement. It's normal; your breasts are transitioning from just making two ounces of colostrum a day to twenty ounces or more of milk per day! Your breasts may feel hard and warm as blood rushes to them and they become engorged with milk. The following tips will help relieve engorgement and make you more comfortable:

- Feed your baby frequently—at least eight times in twenty-four hours.
- Breastfeed from both breasts at each feeding.

Tales from the Trenches: Engorgement

I remember it like it was yesterday: My breasts felt like they were about to burst, and the pump that I'd bought while I was pregnant didn't work. I wasn't up to leaving the house yet, and my husband was working at the time. So I called my friend Jacquie. She was working, too, so I begged her husband, Jeff, to go to the drugstore and buy me a breast pump. The saintly man brought it to me within an hour and saved me from explosion.

- Don't give your baby any supplemental feedings from a bottle.

- Right before you nurse, wrap your breast with a warm towel. This will soften your breast and encourage letdown.

- If your breasts still hurt after a feeding, alleviate the pain with cold compresses, bags of frozen peas, or cold cabbage leaves. You can also take ibuprofen or acetaminophen.

- If your baby can't keep up with your milk production, pump both breasts to ease engorgement.

Milk Supply

Since you can't measure how much breast milk your baby is drinking, it's easy to have concerns about milk supply. This is a big concern of new moms and unfortunately one reason why women stop breastfeeding, often unnecessarily.

Your milk supply is not low if:

- Your baby is growing well. If you're not sure, go to the doctor for regular weight checks.

- Your baby is having at least six wet diapers and three bowel movements a day.

- Your baby nurses frequently. Many women think this is a sign that their baby isn't getting enough; actually, it's totally normal for babies to nurse as often as every ninety minutes.

- Your baby is fussy and cluster-feeds in the evening. This is also very normal. It's often chalked up to baby's immature nervous system and milk flow that's sometimes slower in the evening. (Formula-fed babies are also often fussy in the evening.)

- When you pump, very little milk comes out. This isn't a good indication of milk supply, because pumping output varies with your skill and experience as well as your pump's performance.

- You feel little or no letdown. Some women don't, and this is normal.

- Your baby seems to gulp down a bottle right after nursing. It may seem that your baby is still hungry, but he or she may just be caught in an awkward position. Your baby's got a bottle filling his or her mouth with liquid, which your baby must swallow, which encourages more sucking and then another swallow. Liquid flows fast from a bottle, so the bottle empties quickly.

If you still think your milk supply isn't optimum, consider some of these possible causes:

- Skipped feedings
- Supplemental bottles of formula
- Pacifier use
- Keeping a feeding schedule
- Having a sleepy baby who doesn't wake up regularly to nurse

If you still think you have low milk supply, contact a lactation consultant or a La Leche League leader.

Letdown Problems

Your baby's suckling stimulates your pituitary gland to release oxytocin and prolactin, which in turn triggers a letdown reflex. This reflex squeezes milk outward through your milk ducts to make it accessible to your baby. You have several letdowns per feeding, but you probably feel only the first one—or you may not feel any of them. Moms who feel letdown describe it as a hormonal rush, followed about ten seconds later by a swelling, tingly feeling.

Slow Letdown

Many things can disrupt letdown. Pain, stress, anxiety, and embarrassment are common culprits. They make your body release extra adrenaline, which can reduce or block the oxytocin and prolactin release. Other causes are cold, excessive caffeine, smoking, alcohol, and some medications. Finally, moms who've had breast surgery may have nerve damage that interferes with letdown.

Slow letdown can trigger a vicious cycle: Baby fusses and detaches with frustration, which makes mom tense up, which slows letdown even more, and so on. To break this cycle, use relaxation techniques. Nurse in a quiet, calm, comfortable location. Try to reduce distractions and add things that soothe you—perhaps some relaxing music or a burning candle. If your slow letdown persists, contact your doctor or a lactation consultant to help you figure out the cause and deal with it.

Fast Letdown

Fast letdown (also called forceful or overactive letdown) is often associated with having too much milk (oversupply). If your baby does any of the following things, your letdown may be too fast for your baby to handle.

- Your baby gags, chokes, strangles, gulps, gasps, or coughs while nursing.
- Your baby often detaches while nursing.
- Your baby clamps down on your nipple at letdown.
- Your baby makes a clicking sound while nursing.

Maternal Weight and Milk Production

If you're overweight and are having trouble with milk supply, the two situations might be related. One study found that overweight women produce significantly lower levels of prolactin—a hormone necessary for full milk production—than do women of normal weight.[27] Talk to a lactation consultant if you suspect you're having this problem. You may be able to compensate for low prolactin by nursing for longer periods of time.

- Your baby spits up a lot or is very gassy.
- Your baby occasionally refuses to nurse.
- Your baby doesn't seem to like comfort nursing.

Sometimes fast letdown is just an inconvenience. If, however, you think it's damaging your nursing relationship, you should address it. There are two ways you can remedy fast letdown: by helping your baby deal with it and by reducing your supply. You'll probably need to do both, since fast letdown is usually a result of oversupply. It may take a couple of weeks to see results from interventions for oversupply, so try to be patient and keep working on it.

To help your baby deal with fast letdown:

- Position your baby with head and throat higher than your nipple.
- Burp your baby often.
- Nurse often to keep your breasts from getting too full.
- Nurse when your baby is sleepy and more likely to suck gently.
- Detach your baby at letdown and catch the milk in a towel. When the milk flow slows, relatch your baby.
- Pump or hand-express until the milk flow slows, then latch on your baby. (Do this only if nothing else works, as it stimulates additional milk production.)

To reduce your supply:

- Nurse your baby from only one breast per feeding. If your baby detaches (to burp, for example) and then wants to nurse more, nurse on the same breast again. If the other breast gets uncomfortably full, express a little milk from it, then use cool compresses on it.
- Avoid extra breast stimulation (for example: unnecessary pumping, long warm showers, or wearing breast shells).
- Between feedings, use cool compresses on your breasts to discourage blood flow and milk production.
- If nursing on one breast per feeding isn't working after a week or so, try block nursing: nursing on one breast for a certain period of time (including more than one feeding) before switching breasts. Start with two- or three-hour blocks and increase in half-hour increments if needed. If the other breast gets uncomfortably full, express a little milk from it, then use cool compresses on it.
- If you have a severe case of oversupply, talk to a lactation consultant about using cabbage leaf compresses and herbs.

Sore Nipples

Sore nipples are common the first few weeks of breastfeeding; it takes time for your sensitive breasts to get used to this new function. But your nipples shouldn't be persistently sore. Chronic soreness usually has an identifiable cause—typically improper latch or positioning. The first step you should take to prevent (or remedy)

Sore Nipples Troubleshooting Guide

Problem	Solution
Your breast is engorged, stretching your nipple and areola so they're hard and flat. Your baby has a hard time latching properly because the nipple is misshapen.	Before feeding, manually express a little milk and apply warm compresses to soften the nipple and areola.
The tip of your nipple is sore. If you both breastfeed and bottle-feed, your baby may have developed a poor latch or a habit of tongue thrusting while bottle-feeding.	Discontinue bottle-feeding for three or four weeks or until breastfeeding is well-established.
The bottom of your nipple is sore, and you notice that your baby's lower lip is tucked in over the lower gum.	Make sure your baby's mouth is wide open with lips flanged outward before latching your baby to your breast.
The top of your nipple is sore. When you're latching your baby, your nipple is tipped upward and grazes the roof of your baby's mouth.	When you're latching your baby, make sure your nipple is aimed straight at your baby's mouth.
Your nipples feel very tender. Either you have a "barracuda baby" who sucks very vigorously or very sensitive skin.	This problem has several possible solutions: • Expose your breasts to air as often as possible (at least after each feeding). • Use only breathable nursing pads. • In humid climates, apply dry heat using an electric hair dryer for two to three minutes, fanning your breast from six to eight inches away. • In dry climates, leave excess milk on your skin after feedings and let it air-dry.
You feel a burning or stabbing pain that radiates through your milk ducts. You or your baby may have taken antibiotics recently.	This type of pain is associated with a yeast infection (also called thrush). Contact your doctor immediately; both you and your baby must be treated.

sore nipples is to make sure your baby is correctly aligned and latched. (See page 39 for a step-by-step guide to positioning.) Next, check out the above troubleshooting guide for common problems and solutions:[28]

Comfort Measures

Even after you've figured out and addressed the cause of your sore nipples, you may need comfort measures until your nipples heal. Routine use of nipple cream isn't recommended, because it can block glands in the areola and nipple. Using anesthetic cream or ice to numb the pain is also discouraged because this can interfere with letdown. Warm, moist compresses seem to be the most effective way to relieve pain and speed healing. In some cases, though—especially in very dry climates—a nipple cream of 100 percent modified lanolin is helpful. (See page 33 for more information on nipple creams.) If you have cracked nipples (depending on severity and location of cracks), your lactation consultant or doctor may recommend other therapies. Your doctor may also recommend ibuprofen or acetaminophen right before nursing.

Plugged Ducts and Mastitis

No doubt you've heard at least one horror story about plugged ducts or mastitis. Just as people feel compelled to share tales of childbirth woe with pregnant women, they think it's a duty to regale new breastfeeders with stories of mammary misery. It's certainly true that plugged ducts and mastitis can be painful, but what you may not hear is that these problems are easily solved. Neither is a reason to stop breastfeeding—in fact, *more* nursing is the best thing you can do.

Plugged Ducts

When a milk duct hasn't been completely drained, the milk can coagulate and form a small plug. If you have a tender lump in your breast or nipple, it's probably a plugged duct. If you see a small white blister on your nipple, that means the opening of a duct is plugged.

Here's how to treat a plugged duct:

- **Apply warmth**: Warmth increases blood flow to the area, which helps milk flow through the duct, which in turn helps dislodge the plug. Take a warm shower; soak your breast in a basin of clean, warm water; or place a heating pad, hot water bottle, or warm compress on the plugged area.

- **Massage**: Massage your breast gently but firmly from the plugged area toward the nipple.

- **Nurse or pump often**: Nurse or pump at least every two hours.

- **Change positions**: Nursing with your baby in a variety of positions puts pressure on different areas of the breast. Try to nurse with your baby's chin over the plugged duct. Laying your baby on his or her back and feeding from above uses gravity to help drain your breast.

- **Reduce stress**: Stress can inhibit letdown and weaken your immune system. Let go of housework and any other nonessentials for a few days. Ask your partner, family, and friends for help.

- **Rest**: Exhaustion weakens your immune system, too. A plugged duct is a message from your body to slow down. Take heed and go to bed! Take your baby with you so you can nurse often.

- **Strengthen your immune system**: Along with resting and reducing stress, drink plenty of fluids and eat a balanced diet. Take a multivitamin, too. Wash your hands often.

- **Manage your pain**: Don't just endure pain; it can hamper letdown and make your problem worse. Take ibuprofen or acetaminophen if necessary.
- **Relieve pressure points**: Tight clothing (especially underwire bras) can cut off milk flow. So can carrying a heavy purse or diaper bag that rests on any part of your breast. Toting your baby in a front carrier or sling in a position that puts a lot of pressure on one area can also be a problem. Examine your wardrobe and your habits for any of these suspects.
- **Try alternative treatments**: Adding lecithin to your diet and reducing your saturated fat intake may help with plugged ducts. For more info on lecithin treatment for plugged ducts, see http://www.kellymom.com/nutrition/vitamins/lecithin.html.

Mastitis

If you don't treat a plugged duct, it can quickly turn into mastitis, an infection of the breast. The symptoms of mastitis include body aches, fever and/or a red, swollen, sore, and hot spot on the breast.

Self-care for mastitis is the same as for plugged ducts. In addition, you should:

- See your doctor for an examination.
- If your doctor prescribes an antibiotic, follow the directions carefully and finish the complete course even if you feel better before you've taken all the pills.
- To prevent an antibiotic-induced yeast infection, ask your doctor about taking a probiotic such as lactobacillus at the same time. (For more information about yeast infections, see the following section.)

Yeast Infection (Thrush)

If you feel sudden burning pain in your nipple or breast, you may have a yeast infection there. Women give very vivid descriptions of the pain, such as "liquid fire," "like broken glass," and "stabbing pain."

Yeast infections are caused by a fungus called candida, which is a normal resident of our skin and the mucous membranes of the mouth, intestines, and vagina. Usually yeast lives in balance with other organisms. When the balance is upset—for example, during times of hormonal change such as pregnancy and postpartum and after antibiotic use—yeast become overpopulated and a yeast infection can occur.

Yeast can also grow out of control on other parts of the body that are moist and dark, such as under the arms, under the breasts, and in the diaper area. If a woman has a yeast infection while she's pregnant, she can pass it to her baby during birth. In babies, yeast infections show up as a bumpy red diaper rash, a rash in the moist skin between fat folds, and in the mouth as thrush.

Thrush causes creamy white patches inside the mouth. If you wipe away a white patch, you'll see a red, irritated area underneath. If your baby has thrush, he or she can pass it to you, causing a yeast infection in your breast. Such an infection

Are You at Risk for a Yeast Infection?

If any of the following describe you, the answer is yes.
- You've recently experienced hormonal changes.
- You take birth control pills.
- You've recently taken antibiotics.
- You have moist skin folds.
- You're not scrupulous about washing your hands after changing your baby's diaper or touching infected areas of your baby's body.
- You have diabetes.

can also cause inflammation of the milk ducts, which can lead to plugged ducts and even to mastitis. Unless both of you are treated simultaneously, you'll continue reinfecting each other! (Even if only one of you has symptoms, both should be treated.) If your baby has thrush, he or she may be gassy. Your baby may refuse to nurse or may nurse only briefly because of mouth pain.

It's no problem to use fresh or frozen milk expressed during a thrush episode while you're being treated for thrush. However, you may be advised not to *freeze* milk expressed while you have thrush. That's because freezing doesn't kill the yeast, and you'll probably be using the frozen milk after you're thrush-free. On the other hand, some experts believe that several components in breast milk both protect your baby from a yeast infection and stifle the growth of yeast in the milk. If you do decide to freeze this milk, label it accordingly. When you use it, you can dilute it with other milk or you can heat it to kill the yeast. (For instructions, see http://www.kellymom.com/bf/concerns/thrush/thrush-expressed-milk.html.) Heating your milk will kill its antibodies, but the milk will still be healthier than formula.[29]

If you or your baby has a yeast infection, your doctor will probably prescribe an antifungal medication for your baby's mouth and for your nipple and areola. Be sure to continue the treatment as long as your doctor directs—usually two weeks after symptoms disappear. During this time it's especially important to wash your hands before and after touching your breasts and after changing diapers. Dry your hands with paper towels. Wash anything your baby mouths with hot soapy water. All clothing that touches your breast or your baby should be changed daily and washed and dried in hot temperatures. Changes in your diet could also help; eating yogurt with live cultures or taking probiotics such as lactobacillus can help re-establish the "good" bacteria in your body.[30] Drinking cranberry juice may also prevent yeast infections.[31]

Baby's Sensitivity to Your Diet

Babies cry a lot—and it may or may not be related to diet. Take a lesson from Mary: Her baby had bouts of painful gas; he sometimes stopped nursing in the middle of a feeding because of the pain. Her doctor suggested she give her baby over-the-counter simethicone drops for infants. The doctor also asked Mary to examine her diet for foods that could be affecting her baby. She began slowly eliminating foods—to the point where her diet was very bland and limited—and still her baby had gas. Conclusion? Sometimes babies have gas, regardless of what you or they eat. Luckily, they outgrow it as their digestive systems mature.

Here's a quick look at foods that are commonly blamed for fussy babies. (For more information about your baby's digestive system, see Chapter 6.)

- **Milk**: Milk in mom's diet is sometimes the cause of a fussy or even colicky baby. If you think this might be your problem, stop eating all dairy products. It'll take about two weeks to get all the dairy out of your system. If milk is the culprit, you should see improvement in your baby in four or five days. Many babies outgrow dairy sensitivity, so try adding a little dairy back into your diet in a few months and see if your baby reacts to it. In the meantime, be sure to eat or drink an alternate source of calcium. (See page 63 for other good sources of calcium.)

- **Gassy foods**: Foods that cause gas in adults (cabbage, broccoli, onion, beans, and so on) may or may not cause gas in babies. If you suspect any of these foods, eliminate them from your diet one at a time to see if it helps your baby.

- **Spicy foods**: You may have heard that you shouldn't eat spicy foods (those with garlic, chili peppers, and so on) while you're breastfeeding. It's possible that your baby may not like milk flavored with a touch of garlic, but it's just as likely that your baby will love it! Everything you eat adds flavor to your milk; overall, this is a good thing. Research shows that breastfed babies are more accepting of new foods later because they've tasted these foods through their moms' milk.

> **Food Allergies**
>
> If, after you eat dairy, your baby has symptoms that signal a true allergic reaction (severe colic, abdominal discomfort, a skin rash, vomiting, diarrhea, or difficulty breathing), avoid all dairy products as well as foods that contain milk protein (casein and whey). You'll need to read food labels carefully. Check with your baby's doctor to find out when—or if—you should try to introduce dairy again. The doctor may recommend a dairy challenge in the controlled environment of his or her office.
>
> If you have a strong family history of allergies, staying away from allergenic foods like cow's milk, egg, fish, peanuts, and other nuts may help prevent allergies in your baby. For more information about food allergies, see page 136.

When Your Baby's Sick

It's highly likely that your baby will get sick during the first year, and illness will probably dampen your baby's appetite. If your baby is old enough to be eating solids, don't worry if your baby suddenly loses interest in them. It is, however, important to keep your baby hydrated. Read on to learn how common illnesses may affect your baby's nursing.

- **Ear infection**: Because ear pain often radiates to the throat, it may hurt for your baby to suck when he or she has an ear infection. Ask your baby's doctor for guidance on using a pain reliever to help your baby nurse more comfortably. If your baby takes bottles occasionally, you may want to try a cup instead; cup feeding may be less painful than bottle-feeding.

- **Sore throat**: Your baby's eating will probably take a dive when swallowing hurts. If your baby is younger than six months or not eating solids yet, try to keep his or her breast milk intake as close to normal as possible. If your baby is older than six months and eating solids, offer soothing liquids like warm broth or cool juice. Older babies can also suck on "momsicles" (frozen breast milk pops) or frozen juice pops, or they can be spoon-fed a breast milk slushie, a fruit smoothie, or pureed soup.

- **Congestion**: If your baby's nose is plugged up or your baby is coughing, he or she may not be able to nurse very well. Try these strategies for thinning and loosening mucus:
  - Rub menthol on your baby's chest.
  - Bathe your baby in warm water with a touch of menthol or eucalyptus.
  - Use a cool-mist vaporizer during naptime.
  - Use over-the-counter saline nose drops to help your baby clear his or her nose.

When to Get Help

Whatever nursing problem(s) you and your baby are having, remember: It's never too early or too late to ask for help! If you've just given birth in a hospital, work with a lactation consultant before you leave. Once you're home, you should call your baby's doctor or a lactation consultant if:[32]

- Your newborn is very sleepy and frequently sleeps more than four hours straight.
- After five days, your milk hasn't come in or your breasts don't feel like they're filling with milk.
- You have severe breast engorgement that discourages you or your baby from nursing.
- Your breast still feels full and hard after a feeding.
- You have severe nipple pain.
- Your baby still seems hungry after most feedings.
- You don't hear a rhythmic suck-and-swallow when your baby nurses.
- After seven days, your baby has fewer than five wet diapers and three quarter-size poops a day; your baby's urine is dark yellow or specked with red; or your baby's poops are still thick and tarry.
- After two weeks, your baby is below birth weight.
- After your milk comes in, your baby hasn't started gaining five to seven ounces per week.
- After a week or two, you don't feel the letdown reflex.
- Your baby's feedings are consistently either very short or very long.

Breastfeeding Your Premature Baby

Feeding Method

If your baby is born past thirty-two weeks gestation, you may be able to nurse the way nature intended—with or without an SNS. If your baby has any health problems or is born before thirty-two weeks, he or she will probably have to be fed through a nasogastric or orogastric tube. You baby can also be fed with a feeding syringe. Whatever the feeding method, you'll need to pump your milk. (See page 7 for more information on the importance of breast milk for preemies.)

Pumping for a Preemie

To express your milk successfully for a preemie, you'll need to mimic the breast-feeding your baby would have done under normal circumstances. (See pages 105–106 for more basic information about pumping.) Here are some tips:

- **Starting up**: Begin pumping as soon after birth as possible. This will signal your breasts to start making milk. Don't be alarmed when you see only very small amounts of yellowish milk (colostrum) at first. This is normal! Colostrum is very rich in antibodies and nutrients, and it comes in small amounts because a newborn's stomach (especially a preemie's) is very small. (For more information about preemie colostrum, see page 17.)

- **Equipment**: Use a hospital-grade pump. This type will express milk efficiently from both breasts at the same time. Your hospital's lactation consultant can help you locate and borrow or rent a high-quality pump.

- **Frequency**: You should pump as many times a day as your baby would probably nurse (eight to twelve times a day in the first weeks, or about every two to three hours). Since you won't have your baby's normal feeding cues to keep you on track, stick to a schedule.

- **Duration**: At the end of each pumping session, continue pumping for several minutes after your milk stops flowing. This will tell your breasts to ramp up milk production and will ensure an ample milk supply for your quickly growing baby.

- **Storage**: Label and store your breast milk in containers that meet your hospital's requirements. Labeling requirements usually include your baby's name, the date and time of pumping, and any medications you're currently taking.

Additional Nutrition

Breast milk provides the best possible nutrition for your preemie, but depending on your baby's birth weight and development, he or she may need additional nutrients and calories. Your baby's neonatologist may recommend vitamin supplements and/or a human milk fortifier containing extra calories and other nutrients to meet your baby's special needs.

Learning to Nurse

As your baby matures and stabilizes, naturally you'll want to teach him or her how to nurse. Keep a few things in mind: If your baby has been fed by bottle until now, he or she is now quite accustomed to bottle-feeding. Your baby will probably have an adjustment period while learning how to nurse and may even prefer the bottle. It's nothing personal—it's just much easier to get milk from a bottle! Don't get discouraged; this phase will probably pass. To ease your baby's adjustment, you may want to use an SNS at first. It delivers expressed milk to your baby through a tiny tube taped next to your nipple. It provides a quicker reward for your baby's learning efforts. Eventually you should be able to ditch the SNS and fully nurse your baby.

When to Get Help

- **Before or immediately after birth**: I recommend that you talk to a lactation consultant right after your baby is born. (If you suspect you'll be giving birth prematurely due to health problems or multiple babies, talk with a lactation consultant *before* birth.) A lactation consultant can tell you what to do now and what to expect in the coming weeks and months.

- **When your baby switches from tube- or bottle-feeding to nursing**: You may need expert help making this transition, especially if your baby has been fed through a tube or bottle for a long time.

- **If your baby has suckling problems**: Premature infants sometimes have problems suckling because they have been suctioned or intubated, or have been on ventilators. They may also develop high arched or grooved palates as a result of endotrachial tubes. If your baby has any of these problems, you may need special positioning and other tips to make breastfeeding work.

- **If you have any other problems**: What seems to be a big problem can often be solved easily by a simple change in position or timing. Never hesitate to call a professional! Because breastfeeding is so important for the health of a preemie, medical insurance usually covers the cost of a lactation consultant.

Chapter 3

Power Eating for Breastfeeding

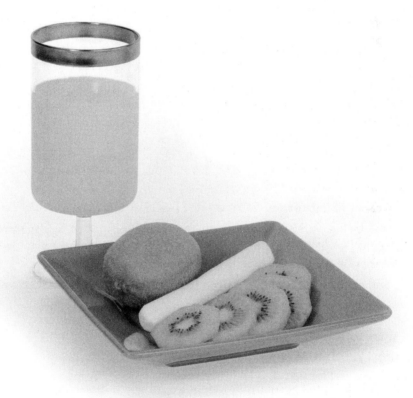

Inside some of us is a thin person struggling to get out,
but that person can usually be sedated with a few pieces of chocolate cake.
—Author unknown

While you're pregnant, you get used to eating three big meals a day plus a few snacks. You don't worry about the occasional ice cream sundae. You may be dreading postpartum, thinking that you'll have to starve yourself to lose your baby fat.

Good news: You don't have to diet when you're breastfeeding, and you still lose weight! In fact, because it takes a lot of energy to run a milk factory, you may need more calories than you did while you were pregnant. While you're exclusively breastfeeding, you may need about the same number of calories per day that you needed at the end of pregnancy—or even up to two hundred more.

Before you heed those visions of doughnuts dancing in your head, remember that you're still eating for two! While you're exclusively breastfeeding, your baby is still depending on you for total nourishment. Must you have a perfect diet? No. Should you eat as well as possible? Yes! A good breastfeeding diet is very similar to a good pregnancy diet, so there won't be any big changes to get used to.

Postpartum Weight Loss: What to Expect

In General

- You should lose ten to fifteen pounds immediately after delivery and usually a few more over the next week or so as your body gets rid of extra fluid.

- Postpartum weight loss varies a lot among women. A few women will fit into their prepregnancy clothes within three months; most will take a year or more to do so. A few women even gain weight postpartum.

- Factors that most influence weight and fat loss are:
  - How much weight you gained
  - Your activity level
  - Your motivation

- Don't be discouraged if it takes longer than you expected to lose your baby weight. Do stick with it and lose the weight, especially if you plan on having another baby.

- Eat high-fiber foods and dairy products; these are associated with weight loss. The fiber can also help with postpartum constipation, and the dairy products can also help prevent or replenish calcium loss from your bones.

When You're Breastfeeding

- After your initial postpartum weight loss of ten to fifteen pounds, you'll naturally lose one or two pounds per month without really trying. In fact, it's best not to do anything special to lose weight the first two months. Just try for a healthy diet.

- After the first two months, it's safe to lose a pound per week. It's best to lose weight by adding exercise to your routine. This will decrease body fat while increasing muscle mass, which burns extra calories.

- Some research shows that nursing women lose the most fat and weight between three and six months postpartum.[1]

- Some nursing moms get back to their prepregnancy weight quickly and need lots of extra calories to maintain their weight. For example, Christine says she went five to ten pounds below her normal weight while "shoveling in tons of food." (Now that's a great problem to have!)

- Some nursing moms will hang on to the last five pounds or so of baby weight until their babies wean.

Ten Tips for Losing the Baby Fat

When you give birth, you have a really good excuse to be a bit chubbier than usual for a while. But this excuse won't cut it for more than two years. Trust me: You don't want to wait too long to get back into shape. I've met many fifty-year-olds who are still carrying their baby fat, and it's really hard to drop those pounds at that point. Don't let it happen to you!

Following are some tips for losing your pregnancy weight. Remember, getting back to your ideal weight means you'll be better able to take care of your children—not to mention being able to run and play with them!

1. **Eat small, frequent meals**: Eating six small meals instead of three (or fewer) big ones revs up your metabolism. It also fits better with your demanding new life as a mom.

2. **Keep healthy food in the house**: If you can't resist the temptation when sweet and salty snacks are around, don't bring them home.

3. **Eat at the table and focus on eating**: If you eat while doing something else, it's easy to forget the food and just keep shoving it in. The next thing you know, you've eaten an entire bowl of popcorn. If your mouth needs something to do while you watch the news, pay bills, or whatever, chew on some sugarless gum.

4. **Keep a food diary**: This can be a real eye opener. Most people have no idea how much and how often they're eating. You may spot some bad habits you didn't know you had, or you may find that you're actually eating great! People who lose weight and keep it off report that this is one habit that really makes a difference. Participants in my weight-loss classes generally lose weight the first week without making any conscious diet changes—they simply keep a food diary!

5. **Think about your drinks**: Many of us don't eat too much—it's our drinks that get us in trouble. If you drink more than a cup of juice or regular soda a day, that's too much! Soda and juice drinks contain about 150 empty or low-nutrient calories per 1½ cups. Doesn't sound like much until you add up the calories from just one extra 150-calorie beverage a day for a year—it would add up to a fifteen-pound weight gain! Some other healthy thirst quenchers include water with a slice of lemon or orange, vegetable or tomato juice, or a juice and club soda spritzer.

6. **Get active**:
   - *Take a walk*: During the first couple of months postpartum (before your doctor okays strenuous exercise), a walk around the block (or two) can start your body on the path to healthy activity.
   - *Join a gym*: If mainstream health clubs give you the willies, you might like an all-women facility. I've tried Curves and Ladies' Workout Express (thirty-minute fitness centers for women) and love them. They both offer a low-key environment and an easy way to combine aerobics and weight resistance in a short workout—and with no class schedules to keep track of.
   - *Join a pool*: Even if you're not a swimmer, walking back and forth across a pool is great exercise. It's easy on the joints, too. If you want to kick your workout up a notch and provide more muscle resistance in the water, a buoyancy belt keeps you suspended in deep water, while dumbbells and resistance cuffs for your ankles or arms increase your cardio workout.
   - *Climb the stairs*: If you have a two-story house, you can create your own training circuit. Combine short aerobic spurts up the stairs with some light weight lifting on each floor.
   - *Dance*: By yourself or with your baby, it's fun and it's free!
   - *Watch a TV workout*: Oh, and you also have to *do* the workout.
   - *Do a slow workout*: Yoga and Pilates are both very effective ways to strengthen your muscles and realign your posture.
   - *Track your steps*: Numbers can be great motivators—get yourself a pedometer and watch your steps pile up! If you walk five thousand steps a day, that's about two miles. Add an extra five thousand steps per day, and that's equal to about an hour of continuous walking, which burns three to four hundred calories, depending on your pace and your weight. That's the calories you need to burn to lose about 2½ to 3½ pounds per month.

7. **Get enough sleep**: That's a joke, right? Nope—it's important to sleep when your baby sleeps. Researchers believe that inadequate sleep affects leptin and ghrelin, hormones that regulate appetite.[2] Also, not getting enough shut-eye appears to increase your risk of overweight, hypertension, and type 2 diabetes.[3, 4, 5]

8. **Don't go too fast**: Your body may not be ready to follow you on a weight-loss adventure. If you feel exhausted from changes you're making, back off a bit. And make sure you don't lose more than two pounds a week.

9. **Eat lots of fruits and veggies**: If you eat at least seven fruits and vegetables in a day, the rest of your diet will fall into place like magic. You'll feel satisfied and energized.

10. **Don't deprive**: Most people think of a diet as a temporary period of deprivation they struggle through to get their favorite foods back. Sound familiar? If so, you'll do much better with an "undiet," a way of eating that includes your favorite foods (in smaller amounts). This type of eating is much easier—and more pleasant—to sustain over the long haul.

Nutrition for Nursing Moms

When you're breastfeeding, it's important to eat well to fuel milk production without depleting your own nutrient stores. Eating well also gives you the energy you need to care for a new baby. This section will explain how to have the best possible diet for both your health and your baby's.

Your baby may not be sitting at the dinner table with you yet, but he or she *is* sharing what you eat. If your diet doesn't supply all the nutrients your baby needs, your body will rob them from your own nutrient stores. It's a good idea to take a multivitamin/mineral supplement while breastfeeding to cover your bases. Some experts recommend continuing your prenatal supplement, and that's a good idea if you're anemic. If you're not anemic and your prenatal vitamin has a lot of iron, you may find it too constipating. (Lactation hormones can also cause constipation.) In this case, you should choose a different multivitamin.

Nutrients You Need More Of

Though multivitamins can help fill nutritional gaps, they aren't magic pills. The best way to nourish you and your baby is by eating nutrient-rich foods. To make milk, your body needs a lot more of certain nutrients than it needed during pregnancy:

Nutrients in High Demand for Nursing

Nutrient	Foods Rich in This Nutrient
Vitamin A/ beta carotene	Organ meats, milk, cheese, orange and dark green fruits and vegetables such as sweet potato, carrots, spinach, kale, vegetable soup, cantaloupe, apricots, papaya, and mango
Vitamin C	Guava, peppers, kiwi fruit, citrus fruit and juice, strawberries, Brussels sprouts, cantaloupe, papaya, broccoli, tomato juice, pineapple
Vitamin E	Wheat germ oil, almonds, sunflower seeds, sunflower oil, hazelnuts, peanut butter, peanuts, wheat germ
Choline	Beef liver, eggs, wheat germ, cod, beef, Brussels sprouts, broccoli
Iodine	Iodized salt, seaweed, cod, potato, milk
Manganese	Raisin bran cereal, pineapple, pineapple juice, instant oatmeal, pecans, spinach, almonds, whole-wheat bread
Selenium	Salmon, shrimp, crab, halibut, pork, chicken breast, brown rice

Foods are listed according to nutrient content, in descending order.

How Diet Affects Breast Milk

You'd have to be really malnourished for your diet to drastically affect your milk. Your body will use stored nutrients to make high-quality milk if those nutrients are absent from your diet. That's not to say that your diet doesn't affect your milk at all—it does—but less than you probably think. (The one part of your diet that can have long term effects on your baby is fat.) Read on to find out more.

- **Volume**: Your rate of milk production varies according to how much your baby sucks. Your milk volume will drop if you're dehydrated or severely malnourished. Ironically, drinking too much fluid can also reduce your milk volume. It's best to drink simply to quench thirst.

- **Protein**: The amount of protein in your milk stays stable regardless of how much protein you eat.

- **Fat**: Your diet doesn't affect the *amount* of fat in your milk, but it does affect the *composition* of that fat. For example, if the fat in your diet is mostly polyunsaturated fat like corn oil, your breast milk will also contain a high percentage of this type of fat. Likewise, if you've been splurging on bakery foods high in trans fats, the trans fat in your milk will increase. The fat you store today could be the fat your baby drinks tomorrow, or the fat baby number two drinks in a few years. Yet another good reason to eat the right kind of fat.

  > ### Trans Fats in Breast Milk
  >
  > Trans fats are produced when liquid oil is hydrogenated (combined with hydrogen to solidify it). Trans fats are found in stick margarine, shortening, and any foods cooked with or in these fats. (Many fried foods and bakery goods are loaded with trans fats.) Research has shown that trans fats can hinder infant growth (and contribute to various other problems in both you and your baby), so read labels and avoid trans fats!

- **Docosahexaenoic acid (DHA) and arachidonic acid (ARA)**: Your baby needs these long-chain fatty acids for brain and eye development, which continues at a fast pace during the first year—and beyond. The amount the body can make depends on the amount of essential fatty acids in the diet and the amount of other types of fat in the diet.

- **Cholesterol**: The amount of cholesterol in your milk stays fairly constant regardless of the amount of cholesterol in your diet. Your baby's body uses cholesterol to build cell membranes, myelin (a protective coating around nerve fibers), and brain tissue.

- **Lactose**: Lactose, the primary carbohydrate in breast milk, doesn't seem to be affected by your diet.

- **Vitamins and minerals**: Does the amount of nutrients in your diet affect the amount in your milk?[6]

  - *Calcium*: No
  - *Phosphorous*: No
  - *Iron*: No
  - *Manganese*: Yes
  - *Zinc*: No
  - *Copper*: No
  - *Sodium*: No
  - *Potassium*: No
  - *Iodine*: Yes
  - *Fluoride*: Yes
  - *Chromium*: No
  - *Vitamin B_{12}*: Yes
  - *Thiamine*: Yes
  - *Riboflavin*: Yes
  - *Niacin*: Yes
  - *Pantothenic acid*: Yes

- *Selenium*: Yes
- *Folate*: No
- *Vitamin C*: Yes

- *Vitamin B₆*: Yes
- *Vitamin D*: Yes
- *Vitamin K*: Probably

Common Questions

Q: What if I don't drink very much milk?

A: That's fine, as long as you have another good source of calcium in your diet. (See the chart below for calcium-rich foods.) Calcium is critical to your bone health and your baby's overall health. To provide calcium for breast milk, your body takes it from your bones, then adds it back later. (Some researchers have found that breastfeeding increases bone density even more than baseline amounts,[7] which is why breastfeeding is ultimately good for bone health.) But if your calcium intake drops below a certain level, you use more of your bone stores than your body can replace, thus decreasing your own bone density.

Another important reason for consuming enough calcium is to prevent lead from leaching into your milk. Ninety percent of the lead in your body is stored in your bones. When your body uses bone as a calcium source, the lead in your bones leaches into your milk. So if you've had significant lead exposure in your life and don't consume enough calcium, the lead level of your breast milk will be elevated.

Food Sources of Calcium

Food	Calcium Content
1 cup (240 milliliters) cow's milk	300 milligrams
1 cup (240 milliliters) soymilk	300 milligrams
1 ounce (30 grams) Swiss cheese	272 milligrams
1 ounce (30 grams) Cheddar cheese	204 milligrams
3 ounces (90 grams) canned salmon with bones	203 milligrams
1 cup (240 milliliters) calcium-fortified orange juice	300 milligrams
½ cup firm tofu made with calcium	250 milligrams*
1 cup (240 milliliters) cooked rhubarb	348 milligrams
1 cup (240 milliliters) cooked frozen spinach	278 milligrams
1 cup (240 milliliters) collard greens	358 milligrams
1 cup (240 milliliters) cooked kale	180 milligrams
2 tablespoons (30 milliliters) blackstrap molasses	344 milligrams
1 cup (240 milliliters) okra	177 milligrams
1 tablespoon (15 grams) sesame seed butter (tahini)	64 milligrams
2 medium (6- or 7-inch) corn tortillas	90 milligrams

The Dietary Reference Intake (DRI) for calcium is 1,000–1,200 milligrams.
Numbers are rounded.
* Varies by brand.

Seven Easy Steps to Fat Balance

1. Use olive or canola oil as your main cooking oil. You can add flaxseed, flaxseed oil, or walnut oil to your diet for extra omega-3 fat. Grapeseed oil, macadamia nut oil, and avocado oil are also good choices. Soybean oil contains both omega-3 and omega-6 fat.
2. If you use margarine, use the soft, spreadable kind that doesn't contain trans fats.
3. Eat fish a few times a week—including a cold water fish like salmon at least once. You can also find a chart with DHA content of over fifty fish species at: www.health.gov/dietaryguidelines/dga2005/report/HTML/table_g2_adda2.htm
4. Round out your other meals with lean meats, pork, poultry, soy, and legumes.
5. Keep your trans fat intake as close to zero as possible.
6. If you don't like to eat fish, consider taking a DHA supplement.
7. Download Keep It Managed, free software that helps you track your omega-6 and omega-3 fats, at efaeducation.nih.gov/sig/kim.html.

Q: What kind of fat should I be eating?

A: Your baby's brain and eyes are made mostly of fat, and both are still developing during your baby's first year. (Your baby's brain will double in size by his or her first birthday!) The most prominent fat in both types of tissue is DHA, a long-chain omega-3 fatty acid. Because your baby gets the fat he or she needs for all this growth from your breast milk, you should try to supply the right kind.

The fat composition of your milk reflects the amounts of different types of fats you eat. Most people eat too many omega-6 fats (found in corn oil, safflower oil, and sunflower oil) and not enough omega-3 fats (found in cold-water fish, fortified eggs, flaxseed oil, walnuts, canola oil, and olive oil.) It's important to balance the two. Since omega-6 fats often sneak into one's diet via processed foods and food preparation, the fat you add in cooking and food prep should be the omega-3 kind. You should also try to eat as little saturated fat and trans fat as possible, since these types of fat, too, hinder your body's ability to make DHA.

Q: Should I take a nutrition supplement?

A: Probably. Even if your diet is close to perfect, a basic multivitamin can't hurt. Ditto for a calcium and/or DHA supplement.

If you have a hard time swallowing pills (especially the notoriously big multivitamin and calcium supplements), try chewable ones. Viactiv makes a multivitamin chew as well as a tasty calcium chew that comes in many flavors. Tums is another chewable—and cheap—form of calcium.

If you want to take a DHA supplement but you're worried about possible seafood contaminants, try one that's not made from fish oil. Expecta Lipil is one good brand. I also recommend Coromega—it's a highly purified fish oil blended in an orange-flavored pudding-like emulsion. Research has shown that this type of fish oil is more bioavailable than other fish oils.

If you have chronic problems with plugged ducts, mastitis, and/or yeast infections (thrush), you might want to take daily probiotic supplements. (See page 126 for more information.)

Q: What about individual vitamins and herbal supplements?

A: It's best to avoid individual vitamins and herbals supplements unless you're taking them under the guidance of a doctor who's knowledgeable about their effects on lactation and on infants. Individual vitamins can disrupt the balance of other nutrients. Many herbal supplements have no clinical research proving their effectiveness or safety.

Q: Why am I always hungry?

A: You're not eating enough! This can happen if you're not taking the time to eat decent meals and snacks or if you're very active and burning up calories like crazy. Your hunger may also mirror your baby's growth spurts. If you notice your baby's nursing a lot more and/or you're getting awfully hungry and thirsty, heed the message from your baby and your body. Eat and drink to appetite and thirst, and keep an eye on your weight, too. Remember: It takes a generous supply of nutrients to fuel a milk factory.

Q: What is a safe rate of weight loss?

A: After the first month or so, losing one pound per week won't affect your breast milk. One study showed that losing up to two pounds a week for a short time (a week and a half) didn't affect breast milk quantity or quality.[8] Most nursing moms will lose two to four pounds a month. If you lose more than that, if you're hungry, if your energy is low (not from lack of sleep), or if your milk supply is insufficient, you probably need to eat more.

Q: What if I lose more than that?

A: Excessive weight loss can reduce the volume and/or nutrient quality of your breast milk. If you lose more than four pounds per month, chances are your diet doesn't contain everything your body needs to make top-quality milk. To make sure your weight loss isn't affecting your baby, monitor your milk supply and your baby's weight gain and eating habits. (See page 46 for more information on low milk supply.)

Q: Should I exercise, too?

A: Yes—definitely! It also does wonders for alleviating baby blues, preventing postpartum depression, improving your energy, and getting you out of the house. And of course exercise will improve your muscle tone and strengthen your bones. When you lose weight without exercising, part of the weight you lose is muscle. You need muscles for strength, obviously, but another not-so-obvious reason to preserve your muscle mass is that muscle burns more calories than fat—even when you're doing nothing. That may not seem like a big deal now, when you're burning calories like they're going out of style, but you'll want that muscle later, when breastfeeding slows down and eventually ends.

If you want to preserve muscle mass and strengthen bones, you need to do weight-bearing exercise (any exercise in which your feet and legs bear your weight, such as walking, stair climbing, or dancing). Try to do a combination of weight resistance (using weights or hydraulic resistance machines) and aerobics. Using soup cans as weights is a great way to get your arms in shape. Other helpful tools you can use at home are an exercise ball and resistance bands. Here's the handiest workout of all: babywearing! Take a daily walk (aerobic exercise) while carrying your baby (weight resistance) in a well-designed soft carrier. Choose one that's lightweight and comfortable for you and also for your baby. (Your baby's weight should be resting on his or her bottom, not crotch.) For even greater intensity, swing your arms or do arm circles at the same time.

A new baby can turn your world upside down; you may not have time for a lengthy workout. If you find it's easier to exercise in smaller sessions throughout the day, go for it! Three or four ten-minute workouts are just as good as a continuous thirty- or forty-minute workout. Increasing fitness through lifestyle changes also helps (parking a little farther away, taking the stairs, hand-delivering messages at work instead of e-mailing them, and so on). (See page 60 for more fitness tips.)

Eating Tips

When you're breastfeeding, eating frequent small meals and snacks is a great way to fit in all the nutrients you need for you and your baby. The next few pages will give you guidance and examples to help you do that.

The Best Breastfeeding Diet

Your daily menu should include at least 1,800 calories and the following numbers of servings from each food group:

- Three servings of calcium-rich foods (dairy, fortified soymilk, or fortified juice)
- Six servings of grains (at least three of them whole grains)
- Six ounces of lean protein foods (including a variety of protein types: fish, beef, pork, poultry, eggs, and legumes)
- Nine servings of fruits and vegetables (two cups of fruit and two and a half cups of vegetables, including one high in vitamin C and one dark green or deep orange)
- Five teaspoons of fat (used in food preparation or found in processed foods)
- Three hundred milligrams of DHA[9] (for example, by eating five ounces of salmon per week)

One-Handed Meals and Snacks

If you keep your kitchen stocked with a variety of healthy foods you can eat with one hand, it'll be much easier to eat well. Nursing a baby can take a lot of time; why not use some of that time to fill up your own tank?

Following is a list of tasty, nourishing foods you can eat while nursing. (Avoid eating hot, very spicy, or highly allergenic foods while holding your baby—if they fall on your baby, you'll have a whole new set of problems to deal with.)

- Fruit and/or yogurt smoothie
- Cheese sandwich with spinach leaves
- Veggie sticks
- Whole-grain crackers and string cheese
- Vegetable juice
- Bean burrito
- Soy dog on a whole-grain bun
- Veggie burger
- Nutrition bar or drink
- Light popcorn
- Vegan "chicken" nuggets
- Sandwich wrap filled with your favorite healthy filling
- Dry cereal
- Granola bar or whole-grain bar

Nutrition Bars and Drinks

Nutrition bars and drinks make good snacks—especially when you're craving sweets. Snack bars and drinks for pregnancy like Oh Mama! are nutritionally tweaked for the needs of expectant moms and work well for nursing moms, too. Some other good-tasting products for nursing moms are Carnation Instant Breakfast and Ensure, which are nutrient-dense enough to replace breakfast. Luna bars, Kashi bars, and others are also tasty snack choices. Those that are a little higher in protein and fiber will keep you full longer. If you choose other nutrition bars or drinks, read the labels carefully and avoid those with caffeine and herbal stimulants like guarana/paullinea cupana, kola nut/cola nitida, and yerba maté.

Sample Menu

The following menu contains about 2,400 calories, the average calorie intake you'd need if you're five feet four inches tall, weighed 140 pounds prepregnancy, and have a low activity level.

Breakfast
- One ounce of whole-grain cereal with one-half cup of blueberries
- One piece of whole-grain toast with one teaspoon of light margarine and one teaspoon of jam
- One cup of 1 percent milk

Snack
- One ounce of string cheese (low-fat mozzarella)
- Two kiwi fruits

Lunch
- Sandwich on whole-grain bread with two ounces of turkey, tomato slices, spinach leaves, red pepper strips, and two teaspoons of mayonnaise
- Carrot-and-raisin salad with two teaspoons of olive oil vinaigrette dressing
- One small or one-half large mango
- One cup of 1 percent milk

Snack

- One-quarter cup of fat-free refried beans
- Salsa
- Two thin avocado slices
- One ounce of baked tortilla chips
- Celery sticks

Dinner

- Tossed salad with romaine or leaf lettuce
- One tablespoon of dressing made with olive or canola oil
- Five ounces of grilled salmon
- One-half cup of carrots and one-half cup of broccoli with one teaspoon of margarine
- One-half cup of brown rice, quinoa, or whole-wheat pasta
- One whole-grain roll with one teaspoon of flavored olive oil for dipping

Snack

- Smoothie with three-quarters cup of flavored low-fat yogurt and three-quarters cup of frozen fruit
- One graham cracker

How Does This Menu Stack Up?

- Grain servings: seven (all whole-grain)
- Protein servings: eight
- Dairy servings: four
- Fruit servings: two and one-quarter cups
- Vegetable servings: two and one-half cups
- Teaspoons of additional fat: seven

Highlights of This Menu

- Salmon provides DHA for baby's brain growth.
- Yogurt provides calcium as well as beneficial bacteria.
- A variety of fruits and veggies provide antioxidants for good health.

Other Considerations

Now you know the role your diet plays in breastfeeding. What else goes into your milk? How might it affect your body or your baby? The following pages should answer all your questions.

Drugs

Whether a drug will adversely affect your baby or your milk supply depends on the drug. Many factors influence how much of a drug enters your milk—and of course every drug and every person is unique—so it's impossible to make a general statement about the safety of drugs while breastfeeding.

The most important thing to remember is that the need to take medication is almost never a reason to stop breastfeeding. Most medications are either inherently safe for your baby or enter your milk in such small amounts that they create no risk. For the few meds that aren't safe to take while nursing, breastfeeding-safe alternatives are almost always available.

Ask your baby's doctor, your lactation consultant, and/or your pharmacist if the medications you normally take (over-the-counter and prescription) are okay to take while nursing. In my experience not all doctors are knowledgeable about breastfeeding-compatible drugs and sometimes ill-advise nursing moms to quit because of medication use. Therefore it's always wise to get a second opinion from someone who is better versed on the topic, or consult one of the accurate and up-to-date resources on drugs and lactation I've listed below. Don't settle for an answer straight out of the *Physician's Desk Reference*, which *does not* contain complete information on this topic.

- Drugs and Lactation (LactMed) Database at http://toxnet.nlm.nih.gov/cgi-bin/sis/htmlgen?LACT
- Search http://www.kellymom.com to find many online references about medications.
- *Medications and Mothers' Milk* by Thomas Hale
- *Drugs in Pregnancy and Lactation* by Gerald Briggs, Roger Freeman, and Sumner Yaffee
- *Drug Therapy and Breastfeeding* by Kenneth Ilett and Thomas Hale
- *Clinical Therapy in Breastfeeding Patients* by Thomas Hale and Pamela Berens
- *Breastfeeding: Conditions and Diseases* by Anne Merewood and Barbara Philipp
- *Breastfeeding: A Guide for the Medical Profession* by Ruth Lawrence and Robert Lawrence
- *United States Pharmacopeia Drug Information*

Smoking

You probably already know the many ways smoking and exposure to secondhand smoke endanger both you and your baby. What you may not know is how smoking affects breastfeeding. Research links smoking to:

- Earlier weaning
- Lower milk production
- Interference with letdown
- Decreased iodine in breast milk, which could lead to a deficiency[10]

Quitting smoking is the ideal, of course. But even if you can't quit, you should still breastfeed! It's riskier for your baby's health to formula-feed than to breastfeed if you smoke. That's because the special immune factors in breast milk help your baby fight illness and counteract some of the negative effects of exposure to smoking.

If you smoke:

- Breastfeed.

- Try to quit smoking.

- If you can't quit smoking, cut back as much as possible.

- Don't smoke right before or during breastfeeding.

- Smoke immediately after you nurse so plenty of time lapses before your next breastfeeding session. It takes about ninety-five minutes for half of the nicotine to leave your body.

- Never smoke or let anyone else smoke in the same room as your baby; ideally, smoke outside.

Artificial Sweeteners

If you buy a sweet, low-calorie food, it probably contains an artificial sweetener—that's a sweetener that contains few or no calories (called a non-nutritive sweetener), that's made in a laboratory, and that's much sweeter than sugar. But it may not be apparent if its chemical name is buried in the ingredient list.

Following is a brief outline of common artificial sweeteners, including their brand names, chemical names, and current recommendations.

The Sweet Sheet

Chemical Names	Brand Names	Recommendations
acesulfame potassium (acesulfame K)	Sweet One, Sunnette	Approved by U.S. Food and Drug Administration (FDA) and Health Canada
aspartame	Equal, NutraSweet	Approved by U.S. FDA and Health Canada, contraindicated for moms of babies with phenylketonuria (PKU)
neotame		Approved by U.S. FDA, not in use by this book's printing
saccharin	Sweet'n Low, Sweet Twin, Necta Sweet (Hermesetas in Canada)	Approved by U.S. FDA, not recommended by Health Canada
stevia		Dietary supplement not approved by U.S. FDA or Health Canada as a sweetener
sucralose	Splenda	Approved by U.S. FDA and Health Canada

A word of caution: Just because a sweetener has been approved by a regulatory agency doesn't mean you should eat a steady diet of it. The Center for Science in the Public Interest (CSPI), a consumer watchdog group, has raised a red flag on the use of saccharin (safety issues) and acesulfame K and stevia (inadequate testing issues). The CSPI gives Splenda and Neotame a green flag for safety; aspartame is listed as probably safe. One or two servings a day of any artificial sweetener is a reasonable approach. For small amounts, I think it's just fine to use real sugar. It has only sixteen calories per teaspoon; a few teaspoons here and there aren't going to derail a healthy diet![11]

Nutritive Sweeteners

There's another type of sweetener found in food: sweeteners that contain calories, but fewer than sugar. These sweeteners are called sugar alcohols or polyols. They occur naturally in some fruits and vegetables but are manufactured in large amounts from common sugars. (No doubt you've seen them on chewing gum and sugar-free candy labels. Their names usually end in *ol—zylitol, sorbitol, mannitol,* and so on.)

Sugar alcohols average half the calories of sugar and aren't metabolized the same as sugar, so they have little effect on insulin and blood sugar levels. They're also better for teeth. Most sugar alcohols are used in small amounts in food products because too much can cause digestive effects like diarrhea.

However, one sugar alcohol, erythritol, does not cause digestive side effects like the other sugar alcohols, so it can be used in reduced-calorie and sugar-free foods with no worries. A relatively new sweetener on the market made from erythritol is sold in the U.S. as Zsweet. See the sidebar for more Zsweet info.

Sugar alcohols approved for use in the U.S. are sorbitol, mannitol, zylitol, erythritol, D-Tagatose, Isomalt, Lactitol, Maltitol, Trehalose, and hydrogenated starch hydrosylates (HSH). Sugar alcohols approved for use in Canada are HSH, isomalt, lactitol, maltitol, maltitol syrup, mannitol, sorbitol, sorbitol syrup, xylitol, and erythritol.

> **Sweet News about Zsweet**
>
> I'm very excited to see a new player coming onto the sweetener market: Zsweet. I recently tasted Zsweet on strawberries. It tastes like sugar (but slightly less sweet), looks like sugar, has no aftertaste, and is naturally produced. The really good news is that Zsweet is virtually unabsorbed, so it has zero calories, doesn't cause digestive problems in large amounts like other sugar alcohols can, doesn't raise blood glucose or insulin levels, and doesn't cause cavities. For more info, see http://www.zsweet.com.

Lead

Lead is toxic to the developing brain. At high levels it causes numerous poisoning symptoms, and at low levels it subtly hinders learning, memory, and attention span. Because your baby's brain is still developing rapidly for several years after birth, lead exposure during early childhood can be particularly harmful.

Naturally you hope that lead isn't a regular part of your diet (or your environment), but it may be. See page 207 for common sources of lead exposure and advice on minimizing your lead exposure.

If you've had lead exposure, the lead is stored mostly in your bones. If you don't get enough calcium while breastfeeding, calcium stored in your bones—along with any stored lead—will be released into your bloodstream. You can minimize your baby's lead exposure by making sure you get plenty of calcium while breastfeeding. (See page 63 for more information.)

Mercury

Mercury is another potent neurotoxin in the environment, and it can be passed from mother to child through breast milk. It enters our food supply mainly via fish. See page 208 for detailed advice on minimizing mercury exposure in your diet.

Other Chemicals

You're probably aware of other chemicals, like persistent organic pollutants (POPs), growth hormones, and pesticides in the food supply as well. Buying organic meats, milk, grains, and produce can reduce your exposure (and thus your baby's exposure) to these contaminants significantly.

Buying organic is a sure path to fresh, healthy, tasty food, but it can also be expensive. If organic eating is busting your budget, go organic selectively. Choose organic for produce that tends to have high pesticide residue. And be sure to check out locally grown foods. If you buy locally, you avoid chemicals used for shipping: wax, post-harvest pesticides, and other preservatives. Local foods also tend to be cheaper because they don't incur the cost of traveling great distances.

Another easy way to improve the quality of your diet and minimize your exposure to contaminants is to eat a wide variety of foods and eat all foods in moderation. (In other words, even if you adore broccoli, you shouldn't eat a pound at a time!) You can also scrub fruits and vegetables thoroughly or use a produce wash to remove surface contaminants. (See page 204 for more information.)

Allergenic Foods

Your baby is at higher risk for allergies if either parent has any type of allergic disease. If one parent has an allergies, your baby's risk of allergies is about 48 percent; the risk can increase to 70 percent if both parents have allergies.

As a breastfeeding mom, you're already doing your part to delay or prevent allergies in your child—good for you! Some research has shown that avoiding highly allergenic foods like cow's milk, egg, fish, peanuts, and tree nuts until your child weans may also help postpone or prevent eczema, asthma, and respiratory allergic symptoms.[12, 13, 14, 15] This is because proteins from some foods can make their way to breast milk and can potentially sensitize your infant to the allergenic food. You can try this strategy, but be aware that as of this book's printing, it's not recommended by the American Association of Allergy, Asthma and Immunology[16] or the Australian Society of Clinical Immunology.[17]

To find out current advice in your area, go to http://www.worldallergy.org and click on global allergy links. And ask an allergist about the current recommendations on allergy prevention.

- **Peanuts**: The jury's still out on whether nursing moms should lay off peanuts completely. But we do know that peanut protein has been found in breast milk and can sensitize a young infant. Peanut protein can also find its way to your baby from your clothes after you eat peanut products. Because of the explosion in peanut allergies—and also their severity—you may want to consider avoiding peanuts for a while even if you don't have a strong family history of allergies.

- **Dairy**: Cow's milk protein allergy in breastfed infants is rare—only 2 or 3 percent of breastfed babies have it. You don't need to avoid cow's milk unless your baby reacts to it with symptoms like severe colic, abdominal discomfort, rash, vomiting, severe diarrhea, or difficulty breathing. (Recent research has shown that avoiding high-allergen foods does reduce colic symptoms. See page 140 for more info.) If you notice these symptoms, talk to your baby's doctor right away to determine if your baby is allergic to cow's milk protein. Then see a dietitian to learn how to avoid it while eating well.

See page 136 for a primer on allergies and page 138 for advice on coping with food allergies.

Caffeine

If you think breastfeeding is going to require you to give up your morning coffee, don't worry! A little caffeine is okay for nursing moms, but since it does show up in breast milk, don't overdo it. Your baby's body (especially as a newborn) takes longer to metabolize caffeine than yours does, so caffeine can make your baby even more jittery than it makes you. Limit your caffeine to two or three cups of regular brewed coffee (three to five hundred milligrams per day[18])—or less if your baby seems sensitive to that amount. Caffeine content of coffee varies widely depending on the coffee, method of preparation, and so on. Beware of energy drinks, because they often have an unknown amount of caffeine added.

If you're struggling to stay awake while caring for your baby, try to catnap when your baby's sleeping or nursing instead of relying on caffeine. If that doesn't work, drink caffeinated beverages in small doses. A few ounces at a time every few hours is better for improving alertness (and reducing jitters) than a big wallop all at once.

> **What Contains Three Hundred Milligrams of Caffeine?**
>
> - Two eight-ounce cups of brewed coffee
> - One nine-ounce Starbuck's coffee
> - Six eight-ounce glasses of iced tea
> - Eight twelve-ounce servings of soda
> - Sixty eight-ounce cups of hot cocoa

Herbal Teas and Supplements

Not all herbs are safe while nursing. See page 128 for advice on using herbs while breastfeeding and page 155 for more information on herbs and children.

Alcohol

There's no need to skip happy hour just because you're nursing—just sip smartly. While your baby will share a bit of your margarita or Merlot, only 2 percent of the alcohol you drink reaches your blood and milk.

Alcohol peaks in your blood and milk about one-half to one hour after you drink it. It isn't stored in your milk; as your body metabolizes the alcohol from your blood, the alcohol also disappears from your milk. One drink (a twelve-ounce beer or wine cooler, five ounces of wine, or one and a half ounces of liquor) is usually completely metabolized in about two hours.

In short: You needn't be a teetotaling saint to breastfeed, but you should employ common sense when using alcohol as a nursing mom. Lactation consultant Kelly Bonyata notes on her excellent website (http://www.kellymom.com) that "In general, if you are sober enough to drive, you are sober enough to breastfeed." According to the American Academy of Pediatrics (AAP), "One alcoholic drink...will probably not harm your baby. However there are concerns about long-term repeated exposures to alcohol through breast milk."[19]

Remember that the younger the baby, the longer it takes for your baby's liver to break down alcohol. If you choose to have an occasional drink while breastfeeding:

- Don't drink while you're nursing.

- Wait two to three hours after drinking before your next feeding or pumping session. This way, most of the alcohol will be gone from your milk.

- Limit your alcohol intake to one or two drinks at a time, no more than once or twice a week.

Beer and Breastfeeding

You may hear that drinking beer will increase your milk supply. It won't. In fact, a recent study found that alcohol lowers levels of the hormones prolactin and oxytocin, both needed for the production and flow of breast milk. The women in the study experienced slower letdown after drinking and produced less milk overall.[20]

U.S. Breastfeeding Help Line

Do you have more breastfeeding questions but no one to answer them? Call the National Women's Health Information Center help line at 800-994-9662 Monday through Friday from 9:00 A.M. to 6:00 P.M. La Leche League–trained peer counselors will answer your questions in English or Spanish.

Chapter 4

Formula-Feeding

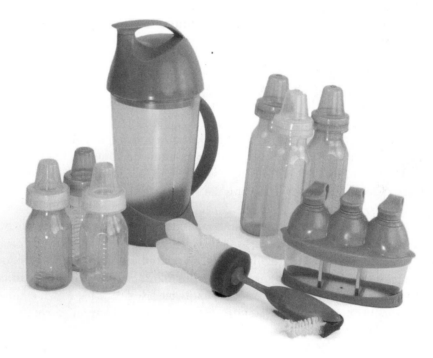

Every baby needs a lap.
—Henry Robin

Many babies will never have a drop of formula cross their lips. Some babies will drink both breast milk and formula. Others will have nothing but formula from day one. Even if you've decided against breastfeeding, I encourage you to read the breastfeeding information in this book (especially pages 20–24) to make sure you've got all the facts you need to make the best possible decision for your family.

If you do choose to feed your baby formula, this chapter will help you do it right. On the following pages you'll learn what's in formula, the types of formula available, what gear you might need, and how to formula-feed your baby safely and lovingly.

Formula Facts

While formula manufacturers will never be able to duplicate breast milk, the gold standard for infant nutrition, they're constantly researching ways to make formula as close as possible to breast milk. This section will tell you what's in the various kinds of formula and why.

How Is Formula Regulated?

Formula has come a long way since mothers used to make their own with canned evaporated milk (a practice that, of course, is no longer recommended). Today, infant formula is the most highly regulated food on the market.

Around the world, formula is regulated by the Codex Alimentarius (food code), which was developed by the Food and Agriculture Organization of the United Nations (FAO) and the World Health Organization (WHO). The Codex establishes minimum amounts of nutrients that formula must contain. In the United States, the Food and Drug Administration (FDA) regulates formula ingredients, manufacturing, and packaging by enforcing the Infant Formula Act, a U.S. law that follows the Codex.

The Infant Formula Act of 1980 (amended in 1986) provides detailed requirements for formula ingredients, manufacturing practices, nutrients, caloric value, labeling, and more. The regulations are updated annually and can be found at: http://www.access.gpo.gov/nara/cfr/waisidx_02/21cfr107_02.html. Health Canada provides similar guidance in its Food and Drug Regulations, which can be found in Division 25 of the document at http://www.hc-sc.gc.ca/fn-an/alt_formats/hpfb-dgpsa/pdf/legislation/e_d-text-2.pdf.

Because knowledge about infant nutrition is rapidly expanding, formula manufacturers often request to add new ingredients. Scientific practice is also ever-changing, and regulatory agencies have realized that existing guidelines for evaluating the safety of conventional food ingredients don't adequately address the myriad new formula ingredients proposed or the unique needs of infants. To solve this problem, the Institute of Medicine formed the Committee on the Evaluation of the Addition of Ingredients New to Infant Formula. This committee has written a book that standardizes the safety assessment of new formula ingredients.[1]

Form

Infant formula is packaged in three different forms: powder, concentrate, and ready-to-feed.

- **Powder**: Powdered formula is prepared by mixing one scoop of powder with two ounces of clean water. One of the best features of powdered formula is its price; it's about ⅓ to ½ the price of ready-to-feed formula. Another attractive feature is its flexibility. You can prepare any amount you like, from a very small bottle to a day's worth. Powdered formula is also the most environmentally friendly option because it requires the least packaging.

- **Concentrate**: Concentrated formula is prepared by mixing it with an equal amount of water. It comes in thirteen-ounce cans that make a total of twenty-six ounces of prepared formula. Some parents find concentrated formula a bit easier to prepare than powdered and feel it's worth the small extra cost.

- **Ready-to-feed**: Ready-to-feed formula comes in eight-ounce cans or thirty-two–ounce jugs. You simply open the container and pour the formula into a feeding bottle. If you're super-busy or prone to mixing-and-measuring mistakes, and you don't mind the 25-percent cost increase, ready-to-feed formula is the best choice for you.

Composition

Types of Formula

There are three basic types of formula: cow's milk–based, soy-based, and hypoallergenic. Among these three basic types, there are also lactose-free formulas and formulas tweaked for other problems your baby might have.

- **Cow's milk formula**: This is the formula of choice for most healthy, full-term babies when breast milk isn't available. (Always consult your baby's doctor before switching from cow's milk formula to a different type.) The cow's milk in this formula has been heated and altered to make its protein easier for human babies to digest.

- **Soy formula**: There's much confusion about the appropriate use of soy formula. Following I've summarized the view of the American Academy of Pediatrics (AAP) Committee on Nutrition regarding soy formula. Soy formula can be used for:
  - Term infants whose nutritional needs are not being met by breast milk or cow's milk formula (In other words, if breast milk isn't available and your baby has a documented allergy to cow's milk protein or other cow's milk intolerance, soy may be better.)
  - Infants who have galactosemia (a rare metabolic disease), hereditary lactase deficiency, or lactose intolerance
  - Infants who are being raised vegan

Soy formula *should not* be used for:

- Preventing or treating colic
- Preventing allergy in either healthy or high-risk infants (Breast milk and extensively hydrolyzed formula would be the first and second choices.)
- Infants with documented cow's milk protein–induced enteropathy or enterocolitis (These infants should be given breast milk or a hypoallergenic formula.)
- Any infant born prematurely or weighing less than four pounds

- **Hypoallergenic (extensively hydrolyzed or protein hydrolysate) formula**: Most hypoallergenic formulas (such as Alimentum and Nutramigen) are made from cow's milk protein (casein), but the protein is broken down into smaller particles (hydrolyzed). These smaller particles are more digestible, and a baby's immune system doesn't react to them. Another type of hypoallergenic formula (such as Neocate) is completely milk protein–free; the protein is in the form of 100-percent free amino acids–which is especially helpful for babies with intolerance to multiple food proteins. Hypoallergenic formula isn't usually the first formula a baby tries. It's typically introduced because a baby isn't tolerating regular cow's milk formula or soy formula. (However, non-breastfed babies who are at high risk of allergy sometimes eat hypoallergenic formula from the start.) Hypoallergenic formula is also helpful for babies with absorption disorders. Sometimes it's recommended for treatment of severe colic. Hypoallergenic formulas are very expensive and sometimes have an unpleasant smell, but babies introduced to them before four months like them just fine!

- **Formula for premature and low–birth weight babies**: Preemies and low–birth weight babies have smaller nutrient stores as well as underdeveloped digestion, but they're also growing rapidly. When breast milk isn't available to these babies, special formula is their best bet. This type of formula typically has more calories, protein, vitamins, and minerals than standard formula. It also contains a more easily absorbed type of fat: medium-chain triglycerides.

- **Human milk fortifier**: Human milk fortifier is a nutrient preparation usually used to meet the special growth needs of low–birth weight breastfed babies. Some types are mixed with breast milk and other types are fed alternately with breast milk.

- **Other special formulas**: Babies who have inborn errors of metabolism or low birth weight or who have other unusual medical or dietary problems sometimes need special formulas. For example, metabolic formulas are made for infants who have metabolic disorders that prevent them from digesting one or more common formula ingredients, such as a specific amino acid.

- **Follow-up formula**: Follow-up formula is geared toward older babies and toddlers nine to twenty-four months old. Compared to whole cow's milk, it contains more of certain vitamins and minerals (calcium, zinc, iron, and vitamin E) that some toddlers don't get enough of. If your older baby or toddler is a very picky eater and isn't breastfed, a follow-up formula can fill any nutritional gaps.

Formula Ingredients

Because formula is a substitute for breast milk, manufacturers try to make it as much like the real thing as possible. Formula's nutrient profile is similar to breast milk's, but not identical. (See pages 16–20 to learn which breast milk nutrients are *not* found in formula.) Because many nutrients aren't absorbed as well from formula, formula contains higher amounts of them.

Since formula is so heavily regulated, aren't all formulas the same? Yes...and no! Regulations require minimum amounts of most nutrients in formula and maximum amounts of some, but there's still a lot of room for tweaking. And because the law doesn't specify nutrient sources, these can also differ among brands. (For example, a standard cow's milk formula usually contains lactose as the carbohydrate source; a soy or lactose-free formula may contain corn maltodextrain and/or sucrose as its carb source.) The manufacturers' varying philosophies and studies result in slightly different formulas. The next few pages discuss the main ingredients in formula and how these ingredients can vary among brands.

Protein

Formula contains about twice as much protein as breast milk, because babies don't absorb protein as well from formula. The protein in formula comes from either cow's milk or soybeans.

The two types of protein in cow's milk are casein and whey. You may see one or both on a cow's milk formula label. Many cow's milk formulas try to match the protein ratio in breast milk (60 percent whey to 40 percent casein); at least one cow's milk formula contains 100 percent whey protein that

> ### Essential Fatty Acids in Formula
>
> Essential fatty acids (EFAs) are fats that can't be produced in the body, so they must be consumed in the diet. Linoleic acid and alpha-linolenic acid are EFAs required by both infants and adults. The body converts linoleic acid into arachidonic acid (ARA) and alpha-linolenic acid into docosahexaenoic acid (DHA).
>
> ARA and DHA are critical for babies' brain and eye development. Breast milk contains preformed DHA and ARA (in amounts that depend on the mother's diet). Research shows that blood levels of DHA and ARA are higher in breastfed infants than in infants fed formula that doesn't contain preformed DHA and ARA. The higher IQs of some breastfed infants may be the result of their higher blood levels of essential fats.
>
> In 2002, the FDA and Health Canada allowed the addition of DHA and ARA to infant formula. Does the addition of DHA and ARA help brain and eye development in formula-fed babies? The short answer: There's not enough evidence to support the idea conclusively. The long answer: Studies show mixed results, depending on the formula used and the breast milk levels of DHA and ARA that served as controls.
>
> Bottom line: The goal is for infant formula to be as close as possible to breast milk to provide all infants similar potential for optimum growth and development. Adding DHA and ARA to all formulas may level the playing field for all formula-fed infants, regardless of the brand they drink. Preterm infants may benefit most of all from the added DHA and ARA because their immature nervous sytems and vision are developing more rapidly.

is *partially* hydrolyzed. (This isn't the same as a hypoallergenic—or extensively hydrolyzed—formula.) Hypoallergenic (extensively hydrolyzed) formulas contain casein protein only with additional amino acids, or 100 percent amino acids.

Fat

Breast milk contains a mix of monounsaturated, polyunsaturated, and saturated fats; formula manufacturers try to match this with a combination of plant-based oils. By U.S. and Canadian law, fat can provide anywhere from 30 to 54 percent of the calories in formula. However, the sources of fat (coconut oil, palm oil, palm olein oil, safflower oil, sunflower oil, soybean oil, and corn oil) can vary. The law also requires baby formula to contain linoleic acid, an essential fatty acid that can be converted into arachidonic acid (ARA). (See the sidebar on page 79 for more information on essential fatty acids in formula.) Special formulas for premature infants and babies with malabsorption problems contain medium-chain triglycerides, a type of fat that's more easily digested.

Are some fat sources better than others? Yes—or more accurately: One fat source seems to be worse than the others. Several studies have shown that adding palm or palm olein oil to formula decreases a baby's absorption of fat and calcium. The molecules of palmitic acid in formula are arranged in a way that causes some of the fat to combine with calcium in an unabsorbable "soap." Further studies show that reduced calcium absorption results in decreased bone mineralization.[2, 3] It's not known conclusively if this effect remains later in childhood.

Carbohydrate

There's no minimum or maximum amount of carbohydrate added to formula. Like breast milk, most formulas provide about 40 percent of their calories via carbohydrates. Also like breast milk, cow's milk formulas generally contain lactose as their primary carbohydrate source. Some other carbohydrate sources are corn syrup solids, sucrose, maltodextrine, and modified cornstarch.

Vitamins and Minerals

Most of the long list of unpronounceable ingredients on a formula label are vitamins and minerals. For example, niacinamide is also known as niacin or vitamin B_3. Cupric sulfate is a form of the mineral copper. Ferrous sulfate is better known as iron. Following is a list of vitamins and minerals that baby formula must contain according to the Infant Formula Act, revised most recently in 2002:

- Protein
- Fat
- Linoleic acid
- Vitamin A
- Vitamin D
- Vitamin E
- Vitamin K
- Thiamine (vitamin B_1)
- Riboflavin (vitamin B_2)
- Vitamin B_{12}
- Niacin
- Folic acid (folacin)
- Pantothenic acid
- Biotin
- Vitamin C (ascorbic acid)
- Choline
- Inositol
- Calcium

- Vitamin B_6
- Magnesium
- Iron
- Zinc
- Manganese
- Copper
- Phosphorus
- Iodine
- Sodium
- Potassium
- Chloride

Other Ingredients

- **Nucleotides**: Nucleotides are building blocks of deoxyribonucleic acid (DNA) and ribonucleic acid (RNA), which carry the genetic information in cells. Nucleotides help your baby's cardiovascular and neurological systems and also aid in the metabolism of carbohydrates, fats, and proteins. They're well-known for their part in defending against bacteria, viruses, parasites, and some cancers.[4] Nucleotides are found in all living cells, in food, in breast milk, and in formula at varying levels.

- **Dietary fiber**: Some formulas contain added fiber to help babies with diarrhea. Consult your baby's doctor before using this formula.

- **Rice starch**: Some formulas contain added rice starch to reduce frequent spit-up or gastroesophogeal reflux disease (GERD). Consult your baby's doctor before using this formula, especially if your baby is younger than four months.

Iron

Although iron is just one ingredient in formula, it's notable because it's on the front label. Iron is very important for your baby's rapid growth and development. The inclusion of iron in formula during the last several decades has dramatically reduced iron deficiency anemia, which can have long-lasting effects on cognitive development. The AAP recommends that all infants not breastfed or only partially breastfed receive an iron-fortified formula until one year of age. Low-iron formulas are available, but you shouldn't use them unless your baby's doctor recommends it.

The Bottom Line

Formulas change, and their advertising does, too. It can be hard to keep track of all the changes and even harder to tease out the facts from the marketing lingo. The best way to figure out which formula is best for your baby is to ignore the ads and look at the science instead. Discuss the differences among formulas with your baby's doctor. You can also seek out research published in peer-reviewed journals like *Pediatrics* and *The American Journal of Clinical Nutrition*. While most studies of infant formula are subsidized by formula companies— after all, who else would pay for them?—their research methods and analysis must meet rigorous protocol to be published in peer-reviewed journals.

Gearing Up

As with all things baby-related, there's a lot of formula-feeding gear to choose from. You may find yourself trying a number of products before you find the one that's just right for your baby.

The Basics

Here are the basics you need:

Bottles

Our parents had little choice when it came to bottles. Today, you could spend hours researching the merits of different bottle types! The following list outlines the advantages of various bottle features.

- **Material**
  - *Glass* bottles are heavier than plastic ones and are breakable, but they're also more stable. Glass won't deteriorate over time as plastic will, nor will it leach chemicals.
  - *Plastic* bottles are made of either polyethylene (EVA) or polycarbonate. Plastic bottles are very lightweight and break-resistant, but research shows that a chemical called bisphenol A may leach from polycarbonate. The FDA says polycarbonate bottles won't leach under normal use with no extreme temperatures. If you do use plastic bottles, avoid overheating them, and if the plastic changes color or becomes cloudy, toss it. Disposable bottle liners are also made of plastic. They're presterilized and contain no bisphenol A.

- **Shape**
  - *Straight* bottles are cheap and easy to clean.
  - *Angled* bottles have a forty-five-degree bend that keeps the nipple filled with liquid to reduce baby's air swallowing and makes it easier to hold a baby upright, which prevents liquid from washing into baby's middle ear (a cause of ear infections).

- **Usage**:
  - *Reusable* bottles are economical and environmentally sound because they can be used throughout your baby's bottle-feeding stage and create no waste. They also allow accurate measurement of the bottle's contents.
  - *Disposable* bottles require less cleaning because the milk is drunk from a presterilized plastic liner, which is thrown away at the end of the feeding. This bottle type may minimize baby's air swallowing (and thus prevent gassiness) because you can squeeze air out of the liner before feeding; also, the liner collapses as baby feeds, which prevents additional air bubbles from entering. Disposable liners also come in a firmer version preformed to fit in a bottle, which is easier to manipulate with one hand.

- **Size**
  - *Four-ounce* bottles are practical for newborns, who may drink only a small amount at each feeding.
  - *Eight- or nine-ounce* bottles are practical for older babies with bigger appetites. They can be used for a baby of any age and are therefore more versatile and long-lasting.
- **Other features**
  - *Bubble-free* bottles are ideal for gassy babies who don't like disposables. They let air in through the bottom of the bottle, which prevents it from mixing with the milk and being swallowed. Because both ends screw off, cleaning is easy.
  - *Chambered* bottles are great for traveling. They have separate compartments for premeasured powdered formula and water. At feeding time, you twist the top and the formula mixes with the water.
  - *Hands-free* bottles are useful in a pinch, when young multiples who can't hold bottles yet need feeding simultaneously, and there aren't enough hands on deck for the usual holding and cuddling. The bottle fastens to a car seat or stroller, and a tube extends from the top to a pacifier-like nipple.

Nipples

There are just as many nipple types as there are bottle types. You may want to buy a sample of each type in the beginning, then let your baby and your budget help you decide which to stock up on. When nipples become hard, stiff, or sticky after use, it's time for new ones.

- **Material**
  - *Latex* nipples are softer and more flexible than silicone nipples. Avoid latex nipples if your baby has other allergies, has had multiple surgeries, or has spina bifida; infants in these situations are at higher risk for latex allergy.
  - *Silicone* nipples are firmer and hold their shape longer than latex ones. They're less porous than latex and thus less prone to bacteria. They typically last three to four times longer than latex. They're also heat-resistant and can withstand dishwashers.

Nipples of Note

If you're both breastfeeding and formula-feeding, take note of the nipples listed below, which may help you avoid latch and suckling problems. These nipples all share a round, broad base that encourages tongue and jaw motions similar to breastfeeding.[5, 6]

- Gerber Comfort Latch is designed to feel "more like mom" and also has vents that are supposed to reduce air in your baby's stomach.
- Many moms report that Avent's Newborn Nipple works well for their breastfed babies.
- Playtex Natural Latch slow-flow nipples are textured to help babies latch on to them.
- The First Years Breastflow nipple comes in two parts: a soft outer nipple and a firm inner one. It requires both suction and compression and "lets down" after baby's initial suckling.

- **Shape**
  - *Bell-shaped* nipples are inexpensive and widely available.
  - *Flat-topped* nipples mimic the shape of a mother's nipple.
  - *Orthodontic* nipples are elongated, flat on one side, and indented in the center to encourage the tonguing action of breastfeeding. They may help reduce tongue thrusting and bite problems caused by standard nipples.
- **Flow**: Nipples come with varying numbers and sizes of holes for varying flow speed. Here's a quick guide to choosing the right flow.
  - Always use newborn (slow-flow) nipples for a breastfed baby of any age.
  - The following guidelines apply to exclusively bottle-fed babies. For a newborn, the nipple size is right if the milk drips steadily when you turn the bottle upside down. For older babies: If your baby is sucking hard, fussing, then sucking hard again, you probably need a faster-flow nipple. If your baby is sputtering and gulping, you may need a slower-flow nipple.

Other Essentials

- **Bottle brush and nipple brush**: These tools make it easier to thoroughly clean the many nooks and crannies of bottles and nipples.
- **Bottle drying rack**: A rack provides a clean place for all your feeding gear to dry. Using a rack also speeds up the air-drying process.
- **Burp cloths**: Any soft, absorbent cloth will do, but many parents find cloth diapers (the flat kind) to be perfect for soaking up spit-up. If you have an especially drooly or spitty baby who tends to "decorate" your clothes at the most inconvenient times, you might want to check out the Mommy Bib. It covers your whole front and shoulders and part of your back. (See http://www.mommybib.com.)
- **Measuring cups**: You might want to use a measuring cup for water if the markings on the bottle are not clear—or just to be sure they're accurate.
- **Can opener**: You may need one if you're planning to use canned formula. Make sure your can opener is clean and rust-free.

The Extras

These items are nice to have, but not crucial:

- **Funnel**: A funnel makes it easier to pour prepared formula into feeding bottles.
- **Bottle warmer**: A bottle warmer takes the guesswork out of heating your baby's formula by alerting you or shutting off when the proper temperature is reached. It also provides a convenient way to warm a bottle anywhere (using an electrical outlet, car adapter, or batteries). Some bottle warmers can be used for baby food jars, too.
- **Steam sterilizer**: If you have clean tap water and a dishwasher, it's not necessary to sterilize bottles and nipples—but some parents do prefer it. You may

want to seriously consider getting a sterilizer if you'll be traveling a lot with your baby. Avent makes an electric sterilizer and a microwave one that are both highly rated.

- **Powdered formula dispenser**: If you often find yourself away from home when your baby is hungry, this handy container can make feeding on the go easier. It has three compartments to hold powdered formula for three feedings.
- **Powdered formula packets**: These packets are also great for feeding on the go. Each premeasured packet makes four ounces of prepared formula; just keep a few in your diaper bag.

The First Two Weeks

The First Few Days

If you plan to give birth in a hospital and feed your baby only formula, you may be tempted to have your baby stay in the nursery so you can rest. However, research shows that mothers who do this don't get any more sleep! Rooming-in has been shown to improve attachment between mothers and newborns. Share your room with your baby so you can get to know each other!

On Your Own

Buying, Preparing, and Storing Formula

Everything you need to know about what's in a formula or how to prepare it is on the label. You'll find ingredients, nutrient content, directions, and a use-by date. All this information is provided to help you choose the best possible formula for your baby and to help you prepare and store the formula safely. Please read the label carefully!

Buying Formula

- Buy formula that's not expired. Check the use-by date on the can or bottle. Use the formula by the first day of the month shown.
- Choose formula containers that aren't dented or otherwise damaged. Dented containers can have small openings that allow contamination of the formula.

Preparing Formula

Cleaning Up

- Wash your hands well with soap and warm water for ten to fifteen seconds.
- Make sure all utensils, bottles, and nipples are clean:
  - Simply wash them in the dishwasher or in hot soapy water and rinse them well. Let bottles and nipples air-dry. (See the next bullet to find out whether you should be sterilizing instead.)

- If your baby's doctor has instructed you to sterilize feeding gear or if your water is nonchlorinated or otherwise questionable, sterilize instead of just washing. You can use a steam sterilizer (see page 84) or place bottles and nipples in boiling water for five to ten minutes.[7]

- Individually wrapped nipples you get at the hospital or doctor's office are presterilized. However, they're meant for one-time use; don't wash and reuse them.

Checking Your Water

If you're using concentrated or powdered formula, you'll need to think about your water source. This section will help you figure out the safest water to use in your situation. Your baby's doctor may also provide special instructions depending on the water in your area and the health of your baby.

Too Much Fluoride

Recent studies have raised the possibility that babies might receive more fluoride than they need from formula mixed with water containing too much fluoride. This could make their developing teeth susceptible to enamel fluorosis. Fluorosis is a cosmetic discoloration of the enamel; it has no known health consequences. The American Dental Association offers this advice for formula-fed infants:

- Ready-to-feed formula is preferred to help ensure that infants don't exceed the optimal amount of fluoride.
- If concentrated or powdered formula is used, it can be mixed with low-fluoride or fluoride-free water to reduce the risk of fluorosis. Examples are water that's labeled purified, demineralized, deionized, distilled, or reverse osmosis filtered water.
- The occasional use of water containing optimal levels of fluoride should not appreciably increase a child's risk for fluorosis.
- Ask your physician or dentist about the need for a fluoride supplement beginning at six months.

Tap Water

The water supply in North America is one of the safest in the world. It's protected by the Clean Water Act in the U.S. and by the Guidelines for Canadian Drinking Water Quality in Canada.

The taste and quality of tap water are affected by its source, mineral content, and treatment. How's the water from *your* tap? Each year local water utilities provide an annual report about water quality. Look up your local water here: http://www.epa.gov/safewater/dwinfo/index.html.

If your water comes from a source other than your local water department (such as a well), you should have it tested for nitrates and bacteria before using it to feed your baby. The AAP estimates that two million families in the U.S. (including forty thousand babies six months and younger) drink from wells that have nitrate levels above ten parts per million (ppm), the government limit.[8] The Environmental Protection Agency (EPA) recommends annual testing. See http://www.epa.gov/safewater/labs/index.html for a list of state officers who certify labs that test drinking water.

Generally speaking, tap water is fine to use in preparing formula. It's not necessary to boil it first, but if you feel more comfortable doing so, if you have well water, or if you're otherwise concerned about your water's safety, go ahead. Some parents boil formula water for the first one or two months, when their babies' immune systems are immature.

If you do decide to boil your tap water, boil it for one minute (or three minutes at altitudes over one mile) only. Excessive boiling (over five minutes) can concentrate impurities (such as lead) in the water.[9] Cool the water before mixing it with formula.

If you live in an older building, your water supply could contain too much lead. To find out, have it tested. Otherwise, use bottled distilled water or ready-to-feed formula.

Bottled Water

In the U.S., bottled drinking water must meet FDA standards for physical, chemical, microbial, and radiological contaminants. In most cases, the standards match EPA standards for tap water. However, bottled drinking water (and tap water, for that matter) may still contain trace amounts of many contaminants—ranging from heavy metals to pesticide residues.

The taste and quality of bottled water, like tap water, are affected by its source, mineral content, and treatment. If you use bottled water, be aware of the differences among the types you may find at the store:

- **Drinking water**: This water meets water quality standards for tap water, but it may be treated with ozone instead of chlorine to kill microbes. It may also contain added fluoride.

- **Distilled water**: To create distilled water, steam from boiling water is condensed and bottled. This process removes microbes and minerals.

- **Purified water**: This water has been treated to remove all chemicals. If it's treated by distillation or reverse osmosis, it's also free of microbes.

- **Sterile water**: Sterile water has been treated to remove all microbes. This type of water is used for medical procedures and is only available at medical supply stores.

Water Treatment Primer

If you plan to use bottled or home-filtered water for your baby's formula, get familiar with the different ways water is treated to remove impurities, minerals, and microbes:[10]

- **Distillation**: Water is boiled, and the steam is condensed. This process removes salts, metals, minerals, asbestos, particles, and some organic materials.

- **Micron filtration**: Water is filtered through screens with microscopic holes. The smaller the holes, the more contaminants are removed. Good filters can remove most chemical contaminants and microbes. Filter holes are measured in microns. (To give you an idea of how big a micron is: The period at the end of this sentence is five hundred microns.) When considering filters, look for an absolute rating (which tells you the size of the largest hole), not a nominal rating (which tells you the average hole size). An absolute rating of one micron is needed to remove *Cryptosporidium* (an intestinal parasite that can cause severe diarrhea).

- **Ozonation**: Water is disinfected using ozone, which kills most microbes (depending on dosage applied).

- **Reverse osmosis**: Water is forced through a membrane, leaving contaminants behind. This process removes all microbes, minerals, color, turbidity, and organic and inorganic chemicals.

- **Ultraviolet (UV) light**: Water is passed through UV light, which kills most microbes (depending on dosage applied).

Don't Forget to Change the Filter!

So, you've got filtered water in your fridge—great! But when was the last time you changed the filter? If you have to think about it, it's probably time to put in a new one. Your water filtration system is only as good as its filter, which needs to be replaced regularly. Pay attention to the filter change indicator or manufacturer's directions. In the case of a refrigerator filter, which doesn't have an indicator, replace it about every six months.

If you use bottled water, choose distilled or purified water; bottled water labeled simply "drinking water" may be no better than tap water. You may want to check out Nursery Water (http://www.nurserywater.com), a distilled water with added fluoride.

Home-Filtered Water

If you'd like to use tap water but would like an extra level of protection from contaminants, consider home water filtration. A home water treatment device can be free-standing (such as a pitcher), attached to a tap, plumbed in with a dedicated faucet (also called a point-of-use device) connected to a refrigerator's water and ice dispensing system, or centrally attached to treat all water entering a house (a point-of-entry device). The system that seems the cheapest is the pitcher; however, over time the cost of replacement filters can make it more expensive than a more complex system.

Following is a look at the simplest systems. For a more comprehensive explanation of home water filtration, visit http://www.epa.gov/safewater/faq/pdfs/fs_healthseries_filtration.pdf. To compare the cost and performance of various brands, see http://www.waterfiltercomparisons.net/WaterFilter_Comparison.cfm.

- **Pitcher systems**: Basic pitcher systems remove chlorine, heavy metals like lead and mercury, and solvents like benzene but don't remove bacteria. Some filters also remove asbestos and the insecticides chlordane and toxaphene. Others remove even more chemicals plus the microbes *Cryptosporidium* and *Giardia*.

- **Faucet-mount systems**: These typically offer another layer of filtration, removing the same contaminants as pitcher systems as well as many other chemicals, such as asbestos and volatile organic chemicals. These systems also remove *Giardia, Cryptosporidium*, and total trihalomethanes (byproducts of disinfection found in tap water that are linked to increased cancer risk).

- **Refrigerator systems**: Refrigerators with filtration built into their water and ice dispensing systems are a convenient choice. Refrigerator filtration systems provide contaminant removal similar to pitcher or faucet-mount systems (depending on the type of filter).

Mixing

Note: If you're using ready-to-feed formula, no mixing is necessary. The following instructions apply to powdered or concentrated formula.

- Shake the formula container well and wash the top with soap and water before you open it. If you're using a can opener, make sure that, too, is clean.

- Open the container and carefully follow the preparation directions on the label.

- If you're using tap water, use cold water only. Run the cold water for a few minutes to flush out water that's been sitting in the pipes. Both of these steps will help reduce lead in the water.

- If you boil the water, let it cool before mixing it with formula.

- Mix formula and water in the exact amounts specified on the formula label. Adding more or less water than recommended can be harmful to your baby. Too much water dilutes the formula so it provides inadequate calories, protein, and fat. Not enough water can concentrate nutrients—which can lead to diarrhea or dehydration. It's convenient to use the measurement lines on bottles, but check their accuracy first by using a measuring cup.

- Don't add honey to your baby's formula (or anything else that goes in your baby's mouth). Honey can cause infant botulism.

Storing Formula

Following are general formula storage guidelines. Be sure to read the label on your baby's formula for more details.

Unprepared Formula

- Store unopened formula in a cool place, ideally between 55°F and 75°F (between 13°C and 24°C). Keep formula away from your stove, heating vents, direct sunlight, and hot water pipes. High temperatures can degrade ingredients and nutrients.

- Store opened liquid formula in the refrigerator for up to forty-eight hours.

- Store opened powdered formula in a cool, dry place—but not the refrigerator, because refrigeration causes clumping. You can keep powdered formula for one month after opening.

Prepared Formula

- Pour prepared formula into clean bottles. (See page 85 for cleaning tips.) Assemble bottles as directed by bottle manufacturer.

- Label bottles with the date and time you prepared the formula. If the bottles will be accompanying your baby to daycare, also include your baby's name.

- Store prepared formula in the back of the refrigerator (the coldest area) for no longer than forty-eight hours—or whatever the formula label recommends.

Other Storage Tips

- Never freeze formula.

- Discard any formula left at room temperature for more than one hour.

- Once your baby starts drinking from a bottle, discard its contents after one hour. It's tempting to save leftovers for the next feeding, but bacteria from your baby's mouth can multiply to hazardous levels in the leftover formula.

- Once you've warmed a bottle of formula, don't refrigerate it again. You need to discard the formula.
- Don't reuse disposable plastic bottle liners.

Feeding Formula

Feeding is a special time to get acquainted and bond with your baby. Pay close attention to your baby during feedings so you can learn to recognize his or her signs of fullness. When you recognize and respond to your baby's cues, you show that you can be trusted and you help your baby feel secure. When you hold your baby close during and after feedings, you help develop your baby's senses of smell, sight, and touch. Best of all, it gives you a chance to enjoy your baby.

During the first few days, your baby may not eat very much. Don't worry; this is normal. Your baby may drink just a few ounces at a time, but may get hungry often. Remember: Your newborn has a tiny stomach that fills up and empties quickly!

Feeding Tips

- **Warm the bottle (or not)**: Some babies drink cold formula just fine. If your baby prefers warm formula, hold it under hot running water or place it in a bowl of hot water or a bottle warmer. (*Don't* microwave it. Microwave ovens heat liquid unevenly and can cause hot spots in the formula that burn your baby's mouth. Also, covered bottles can explode in the microwave.) Warm a bottle just before feeding. To check the formula temperature, shake a few drops on your wrist. It should feel neither warm nor hot, but the same temperature as your body.

- **Get comfortable**: Sit on a comfortable chair or couch with a soft, low armrest. Hold your baby in one arm in a semi-reclining position. Alternate arms from feeding to feeding to help your baby's neck and eye muscles develop equally on both sides. This will also help you avoid muscle fatigue.

- **Introduce the bottle**: To begin a feeding, gently stroke your baby's cheek on the side closest to you, either with your finger or the bottle nipple. Your baby will turn toward you. Then touch the nipple to your baby's lip—if your baby's mouth isn't already open, he or she will open it.

- **Hold the bottle**: Hold the bottle firmly and steadily to help your baby establish good suction. Hold the bottle at about a forty-five–degree angle so milk always fills the nipple. Don't prop the bottle. Propping can cause choking and deprives your baby of the cuddling, bonding, and responsiveness your baby needs to develop normally.

- **Watch your baby**: If your baby seems frustrated while feeding, the nipple hole may be too small. If your baby sputters or chokes while feeding, the nipple hole may be too big. Experiment with different types of nipples until you find one that that works well for your baby. While you feed your baby, also watch carefully for signs of fullness. (See the following page for more information.)

- **Burp your baby**: Take a break in the middle of a feeding for a burp. This gives your baby a rest and a chance to bring up any gas that may be causing uncomfortable pressure. Your baby may or may not need to burp again after finishing the feeding, but it doesn't hurt to try. To burp your baby, give some gentle pats on the back—no need to pound hard! The traditional method for burping is to place your baby against your chest with his or her chin on your shoulder. You can also sit your baby upright on your lap, supporting his or her chin and chest with one hand, and patting your baby's back with the other hand. You can also lay your baby across your knee—but support your baby's head and make sure it's higher than his or her chest. It's always smart to have a burp cloth under your baby's head to catch spit-up. Most babies stop needing help with burping between four and nine months.

Signs of Hunger and Fullness

Crying may seem to be your newborn's only mode of communication. You know crying is a sign of discomfort, but what kind of discomfort? Only trial and error will tell. Isn't there a better way to meet your baby's needs?

Yes, there is. If you watch carefully, you'll see that your baby is often trying to tell you something *without* crying. For example, your baby uses many distinct signs to show that he or she is hungry or full. If you heed them, you can minimize the amount of crying in your house—from both you and your baby!

Signs of Hunger

Early Signs
If you feed your baby promptly when you see these early signs of hunger, you'll prevent the fussing and crying that comes next. You'll also teach your baby that you can be trusted to meet his or her needs.

A Word of Caution about Powdered Formula

Unlike liquid formula, powdered formula isn't sterile, and thus can be a vehicle for bacteria—including *Enterobacter sakazakii*, salmonella, and E. coli. Powdered infant formulas containing *E. sakazakii* have been responsible for several fatalities in hospital nurseries. All infants younger than one month are at risk—but premature, underweight, and immunocompromised babies appear to be at greatest risk.[11]

Following is a summary of recommendations about the preparation of infant formula gathered from the WHO,[12] the Centers for Disease Control (CDC),[13] and the American Dietetic Association (ADA).[14] Some of these recommendations were written for healthcare facilities, but it's wise to follow them at home, too, since high-risk infants are often discharged from the hospital while they're still at risk.[15]

- For high-risk infants, when breastfeeding isn't possible, use a commercially sterile liquid formula (ready-to-feed or concentrate). Use chilled, sterile water to mix with concentrate.
- Store open ready-to-feed formula and prepared formula no longer than twenty-four hours.
- Use a new or sanitized container for feeding.
- Reduce risk of bacterial growth by limiting the time formula is kept at room temperature.

- Smacking or licking lips
- Opening and closing mouth
- Sucking on lips, tongue, hands, fingers, toes, toys, or clothing

Active Signs

When you see these signs, it means your baby's getting impatient because you haven't been paying attention!

- Rooting around on whoever's handy
- Fidgeting or squirming
- Hitting you
- Fussing or breathing fast
- Shaking head quickly from side to side

Late Signs

These are signs of extreme hunger and desperation; your baby's wondering if he or she will ever eat again. Be aware that feeding may be difficult or impossible. You'll have to find a way to calm down your agitated baby first.

- Crying
- Refusing the bottle

Signs of Fullness

Just as your baby can show hunger, he or she can also communicate fullness. The signs listed below may also signal a need to pause briefly and burp.

- Spitting out the bottle
- Turning away from the bottle
- Falling asleep

How Much Formula Should Your Baby Drink?

The quick answer to this question is *as much as your baby wants*. It's important to feed your baby on demand; avoid scheduling feedings or insisting that your baby drink a certain amount. Formula-fed babies may be at higher risk of childhood obesity because they're often encouraged to finish a bottle. This leads to overfeeding and teaches babies to ignore their natural instinct to stop eating when they're full. As you can imagine, this can set the scene for disordered eating later in life.

It is helpful, though, to know approximately how much your baby might drink at different ages and sizes. Following is a general guide to babies' formula intake and practical tips for meeting your baby's feeding needs. As you read it, bear in mind that all babies have unique needs.

- Remember that unlike adults, babies don't eat by the clock! Like breastfed babies, formula-fed babies should be fed on demand. After all, nobody knows if your baby is hungry or full except your baby. It's important to watch for signs that your baby is hungry or full. (See above.) Responding to these signs will encourage a trusting relationship between the two of you. Feed your baby whenever you see signs of hunger. Stop feeding whenever you see signs of fullness. Don't encourage your baby to finish a bottle when he or she isn't hungry anymore.

- Here are a couple of tips to manage demand feeding without excessive formula waste:
  - In the early weeks, prepare smaller bottles of formula—about three ounces each. If your baby finishes a bottle and wants more, feed another ounce. When your baby is consistently eating extra ounces, increase the amount of formula in each bottle.
  - Prepare the formula you think you'll use in a day and refrigerate it in a large jug or pitcher. Pour the formula into clean bottles as you need them.
  - Your baby's intake may vary from day to day. If you make all your bottles at one time, make a few extra with just a few ounces of formula each. You can use these extra bottles to top off a feeding when your baby's especially hungry. Or simply prepare extra formula as you need it.
- See the chart below to get a rough idea of how much your baby might drink according to age. Remember: Formula intake varies from baby to baby and from day to day. (If your baby drinks a lot more than the chart suggests for his or her age, that's perfectly okay! Your job is to respect your baby's appetite, regardless of how it compares with your expectations. Only your baby knows for sure what he or she needs at a given moment.)

Formula Intake by Age

Age	Amount Per Feeding	Amount Per Day
Birth to 3 weeks	½ to 1 ounce, increasing to 4 ounces	12 to 24 ounces
3 weeks to 3 months	4 to 6 ounces	24 to 32 ounces
3 to 6 months	5 to 7 ounces	24 to 36 ounces
6 to 9 months	7 to 8 ounces	24 to 32 ounces
9 to 12 months	7 to 8 ounces	24 to 32 ounces

- Here's a guide to how much your baby might eat according to weight. The AAP suggests that "on average, your baby should take in about 2½ ounces of formula a day for every pound of body weight" (about 165 milliliters of formula per kilogram of body weight). So an average three-month-old baby boy who weighs thirteen pounds (six kilograms) might drink thirty-two to thirty-three ounces (about one liter) of formula a day. The AAP also says that "most babies are satisfied with 3 to 4 ounces per feeding during the first month, and increase that amount by 1 ounce per month until [reaching] 8 ounces per feeding."[16]
- If your baby is bigger than average, is drinking more than forty ounces of formula per day, and is older than four months, your baby's doctor (or well-meaning friends or relatives) might recommend that you introduce rice cereal. Waiting

until closer to six months may help prevent allergies. Be sure to discuss this issue with your baby's doctor.

- During growth spurts, which occur around two or three weeks, six weeks, and six months, your baby may seem ravenous. Follow your baby's lead and feed as much as he or she wants.
- Don't give your baby water (or anything else to drink besides formula–or breast milk, if you're also breastfeeding) until he or she is eating solid foods. If you do give your older baby water, make sure it's in addition to–not in place of–formula.

Combining Breastfeeding and Formula-Feeding

If you don't think you'll be able to breastfeed because you need to return to work, think again! First of all, check out Chapter 5, which contains tons of great tips on breastfeeding while working outside the home. Secondly, remember that *any* amount of breastfeeding is very valuable to your baby and you. Even if you can only breastfeed for a few weeks or a few months, or can only continue breastfeeding part-time after you return to work, it's definitely worth the effort.

If your job makes it impossible to pump, if your employer is antagonistic toward breastfeeding, and/or if the laws in your state don't protect your right to pump on the job, you can combine breastfeeding with formula-feeding. Many women find it very satisfying and stress-relieving to nurse their babies before and after work while providing formula for feedings when they're apart. As their babies get older and start eating solid foods, they can sometimes get by with fewer formula feedings.

> **Tales from the Trenches: Teaching, Nursing, and Formula-Feeding**
>
> Maria wanted to breastfeed for as long as she could. But she went back to teaching first grade when her daughter Brittany was three months old, and her rigorous schedule left no time for pumping breaks. Solution? She both breastfed and formula-fed. She nursed Brittany in the morning before work, as soon as she got home, and at bedtime. Her daycare provider fed Brittany several bottles of formula during the day but would hold off as it approached four o'clock, when Maria came home from work.

Common Questions

Q: I just weaned my baby from breast milk to formula. His poop is much different; is that normal?

A: Yes. You've probably gotten used to the soft, frequent, yellowish, inoffensive poop typical of breastfed babies. Formula-fed babies' poop is a bit firmer or much firmer depending on the formula and is more green or brown in color. Now that your baby is formula-fed, you'll also find that he poops less often.

Q: My one-month-old is having a hard time with her formula. We've tried regular cow's milk formula and soy formula. My mother says she fed me goat's milk when I was a baby, and I did fine. Should I try it?

A: We've learned a lot about feeding babies in the last few decades! You may hear *it worked for me–you should try it* a lot, but bear in mind that the baby "it worked for" may have avoided ill effects by pure luck. Feeding your baby goat's milk or plain cow's milk before one year puts her at a severe nutritional disadvantage and can cause grave problems, including intestinal bleeding, anemia, electrolyte imbalance, and poor growth. Goat's milk protein is similar to cow's milk protein; if your baby has an allergy to one, he or she may react to the other, too. If your baby's not tolerating her formula, ask his or her doctor for advice on switching formulas. She may need a hypoallergenic formula.

Q: I use concentrated formula but recently bought some powdered formula for traveling. I noticed it looks much different after I mix it—is this normal?

A: Yes. Even though the ingredients are the same, the different types of formulas can look different once they're prepared. You may also notice that after mixing (especially shaking) powdered formula, it has a lot of bubbles. Try to wait thirty minutes before feeding it to let the bubbles dissipate, or try mixing powdered formula by swirling it instead of shaking it.

Q: What's the difference between cow's milk and cow's milk formula? Is it okay to give my baby whole cow's milk every once in a while?

A: When cow's milk is made into infant formula, it's tweaked to provide a nutrient profile closer to human milk. For example, straight cow's milk is higher in protein, sodium, and potassium and lower in vitamin C and iron than human milk. Both the excess of some nutrients and the deficit of others can cause problems. Too much protein, sodium, and potassium stresses a baby's kidneys. Regular cow's milk can irritate a baby's digestive system to the point of internal bleeding, which can lead to anemia. By contrast, the protein in formula has been heated and partially broken down so it's easier for babies to digest. You may hear that if your baby is older than nine months, an occasional serving of milk or other dairy products is probably okay. It's true: Most babies will tolerate dairy just fine after nine months or so; but introducing it before one year does raise their risk of allergies. Why take the risk?

Q: My baby is a grazer. He drinks an ounce or two, takes a break or a short nap, then wakes up twenty minutes later wanting to finish his bottle. Do I have to discard the formula between his mini-feedings?

A: No, a bottle of formula can be left at room temperature for an hour. After that, it's best to discard it. Bacteria from your baby's mouth has come in contact with the formula and can grow to dangerous levels if you leave the partially-drunk bottle at room temperature too long.

Q: I hate to throw formula away that my baby doesn't drink. Is it really necessary?

A: Formula can be really expensive, and naturally you want to avoid unnecessary waste. But you also want to avoid making your baby sick by using formula that contains too much bacteria.

Q: I have some unopened formula that's about to expire. Can I freeze it?

A: No, formula shouldn't be frozen. Extremes in temperature—very cold or very hot—can affect the nutrient content of the formula as well as the consistency. When you buy formula, check the use-by date carefully and store containers so you use the oldest formula first.

Q: My friend says formula with iron will constipate my daughter. Should I buy the low-iron type?

A: No. Although extra iron supplements can be constipating, the iron added to most formulas is easier on the system. The AAP says that the only acceptable substitute for breast milk is iron-fortified formula. In the first year, your baby grows at an amazing rate, and he definitely needs the iron in his formula to fuel all that body-building and prevent anemia. Severe anemia during the first year of life can have effects on brain development that last for a decade.

Q: We have so many formula stains on our clothes! What works to get the stain out?

A: Try these tips:

- Soak the stained garment in cold water as soon as possible.
- Don't use bleach; it sets formula stains.
- Before washing the garment, treat it with a prewash stain remover like Axion, Biz, or Era Plus.
- If you think the stain is caused by iron, try Iron-Out.

Chapter 5

Going Back to Work

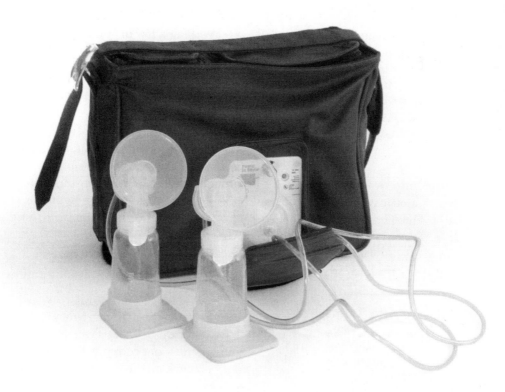

The phrase working mother *is redundant.*
—Jane Sellman

Decisions, Decisions

A baby can rock your world. You may have been intent on climbing the career ladder just a few months ago, but now that you've had your baby, your perspective is totally different. You may not want to go back to work at all! Or perhaps you thought that having a baby would kill your ambition, but you now find that you're even more motivated to do well at work for your baby's sake. Maybe your job is just a job to you—but you need it to make ends meet.

Whatever you're feeling, you know the day you return to work will be bittersweet if not downright miserable. Is there a way around this misery?

As a matter of fact, yes. If necessity is the mother of invention, then mothers are the supreme inventors! Here are some ways moms tweak their working lives to fit better with the demands of motherhood:

> **Work Options**
>
> Your boss is more likely to accept a new work plan if you show him or her a proposal that details your desired schedule and explains how your responsibilities will be covered, both during your leave and after your return. For lots of ideas and downloadable templates, visit http://www.workoptions.com/newmoms.htm.

- Taking an extended leave
- Starting a home-based business
- Working a few days a week at home
- Working a few hours a day at home
- Working longer but fewer days
- Working part-time instead of full-time
- Job-sharing

If these options intrigue you, now's the time to check them out! And if you plan to return to work after your baby's born, it's best to read this chapter while you're pregnant. Your maternity leave will fly by, and it's easier to make arrangements for your baby's care and feeding now, when you're not also recovering from birth, battling sleep deprivation, and mothering a newborn.

You *Can* Keep Breastfeeding

> **Tales from the Trenches: Nancy and Gracie**
>
> Nancy, a nurse manager, went back to work when her daughter, Gracie, was three months old. She nursed in the morning, pumped in her office at noon and five o'clock, then nursed again at seven or eight o'clock. She used the Medela Pump in Style, which emptied both breasts in about ten minutes. Her advice to other moms: "Breastfeeding is hard work, but do the best you can.... Any amount of breastfeeding is beneficial."

Many women choose not to breastfeed—or stop breastfeeding—because they know they'll have to return to work. They don't realize that most women *can* continue to breastfeed after they go back on the job—even if their workplaces aren't supportive of breastfeeding.

If you want to continue breastfeeding, you can:

- Continue nursing exclusively without pumping by:
  - Working at home
  - Hiring a babysitter who can bring your baby to you for nursing

- Choosing a daycare very close to your workplace so you can go there to nurse your baby
- Seeking a workplace that has on-site daycare
- Working part-time (Your baby may decide to just sleep while you're away and wait till you return to feed.)
• Continue nursing exclusively while pumping at work:
  - Stockpiling frozen milk so your baby has milk when you go back to work.
  - Pumping during lunch breaks or while working at your desk.
  - Working a reduced schedule
  - Working an extra hour a day to make time for pumping.
• Doing a combination of breastfeeding and formula feeding:
  - Nursing the baby before and after work and on days off.

This chapter will walk you through the details of breastfeeding while working outside the home, show you how to start a lactation program at your workplace, and give you tips on combining breastfeeding and formula-feeding. It will also give you inspiring examples and advice from real moms who've been there.

Pumping at Work

Doing Your Homework

If you want to continue nursing after you return to work, you need to look into pumping on the job. While it's possible that your baby will reverse-cycle, or sleep while you're apart and get all the milk he or she needs while you're together, you can't count on it.

First, find out if your employer has a lactation program. If there's no official program, ask human resources what policies are in place to support breastfeeding mothers. Large corporations sometimes have policies that middle managers don't know—especially if they're men! Human resources will also be able to tell you whether your insurance plan provides lactation support benefits.

Breastfeeding and Work around the World

If you work for a multinational company, find out how your breastfeeding colleagues in other countries fare. It might provide ammunition for change at your North American work site. For example:[1]

• More than half the countries around the world provide routine nursing breaks.
• In France women may take up to two hours per day for nursing breaks.
• In Israel women can take one hour per day of paid time for nursing breaks during the first four months.
• In China women may take two half-hour breaks each day for nursing until their babies turn one. Other support includes breastfeeding rooms and health centers.
• In Norway mothers get two hours daily to breastfeed at work.
• In Russia women get thirty-minute breaks at least every three hours.
• In Japan full-time employees receive two thirty-minute nursing breaks and part-time employees receive one thirty-minute nursing break per day *in addition to normal work breaks*.
• In Argentina moms can take two thirty-minute breaks per day for breastfeeding until their babies turn one.

Another important step is learning your legal rights regarding breastfeeding and work. For example, Minnesota and California both have laws that require employers to provide break time and a private, non-bathroom area for pumping. Check out your state's laws at http://www.lalecheleague.org/Law/LawBills.html or http://www.ncsl.org/programs/health/breast50.htm. You can find info on federal legislation in the United States at http://maloney.house.gov. (Search for *women's issues* under *issues and legislation*, then click on *breastfeeding*.) To learn about breastfeeding rights in Canada, visit http://www.infactcanada.ca/Breastfeeding_Rights.htm.

After doing your homework, you'll probably find yourself in one of the situations listed in the following chart.

Different Workplace Scenarios

Your Situation	How to Proceed
Workplace has a lactation program.	Count your blessings and sign up!
Workplace has no lactation program but is open to one.	Talk to your boss or human resources about starting one. Pitch the benefits for the company. Find out if your company's health plan would contribute support for lactation consultant services or breast pumps.
Workplace (usually a small one) won't start a formal program, but is willing to support a breastfeeding mom's needs.	Figure out what time, space, and/or other accommodations you need, and work with your company to meet those needs.
Workplace doesn't support breastfeeding.	Where there's a will, there's a way! First, double-check your state's breastfeeding laws. (See above.) If your company is breaking the law, help bring it into compliance. If your rights are not well-protected, try a "don't ask, don't tell" strategy—you may very well be able to pump successfully without anyone knowing.
Your schedule or location makes pumping impossible.	You can still nurse your baby in the morning, at night, and on weekends. You'll be amazed at how your body adapts!

Selling Your Boss on Breastfeeding

Whatever your situation, it's best to proceed with a smile and a positive, cooperative attitude. If you want your employer to be flexible with you so you can continue breastfeeding, your best bet is to explain how it will help *the company*, not you. Here's how employers benefit from supporting breastfeeding:[2]

- Reduced staff turnover
- Higher productivity and employee satisfaction

- Reduced sick time and/or personal time
- Reduced health care and/or insurance costs
- Added retention and/or recruitment incentive for female employees
- Enhanced reputation as a progressive company

Aetna found that for each breastfed baby in their company, the company saved $1,400 in medical claims and three days of sick leave. At Cigna, breastfeeding moms saved the company $60,000 in absentee pay and $240,000 per year in healthcare expenses.[3] In a large study published in the *American Journal of Health Promotion*, researchers found that of all the infants that never got sick, 86 percent were breastfed; among mothers who were absent due to a sick infant, 75 percent were formula-feeding.[4]

> **Walking the Talk**
>
> If you like to support businesses that do the right thing, you'll be happy to know that the publisher of *Baby Bites* supports breastfeeding moms. The editor of this book, Christine, has a one-year-old daughter, Maria, who's never had a drop of formula—thanks not only to her own dedication but also to the support of her employer, Meadowbrook Press. She had a generous maternity leave and now has a flexible work schedule, time to pump, and a little-used photo studio for her pumping sessions. If only all employers could be that supportive!

Starting a Workplace Lactation Program

So there's no lactation program at your workplace. What to do? Start one! If you have a boss who's even somewhat supportive, you can most likely sell the idea. (Alternatively, if you're currently job-hunting, look for a company that has a lactation program. Check out http://www.workingmother.com, where you'll find an annual list of the one hundred "family friendliest" companies in America.)

Breastfeeding helps an employer's bottom line, which is why many companies have established on-site lactation programs for their moms returning from maternity leave. They include Cigna, Aetna, Procter and Gamble, The Home Depot, PriceWaterhouseCoopers, Kodak, Lilly, the Los Angeles Department of Water and Power, the American Academy of Pediatrics, the U.S. Department of Agriculture, the University of Minnesota School of Nursing, the Kentucky Cabinet for Health and Family Services, and many, many more.

A lactation program can consist of minimal support that includes a flexible work schedule with breaks, or it can include a

> **Tales from the Trenches: Kacey and Romey**
>
> Kacey works at Ross Products, maker of Similac formula. Ross has a lactation room with a pump, sink, and refrigerator. Kacey pumps twice a day. She says, "At first I felt guilty taking time off to pump, since I had just come back from maternity leave and had so much catching up to do. But finally I realized that the break time was a small price to pay for all the benefits. Now that I've gotten better at pumping, I can read over work materials while I pump."

Hats Off to Carolyn Maloney, New York Senator

Politicians get a lot of bad press, but here's some good news for a change: New York senator Carolyn Maloney is a great advocate for breastfeeding moms. She's been introducing bills to support breastfeeding since 1998. In 2005 she hosted a nurse-in on Capitol Hill to call attention to her reintroduction of the Breastfeeding Promotion Act, federal legislation that would shield mothers from discrimination for breastfeeding and encourage new mothers to breastfeed.

gamut of services like a lactation room with pump rental, a refrigerator and sink, and free phone consultation with a lactation consultant. If you want to help your company start a workplacee lactation program, check out these helpful resources on the Internet:

- http://www.medela.com/NewFiles/corplactprgm.html
- http://www.wicworks.ca.gov/breastfeeding/EmployerResources/bf_bestinvestment.pdf
- http://www.breastfeedingtaskforla.org/BFWork.htm

Pumping Checklist

Read on to find out what you need to express milk effectively at work. You'll also learn how you can get by without certain items.

- **Regular breaks**: To maintain adequate milk production, you need pumping breaks at fairly regular times during your workday, ideally no more than three hours apart. If you can't have your lunch until two o'clock and your break until four o'clock, you'll have a hard time staying comfortable and producing enough milk. You also need enough time to empty both breasts. Time needed varies from woman to woman and from pump to pump, but a fifteen-minute break is the bare minimum most women need for each pumping session. If you're a quick pumper and your job already allows you regular breaks, you may be able to use your normal breaks and lunches with no modification. If you're having trouble fitting pumping into your work schedule, see the following ideas.

  - If your boss is strict about length of breaks and you need more time than you're allowed, ask if you can come to work earlier or stay later to make up the time.

  - Ask if you can split your lunch break in two and take a short break in the morning and another in the afternoon (say, at eleven o'clock and three o'clock.

  - Trade lunch or break times with willing coworkers.

- **Privacy**: You'll be most comfortable pumping in a clean, private place with a lockable door. If you have your own office, that's perfect. If not, you could use another room that's available a couple of times a day. Think creatively! Check out all the nooks and crannies of your workplace and chances are, you'll find a spot that suits you: a conference room, an empty office, a storage room, or the like. If you can't find an ideal room, you still have options: your cubicle with a sheet tacked across the doorway, your vehicle, or even the restroom. (Note: The bathroom is a last resort! Pumping in your car with the appropriate power adapter would be far more sanitary and pleasant. And if you set sunshades up inside your windows, it'd be private, too.) If your chosen location isn't lockable, make a sign for the door. Your coworkers really don't want to interrupt you—so make it obvious when they shouldn't!

- **Cooler and/or refrigerator**: It's nice to have a fridge for storing pumped milk till you go home, but not critical. A cooler will do. Many pumps have built-in insulated storage space for expressed milk; all you need to remember are ice packs. Another option is an insulated lunch bag. (See page 113 for breast milk storage guidelines.)

- **Electric breast pump**: This is a must if you need to pump daily in a short amount of time. Most manual and small battery-operated pumps won't stand up to heavy-duty pumping. (See page 32 for a detailed discussion of pumps.) Pumps that can pump both breasts at the same time are ideal. You can buy or rent them, depending on the model you want. (Rentals are usually from a hospital or lactation consultant.) If discretion is important to you, you'll want a quiet model that doesn't look like a pump when in its case.

- **Collection kit**: If you buy a pump, chances are it comes with a collection kit (including horns that fit over your breasts, bottles to collect milk, tubing to connect the horns to the pump, and other gear). If you're renting a pump, you'll probably have to buy a separate collection kit. (Don't worry; it's cheap!) Make sure the horns in your collection kit are the right size for you. If your nipples are sore, you may need a larger size or a softer horn.

> ### Tales from the Trenches: Karen and Eli
>
> Karen is a hairstylist who wanted to continue breastfeeding after returning from maternity leave. Like many women who work in service jobs, she had nowhere to pump at work. So she got a car adapter for her pump and pumped in her car. While at work she pumps every three hours, expressing about eight ounces in ten minutes. Her routine is to set up the pump and call her mom, who cares for her son, Eli. She asks how his day is going and listens to his voice. This helps stimulate letdown. Her advice for other moms? "Understand it takes about six weeks to establish breastfeeding. It's so important for your baby's development and bonding—just stick with it!"

Getting Ready to Go Back

Once you decide how your baby will be fed when you go back to work, you need to prepare. These ideas will help smooth the transition between home and work.

- Take as long a maternity leave as possible—it'll help you bond with your baby and establish milk production.

- While you're at home with your baby, relax and enjoy it! Don't stress about going back to work—that's a sure way to suck the joy from the time you have together now.

Stockpiling Your Milk

If you plan to have your baby fed expressed milk while you're at work, you'll need at least one day's supply in your fridge or freezer before you go back on the job. Many moms begin pumping once their milk supply is well-established. If you're not already pumping, I recommend that you begin pumping and freezing at least two weeks before returning to work. Most moms find that they can pump an extra ounce or two after the first morning feeding. (See page 32 for more info on pumping.)

- You'll need at least one day's supply of expressed milk in your fridge or freezer for your first day back at work. See the sidebar for more on stockpiling milk.

- If possible, start back to work slowly. Work part-time for a few weeks or work half-days the first week.

- Make your first day of work either a Thursday or Friday. A short first week back eases the transition.

- Plan ahead for meals: Cook ahead and freeze, make weekly menus, and have simple meals in mind.

- Keep a journal to record your thoughts. You may want to refer to them if you have another baby and need to make this transition again.

Supplementing? Time to Try Formula

If pumping at work isn't possible for whatever reason, you'll need to think about introducing your baby to formula. It's a good idea to do this a few weeks before you return to work so you can both get used to it. Breast milk is sweet and tasty, so your baby may be hesitant to give it up for some feedings!

The following list provides a few ideas to help a hesitant baby get used to formula. To find what works, you'll no doubt need to use trial and error and a big dose of instinct!

- Try mixing one part formula with three parts breast milk. When your baby accepts that, increase the ratio to two parts formula and two parts breast milk. Repeat this process until the feeding is all formula.

Tales from the Trenches: Cassandra on Engorgement

"When my milk first came in, I swelled up like a balloon and my breasts were rock-solid. What a pain—but it was well worth it for my son. Breastfeeding was easy for me. I just wish I'd continued for a longer time. When I started to use more formula than breast milk, my breasts engorged again. The switch has to be a slow process to prevent that."

- Some moms have been successful with serving the formula at a temperature different from breast milk—a little warmer, at room temperature, or even cold from the fridge.

- Sometimes babies won't take formula from their moms, so you may have to enlist the help of Dad, Grandma, or friends.

Once your baby is drinking formula well, you'll need to gradually decrease the number of feedings at the breast so your milk supply can adjust to the change. If you cut back on breastfeeding too abruptly, you may end up with plugged ducts.

Expressing Your Milk

If you plan to have your baby fed expressed milk while you're at work, this section will walk you through the process. There are two ways of expressing your milk: with your hands or with a pump. Hand expression is very useful when you're engorged and just want to relieve a little pressure, when you're away from home longer than you meant to be and you're without a pump, or if your pump breaks.

Hand Expression

Some women go the low-tech route rather than deal with the cost and paraphernalia of a pump. Once you've perfected hand expression, you can get just as much milk as a pump, though it usually takes longer.

Before you begin, wash your hands—then relax! Sit down with a warm cup of decaf tea or water. (Or you might want to try expressing for the first time when you're in the bath or shower.) Think confident thoughts. Gently massage each breast like when you do a breast self-exam. To let gravity help you, you can lean forward a bit or stand up and let your breasts droop. Gently shake them to help the milk flow. Then follow these five steps:

1. Place your hand around your breast, with your thumb above and your fingers below and one to one and one-half inches behind your nipple.

2. Push your thumb and fingers into your breast and toward your chest wall.

3. Roll your thumb and fingers forward to squeeze the milk from the milk sinuses, located behind the areola. Don't rub your fingers along your skin; this will cause chafing. Once you see milk squirting in all directions, you've got it!

4. Rotate your fingers and thumb around your breast so you drain all the milk ducts. You can use both hands.

5. Once the milk flow slows down, express from the other breast for a while. When milk flow from the second breast slows down, you can come back to the first breast. The entire process should take twenty to thirty minutes.

The cool thing about hand expressing is seeing how your milk exits the nipple from many little holes—hence the squirting in all directions! Because of this, you'll want to place a towel on your lap while you're learning. Collecting milk while hand expressing will take a bit of practice. You can collect it in a bowl, a wide coffee mug, or a jar. Or you can use a tool made just for this purpose, the Medela Hand Expression Funnel. It's a bowl-shaped funnel that attaches to any standard bottle.

Pumping

If you're still looking for a pump, see page 32 for a detailed discussion of the many kinds. Before you buy one, seek out reviews from other moms (in person or online).

If possible, rent a pump before buying to make sure it's the right one for you. You may not love your pump at first, but you and your pump will be getting along fine before you know it. Some women don't continue with the pump they started with; that's okay, too. Keep looking until you find one that works well for you.

When should you first meet your pump? I recommend starting at least two weeks before you return to work, or sooner if you want to have a larger supply of milk in your freezer. Consider, too, that it may take a few weeks to become an expert at pumping. Here's a step-by-step guide for your first pumping session:

1. Start with a relaxing routine to promote letdown. Sit in a comfy chair with a warm drink. Massage your breasts gently in a circular motion, as if you're doing a breast self-exam. You can also let gravity help by leaning forward a bit or standing up and letting your breasts droop. Gently shake them to promote letdown.

2. Center your nipples inside the horns of your pump. (Some moms moisten the edges of the horns first to create better suction.) If your nipples aren't centered, the suction may be uncomfortable. Don't be discouraged if your horns don't fit well; there are different sizes available.

3. For an electric pump, begin on the lowest speed and suction settings; for a manual pump, start with a slow rhythm. Increase the speed and suction as much as comfort allows. The horns must stay sealed against your breasts to maintain suction, so make sure you don't let them slip.

4. Begin pumping just five minutes per breast at each session. Don't worry if you don't get much milk at first; your volume should improve with practice. (Also, be aware that milk supply is usually greatest in the morning and decreases as the day goes on.) Once you feel comfortable pumping for five minutes, you can increase the time to ten then fifteen minutes. After you turn off your pump, break the suction by using a clean finger to gently push down on each breast right above the horn.

5. Some moms pump one side while nursing baby on the other. Then they let baby finish up on the pumped side so both breasts are well emptied.

Letdown is easy when your baby's at the breast, but you might need a little help when you're apart. First, try to relax. Then look at a picture of your baby. Some women like holding a piece of clothing or a toy that belongs to their baby. Close your eyes and picture your baby nursing, playing, or even crying. Don't watch the collection container. A warm compress (even something as simple as a warm paper towel) placed on your breast right before pumping can help, too.

Expressing on the Job

When

Ideally, you should express at least every three hours to keep up full-time milk production. It's best to put yourself on a schedule so you can send your body a consistent message every day.

If you can't express as often as you want, just try to do it twice (or at least once) while you're at work; that'll go a long way toward keeping up your supply. Nurse your baby more at night and on the weekends; this will help, too. On Mondays your breasts will be fuller than usual, but they'll adjust as the week wears on.

If you find that you're not expressing as much as your baby seems to want while you're apart each day, don't despair. There's nothing wrong with you; pumps are notorious for not emptying the breast as well as babies do. To keep up with your baby's demand for expressed milk, try adding a pumping session after your baby goes to sleep at night.

Where

Here are some common workplace locations pumping moms use:

- Lockable office
- Conference room
- Storage room
- Lounge
- Locker room
- Medical or nurse's office
- Cubicle with a sheet tacked across the entrance
- Vehicle
- Clean restroom (Keep your gear and your milk clean by keeping paper towels between restroom surfaces and you and your gear.)
- Dirty restroom (This is a last resort. If it's your only option but it's just too dirty to stomach, you can pump and dump your milk to prevent engorgement and keep up your milk supply.)

Hands-Free Pumping

Imagine being able to double-pump while catching up on your reading, typing a memo, making phone calls, or even driving. Talk about multitasking! Here are a few ways you can pump hands-free:

- Wear a hands-free pumping bustier. (See http://www.easyexpression products. com.)
- Get an attachment kit for your pump that allows hands-free pumping. (See http://www.medela.com/NEWFILES/ seambraspant.html.)
- Make your own hands-free pump attachment with elastic pony tail holders. (See http://www.kellymom. com/bf/pumping/hands-free-pumping.html.)

Dressing for Expressing

The following clothes and accessories will make expressing on the job as easy as possible.

- **Nursing pads**: Be sure to wear them, and keep plenty of extras on hand at work. Your breasts don't know your baby's not around, and they may let down without warning! (See page 30 for more information on the advantages and disadvantages of different kinds of nursing pads.)
- **Nursing bras**: You're probably wearing nursing bras most of the time already, but if not, consider starting. (You might also want to check out a pumping bustier; see sidebar above for more info.) The easy access they provide can speed up each pumping session.

- **Two-piece outfits or nursing tops**: For double pumping, you'll need a top you can easily lift or open down the middle. If you wear a nursing top, you can pump without lifting or opening your shirt at all. If your pumping location isn't completely private, you might want to tie a shawl or large cotton scarf around your shoulders so your chest is covered. (See page 31 for more info on nursing cover-ups.)
- **Dark or patterned fabrics**: Dark colors and busy patterns can camouflage the inevitable leaks and drips.
- **Spare top**: Keep a sweater or an extra blouse at work so you can change tops or hide a big spill or leak.

Baby Meets Bottle

Whether you continue breastfeeding full-time or supplement with formula after returning to work, your baby will eventually have to learn to drink from something besides you. If your baby is younger than five months, he or she will probably need to feed from a bottle. If your baby is five months or older, you may be able to go straight to a cup. Since most North American women who work outside the home get less than five months of maternity leave, this section will focus on introducing a bottle—but many of these tips apply to introducing a cup, too.

The general consensus is that breastfed babies shouldn't try bottle-feeding until about four weeks to make sure breastfeeding is well-established. Many moms successfully introduce a bottle at three weeks; some believe that if you wait longer than six weeks, it can be more difficult. The keys factors are a good nursing relationship and a good milk supply. Every mom and baby are different. If you feel your milk supply is well-established and your baby has developed a good latch, try the bottle. If you're having latch or supply issues, it might be wise to wait for the bottle until you solve your nursing problems.

Whenever you introduce the bottle, don't give it more than once a day; twice a week is adequate. Be forewarned that your baby may not easily accept an artificial nipple. Your baby is used to snuggling close to you and sucking on a soft, warm human nipple, not a firm, cool latex or silicone one. Following are lots of tips to get you started. Once you're successful, give the bottle regularly—at least twice a week. If you stop giving bottles for a while, don't be surprised if your baby takes a dislike to them.

Five Easy Steps

1. Find a nipple that resembles your own—preferably a soft nipple with a wide base. Nipples that have been used successfully by breastfeeding moms include Avent nipples, Playtex NaturalShape nipples,[5] and Breastflow nipples by The First Years. (See page 82 for more on choosing bottles and nipples.) Whatever brand you choose, make sure you use only the newborn (slow flow) nipple if you intend to switch back and forth between nursing and bottle-feeding.

2. Introduce the bottle when you and your baby are both well-rested and happy and have plenty of time, so you won't feel rushed or stressed.

3. Put slightly warmed breast milk in the bottle and run hot water over the nipple to warm and soften it.

4. Try to get your baby to latch on to the nipple as if it were yours. Tickle your baby's lip or cheek with it and wait for a wide-open mouth.

5. Put your baby in a position that's not usually used for nursing to avoid confusing him or her. Walking or standing with your baby in a sling, setting your baby in a bouncy seat, or holding your baby facing away from you are possibilities.

Practical Tips

- If you introduce your baby to a bottle within the first month, you may be able to introduce it yourself. Some moms even do it right after a nursing session.

- Often it's best if someone else (your partner, a friend, a relative, or a babysitter) introduces the bottle with you out of the room—or even out of the house. Experienced bottle-feeders are good candidates; they've done it before and will get less frustrated.

- Some moms find it helpful to distract their babies. You could try sitting outside, feeding in front of family pictures, or—if all else fails—turning on a children's video.

- Some babies accept a bottle better when they can't see who's feeding them. Have someone else put your baby in a bouncy seat, car seat, or front pack and feed from behind. All your baby sees is a hand and a bottle.

If At First You Don't Succeed

- Remember that your baby has a survival instinct and won't starve! Sooner or later, your baby *will* learn to drink from a bottle or cup.

- Don't let crying escalate too far. If your baby's getting very upset, stop and try again later.

Tales from the Trenches: Ana and Alex

Ana breastfed her daughter, Alex, almost exclusively for the first six months. At three to four weeks, she introduced a bottle of breast milk to Alex. Alex accepted the bottle right away from Ana.

After that, Ana gave Alex a bottle a day of mostly breast milk, and Alex had no problem going back and forth. Ana typically nursed Alex on both sides, then pumped a little milk and gave it to Alex by bottle.

When Alex was six months old, Ana went back to work in the engineering department of a manufacturing company. She pumped in a conference room once a day at lunch. It took about twenty minutes using the Medela Pump in Style. Alex's daycare fed her breast milk plus one or two bottles a day of formula. Ana and Alex nursed often on the weekends.

Ana says, "My advice is to buy a good quality pump. I spent about two hundred dollars on mine, and it was worth every penny."

- Try a change of venue. Go to a friend's house, a mall, outside, or just a different room than the one you usually nurse in.
- Try different times. Some babies will take the bottle better at night, when they're half-asleep—others might take a bottle in the morning, when they're wide-awake and ready for adventure.
- Experiment with different nipples. You may have to try many kinds before you find one your baby latches onto. Some babies are very finicky!
- If your baby won't drink frozen expressed milk, try fresh instead—or vice versa.
- Try a bait-and-switch technique. Start a feeding by nursing, and when your baby pauses or falls asleep, sneak in a bottle.

Tales from the Trenches: Robert and Me

At one point I thought my son Robert would never take a bottle! Because I didn't go back to work full-time after his birth, we didn't introduce a bottle until he was about six months old. I tried, my husband tried, and friends tried...we were all utterly frustrated. Robert had the lungs of an opera singer, and he used them! Finally Oma, the grandmotherly caretaker at Mother's Day Out, finally got him to take a bottle after trying for several days. Luckily the workers were all patient with his screaming!

If Your Baby Hates the Bottle

You may feel ready to pull your hair out, but try to relax—and hang in there! This too shall pass. Here's some advice to get you through this rough patch:

- Be prepared for lots of crying, but don't let your baby get too upset. Trust me: You don't want to find out who's stronger-willed! Stop trying after ten unsuccessful minutes.
- Remember that your baby's really not trying to drive you crazy.
- Some babies are very stubborn; they want mommy and are willing to wait for her! You may have to leave the house all day for your baby to finally give in and take a bottle at the *end* of the day.
- Take a vacation from the bottle for a few days if you and your baby are getting too stressed out.
- If you're severely frustrated and distraught, it might be time to consider other options:
  - If your baby's younger than five months and absolutely refuses a bottle, check out other feeding devices. Medela makes several special feeding devices, including a cup feeder, a SoftFeeder (a type of cup feeder), and a finger feeder. You can also use an eyedropper, a small medicine cup, or a medicine syringe.
  - If your baby's older than five months, you may have more luck introducing a soft-spout sippy cup. (If you're using Avent bottles, Avent makes a soft spout you can attach to any Avent bottle or cup.)

- Instead of struggling with bottles, cups, or other feeding devices, re-evaluate your work and childcare options. For example, investigate telecommuting or seek a daycare provider close to your workplace so you can nurse your baby during your breaks.

- Encourage your baby to reverse-cycle (sleep when you're apart and nurse frequently when you're together). This usually means a lot of night nursing, so cosleeping will help you get as much sleep as possible.

• Keep in mind that as your baby gets older and learns to eat other foods (and drink from a cup), bottle-feeding won't be as much of an issue.

• If you're worried about your baby's growth during this transition, visit your baby's doctor weekly for weight checks.

• To find more advice from other moms who've faced this challenge, visit the Berkeley Parents Network at http://www.parents.berkeley.edu/advice/nursing/bottle.html.

Back-to-Work Countdown

Two to Four Weeks Ahead

Begin pumping after nursing sessions as often as possible to build up a freezer stash of breast milk. When you're cooking dinner, make a habit of doubling recipes and freezing the extra food.

Two Weeks Ahead

Gradually change your pumping schedule to the schedule you'll keep at work. If you're going to replace any feedings with formula, begin doing so now. Replace one feeding at a time. When your body adjusts to the change (usually in five to ten days), you can replace another feeding (if necessary).

One Week Ahead

Go through the motions of a typical workday. Get up when you would for work. Nurse your baby in the morning. Feed a bottle when your baby's daycare normally would. Pump when you would at work.

Four Days Ahead: Dress Rehearsal

Bring your baby to daycare for a trial run. Instead of going to work, give yourself the day off. Run errands, have lunch with friends, or go shopping. Pump at the same time(s) you'll be pumping at work. Pick up your baby when you normally would and nurse briefly. Go home and have a full nursing session. Assess your day and tweak your feeding and pumping plans if necessary.

Feeding the Family When You're Back at Work

In most families, even though moms put in the same number of work hours as dads, they still wear the chef's hat (not to mention many other domestic hats) at home. The first few weeks may find you struggling to do it all. Here are some tips to help you and your family continue to eat healthfully.

- **Call in favors**: Remember all those friends who said, "If you need anything, just call..."? Now's the time. Ask each of them for a home-cooked meal the week you go back to work.
- **Recruit your partner**: If possible, put your partner in charge of as many meals as possible. If you make a weekly menu and plan easy-to-cook meals, even the most hopeless kitchen klutz should be able to manage this job.
- **Give yourself a break**: Plan to eat take-out meals or have pizza delivered once or twice a week.
- **Use a Crock-Pot**: Prep the food in the evening, turn on the Crock-Pot the next morning, and—voilà!—supper's ready when you get home from work. Plus, it's easy to make big batches in a Crock-Pot. Freeze the extra food for later.
- **Start a dinner co-op**: Enlist one or two friends who live close by. When you cook, you make double or triple and they pick their dinner up from you. In return you get one or two great meals with no cooking.
- **Cook on weekends**: Cook several meals on the weekend. Double each recipe, store the food in freezer containers, and label each container with the contents and date. In no time, you'll have a freezer full of meals.
- **Shop with convenience in mind**: Following are just a few easy-to-cook meals you can find at most grocery stores.
  - *Ready-made salads*: Spinach is healthiest.
  - *Cooked, sliced chicken*: This is a versatile ingredient for many quick meals.
  - *Frozen, cooked shrimp*: It thaws quickly for a shrimp cocktail, a main dish salad, or prepared vegetable or minestrone soup.
  - *Family-size deli meals*: Many grocery delis sell heat-and-serve lasagna and other dishes. Or try family-size frozen entrées.
  - *Dinner in a bag*: Usually all you have to add is meat.
  - *Veggie burgers*: Enjoy a burger with all your favorite fixings—and no guilt!

Two to Three Days Ahead

Run last-minute errands. Do your grocery shopping for the week. (See the chart above for tips on feeding your family well when time's in short supply.) If you haven't done so already, prepare and freeze a few extra meals.

One Day Ahead

Have a relaxed day. Enjoy your baby. Get plenty of rest. Assemble all the gear you'll need for the next day—a spare shirt for you, extra breast pads, diaper bag, and so on.

Back-to-Work Day

This is it! You've prepared and practiced, and you're ready. Even if the day doesn't go as you hope it will, know that you've given it your best shot. Remember that you're in control—you can change the plan as you go along.

You may experience a roller coaster of emotions—guilt, sadness, or worry about leaving your baby; happiness about returning to a satisfying job. All these feelings are normal. Undoubtedly you'll miss your baby; pumping can really help soothe that hurt. While you pump, think about how you're giving your baby your best, even when you're apart. You'll probably think about your baby a lot—and this may cause letdown at inopportune times. If you're worried about leaking, cross your arms over your chest.

The first day will be a long one. But your workdays will get better!

Storing Breast Milk

Breast milk is a perishable food. However, because it contains natural antibacterial properties, it doesn't spoil as easily as formula. Refrigerating and freezing may lower the antioxidant activity in breast milk; longer storage time and lower temperatures are related to lower antioxidant levels. So, refrigerate your milk for the longest time possible before freezing it.[6]

The following information applies to healthy, full-term infants. If your baby was premature or has any health problems, ask your baby's doctor if you should take any further precautions when storing your breast milk.

Containers

The simplest way to store your milk—especially if you'll be freezing a lot of it—is in sterile plastic zipper bags or bottle liners made specifically for refrigerating or freezing breast milk. Gerber Seal 'n Go bags and Lansinoh bags are very well rated by moms. Or you might want to check out Avent's Via reusable/disposable storage cups. They attach directly to any Avent pump or nipple. Via cups can be frozen and sterilized several times (until they show signs of wear). After that, you can recycle them.

If you'll be storing smaller amounts of milk, you might prefer to use bottles. Storage bottles should be clean and made of glass or food-grade plastic. It's unclear whether glass or plastic best protects the immune properties of breast milk. Plastic is lightweight and break-resistant, but it can slightly change the taste of breast milk.

If you use storage bags or cups made for breast milk, they're already sterile. If you use bottles or other reusable containers, you'll need to wash them in the dishwasher or hand-wash them with hot soapy water, rinse them well, and air-dry them. If you hand-wash your containers but your water supply isn't clean, you'll also need to sterilize them. (See page 86 for sterilizing tips.)

Storage Instructions

These practical tips will ensure a safe and adequate supply of stored breast milk:

- Store milk in small amounts (two to four ounces) to prevent waste.
- Store some milk in even smaller amounts (one to two ounces) for times when your baby wants just a bit more.

Why Does My Milk Look Funny?

The first time you pump, you may be shocked at its appearance. You might have expected it to look like milk from the grocery store. It can vary in color from white to yellow to pinkish, greenish, or even bluish. Breast milk changes not only with your baby's needs, but also somewhat with your diet:[8]

- Colostrum will look yellow or yellow-orange and thick.
- Mature milk (after two weeks) will look more bluish-white.
- Milk from the end of a feeding (hindmilk) is higher in fat and will look creamier.
- Food or food dyes can give your milk a pink or pink-orange hue.
- Natural green pigments in vegetables, seaweed, and food dyes can give milk a greenish tint.
- Some prescription medications can also color your milk.
- Even if your milk is rainbow-colored, that's no reason to discard it!
- Pinkish milk that has a touch of blood in it from cracked nipples can be safely given to your infant.

You may also notice that your milk has a distinct smell—generally mildly sweet. Milk that has been frozen has been described as having a soapy smell. Because the food you eat flavors your milk, the smell can also change depending on your diet. This is good! Breastfed babies tend to be more accepting of a variety of foods because they've been introduced to more flavors while breastfeeding.

- You can add fresh milk to frozen milk, as long as the fresh milk isn't a bigger quantity than the frozen milk. Cool the fresh milk in the refrigerator first so it doesn't thaw the frozen milk.
- Leave an inch of room at the top of the container; milk expands as it freezes.
- Use bags made specifically for storing breast milk. Ordinary zipper bags aren't sterile and are more prone to ripping and leaking.
- Don't refreeze thawed milk.
- Store milk in the back of the freezer or refrigerator, where the temperature is the most stable.
- Don't store milk in the door of your freezer or refrigerator, where temperatures fluctuate whenever the door is opened.
- Date storage containers and use the oldest milk first.

Storage Time

Breast milk comes complete with antimicrobial factors that prevent spoiling, so you can store it at room temperature much longer than formula or many other foods. Colostrum can be stored up to twelve hours at room temperature! The following guide explains how long you can safely store mature milk at various temperatures.[7]

- At room temperature (Although breast milk can be left at room temperature if necessary, it's best to refrigerate it as soon as possible.)

- At 60°F or 16°C for twenty-four hours
- At 66°F to 72°F or 19°C to 22°C for ten hours
- At 79°F or 26°C for four to six hours
- At 86°F to 100°F or 30°C to 38°C for four hours
- In the refrigerator: at 32°F to 39°F or 0°C to 4°C for eight days
- In the freezer:
  - In a freezer compartment within a refrigerator for two weeks
  - In a self-contained freezer on top of or on the side of a refrigerator for three to four months
  - In a deep freezer for six months or longer

Thawing Breast Milk

- You can thaw your milk in the refrigerator by first running hot water over it or by setting it in a bowl of hot water.
- When you store breast milk, the cream separates and rises to the top. Before feeding it to your baby, gently swirl it to mix the cream back in. (Don't shake it; this damages the milk and creates lots of bubbles.)
- Don't thaw breast milk at room temperature or heat it on the stove. Also, don't microwave your milk; microwaving destroys important nutrients and creates hot spots that may burn your baby.
- Use thawed breast milk within twenty-four hours.
- Discard bottles of thawed breast milk that your baby has partially consumed.

When Caregivers Feed Your Baby

Whether you go back to work full-time or part-time, day shift or night shift, at some point a caregiver will be feeding your baby. Babies spend a lot of their time eating, so how others feed your baby is an important point to consider when you're shopping for a caregiver.

Following are some things to look for when choosing childcare, as well as tips to help you share the job of feeding your baby.

Daycare Centers and Home Daycares

Facility

- Clean refrigerator at proper temperature (below 40°F or 4°C) for storing breast milk, formula, and food
- Clean area for bottle and food preparation (not close to diaper changing area)
- Dishwasher or sink and drying rack dedicated to washing and drying bottles and nipples (or a sink sanitized between uses)

- Sink that's used for hand-washing only
- Way to heat breast milk and formula

Staff

- Adequate staff who have time to feed your baby properly
- Staff who understand the needs of breastfed babies and know how to support breastfeeding
- Staff trained in child nutrition, cardiopulmonary resuscitation (CPR), and first aid for choking
- Staff trained to feed babies properly (Observe the staff and answer the following questions; all answers should be *yes*.)
  - Do they feed babies on demand?
  - Do they respond promptly to signs of hunger and fullness, letting babies eat until satisfied and not coaxing babies to keep eating when full?
  - Do they burp babies during and after feedings?
  - Are they patient and nurturing?
  - Do they discard leftover breast milk or formula that's been out of the refrigerator more than an hour?

Nannies and Grannies

If someone takes care of your baby at your home, this makes life easier in many ways. It's a familiar environment for your baby, and all the supplies and gear your baby needs are in place. All you need to do is give clear instructions. Be aware, though, that both nannies and grannies may come to the feeding table with notions about feeding babies that don't match yours.

Since you're paying a nanny and may even have a contract with her that requires her to care for your child as you instruct, it should be easy to make sure your baby is fed properly by a nanny. Convincing a granny, on the other hand, that your feeding strategy is best may not be so simple.

Older caregivers have much valuable wisdom and advice to offer, but some of it may be out of date. Gently let your granny know the current thinking on feeding babies. If necessary, copy pages from this book and other baby care books for easy reference.

Childcare Info Organizer

If you're daunted by the task of telling your baby's caregiver everything he or she needs to know about your child, check out Kids Klues at http://www.kidsklues.com. This software helps you create a well-organized three-ring binder to inform your caregiver about your child's routine, special needs, how to cope with an emergency, and much, much more.

Giving Instructions

The best way to make sure your baby is fed the way you want is to leave nothing to doubt! It's best to have bottles of breast milk or formula prepared in advance and in the refrigerator. Give a list of clear feeding instructions, including:

- When your baby might be hungry
- Your baby's usual signs of hunger and fullness
- How long a bottle can be left at room temperature safely
- Special instructions, if you have any (for burping, positioning, and so on)
- If your baby is eating solids, a list of foods your baby can and can't eat

Stress

Going back to work, introducing a bottle, changing your nursing schedule, learning to pump, starting daycare—it's enough to make a grown woman cry! And most of us do at some point. Too little sleep and too much change can make you feel like you're coming undone.

Don't worry; it's normal for moms who work outside the home to feel stressed out. Keep in mind, though, that stress and fatigue can negatively impact nursing, triggering a vicious cycle that's hard to escape.

To minimize stress, find support wherever you can. Join a working mom's group; as you share stories and advice, you're sure to find someone who can empathize with you. If your schedule has no room for another club, find support online. Accept help whenever it's offered. Take every opportunity—however brief—to put your feet up, take a walk, chat with a friend, or do anything that lightens your physical or mental load.

You'll be glad you did. And I promise you'll survive this transition. In a few months you'll look back and wonder what all the fuss was about!

Chapter 6

Your Baby's Digestive System

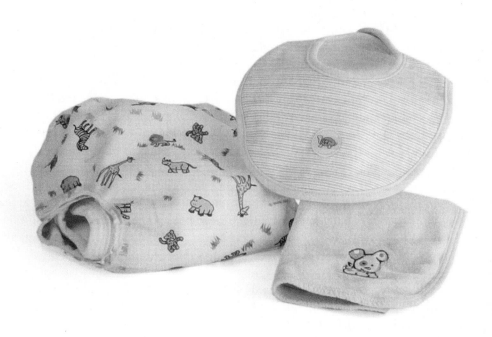

Men who have fought in the world's bloodiest wars...
are apt to faint at the sight of a truly foul diaper.
—Gary D. Christenson

Parents spend so much time pondering what comes out of their babies, we might as well devote an entire chapter to it! In the next 21 pages you'll find everything you've ever wanted to know about pooping, burping, gas, and other delightful digestive topics. If you have questions about your baby that you're too embarrassed to ask, chances are you'll find the answers right here.

The Scoop on Poop

Normal Appearance, Texture, and Frequency

Here's the general scoop on poop during a child's first two years. Remember that all children are different; if you get to know your child's pattern, you'll know better when something's wrong. Grunting and straining is normal at all ages.

For the first twenty-four hours or so, both breastfed and formula-fed babies poop meconium (thick, tarry, black poop that contains cellular debris, mucus, and other material swallowed while in the womb). A transitional poop follows that's greenish and somewhat runny. Around day three or four, the poop changes color and texture. Breastfed babies begin to have loose, golden-yellow poop—often described as looking like mustard with seeds—while formula-fed babies begin to have pasty, yellowish-tan poop.

For the first three or four days, breastfed babies should have at least one poopy diaper for each day of life (one on day one, two on day two, and so on). Formula-fed babies generally poop less often; it can depend on the brand and type of formula.

Toward the end of the first week, babies' poop starts to look the way it'll look for the next several months (until they start eating solids). Breastfed babies begin to have loose, seedy or curdy, mild-smelling yellow poop. The color of breast milk poop may range from greenish yellow to golden yellow to yellowish brown. The smell is like slightly sour milk. Formula-fed babies begin to have firm, pasty, yellowish tan to greenish tan poop. The texture of formula poop is usually like strained peas, and its smell is stronger (and to most people, stinkier) than breast milk poop.

From day four through weeks four to six, breastfed babies should have at least three quarter-size poops per day. Formula-fed babies should poop at least once a day. After four to six weeks, some babies begin to poop less often—as infrequently as once every seven days. Formula-fed babies may poop only every four days. As long as baby continues to gain weight well, this is normal. If your baby poops infrequently, just check to make sure he or she isn't in pain while pooping and that the texture of your baby's poop doesn't indicate constipation. (See pages 122-123 for more info on constipation.)

When babies start eating solid foods, their poop changes a lot. Overall it becomes much stinkier. Solids aren't as easily digested as breast milk and formula, so more waste from solids (undigested fiber and tiny amounts of carbohydrate and fat) ends up in babies' poop. Its color and texture depend on foods recently eaten. It may also contain undigested pieces of food. Here are a few things to keep in mind about your older baby's poop:

- Some foods, like corn, come out whole until your baby learns to chew well and has more digestive enzymes. You may also see other unchewed high-fiber foods in your baby's poop. Ditto for seeds, such as kiwi seeds, berry seeds.
- Foods with a lot of pigment (natural or artificial) will color your baby's poop. For example, if your baby eats large amounts of brightly colored fruits or vegetables such as carrots, raspberries, or beets, their natural pigments will find their way into your baby's diaper. (Beets can color your baby's urine as well.)

> ### How to Change an Old-Fashioned Cloth Diaper: For Baseball Fans
>
> *Spread the diaper in the position of the diamond with you at bat. Then fold second base down to home and set the baby on the pitcher's mound. Put first base and third together, bring up home plate, and pin the three together. Of course, in case of rain, you gotta call the game and start all over again.*
>
> —Jimmy Piersall, former Major League centerfielder

And here are some other factors that can affect your baby's poop:

- **Growth spurts**: When your baby goes through growth spurts—often at two weeks, six weeks, and three months—he or she will eat more, which will ramp up the pooping.
- **New routine or environment**: If you're traveling or have moved recently, your baby's routine may be out of whack. This can throw off your baby's normal pooping pattern; it'll take some time to readjust.
- **Illness**: If your baby is sick, he or she may eat less and also poop less. Antibiotics and other medications can upset your baby's digestion, causing looser and different-smelling poops.

By age two, your child may have one or two large poops per day, or they may be more frequent and smaller.

Worrisome Poops

When Should You Worry?

Your baby's bowels have been working like clockwork; you've come to expect a poopy diaper after almost every feeding. Then you notice your baby's poop pattern slowing down till it settles at once a day. Should you worry?

No. As babies gets older, their digestion naturally slows down a bit, and the normal outcome (no pun intended) is less frequent poops. Keep in mind that less frequent poops may mean larger (read: blowout) poops. Be ready!

Every baby establishes a unique pooping pattern after the first month. A gradual change is normal, but it's time to take notice if your baby's poop changes suddenly. A drastic change in frequency, firmness, or color can signal a problem. The following types of poops may warrant a call to your baby's doctor and/or your lactation consultant as well as a pause to think about what may have caused the change.

- **Tarry poop**: Poop that looks like meconium isn't normal after the first forty-eight hours or so. If you see this type of poop later, it's a sign of blood. Call your baby's doctor.

- **Red-streaked poop**: If you see red streaks, call your baby's doctor. Red streaks are small amounts of blood in the poop, which may be caused by:
  - A reaction to cow's milk formula, or more rarely, dairy products eaten by a breastfeeding mom
  - Tiny tears in baby's rectum from passing hard poops
  - Ingesting blood via a breastfeeding mom's cracked, bleeding nipples

- **Red jelly poop**: This can indicate a bowel obstruction, which is very serious. Call your baby's doctor immediately or visit the emergency room.

- **Green mucous poop**: This kind of poop is a sign of malabsorption, caused either by a virus or by excess saliva from teething. A virus should run its course in several days; you may see this type of poop for up to ten days. If it lasts longer, call your baby's doctor. (Remember that greenish loose stools are normal for some breastfed infants.)

- **Green frothy poop**: In breastfed babies, green frothy poop signals overactive let-down or a foremilk/hindmilk imbalance. A lactation consultant is usually your best bet to analyze the problem and offer a solution. This type of poop may also be a result of lactose intolerance. (See page 133 for more info on lactose intolerance.)

- **Constipation**: Constipation is determined by firmness of poops, not frequency. Remember that a change in eating habits can cause a change in pooping habits. Also, keep in mind that some grunting and straining is normal. (Ever tried pooping while lying down?) Poop that looks like small balls, pellets, or logs signals constipation. Other symptoms of constipation include more straining than usual, signs of pain while pooping, bloated belly (from gas), and abdominal cramping. (It's difficult to tell if your baby has cramping since your baby can't tell you. Symptoms of abdominal cramping include fussiness, arching the back during feeding, and bringing the knees toward the chest. Your baby might also show general signs of discomfort like clenching his or her fists or grimacing.) Following are some ways you can treat your baby's constipation. (Note: Exclusively breastfed babies very rarely get constipated, so these tips are for formula-fed babies and/or babies who are eating solid foods.)
  - If your baby isn't eating solids yet, ask his or her doctor if you can give a small amount of prune juice.
  - If your baby is breastfed and also eats solids, nurse more and try feeding extra fruits and vegetables. If your infant is formula-fed and also eats solids, provide extra fruits and vegetables.
  - If your baby eats rice cereal, try switching to barley or oats, which have more fiber, or try making whole-grain cereal (recipe on page 238). Also assess how often your baby eats cereal—especially rice cereal, which can be constipating in large amounts.

- Do not use home remedies recommended by well-meaning relatives or friends without first running them by your baby's doctor.
- Never give your baby an enema or medication for constipation unless your baby's doctor recommends it.

- **Diarrhea**: Unlike in adults, diarrhea in infants is determined not by texture but by frequency (though babies' poop may also be more watery when they have diarrhea). Frequency doubles or triples with diarrhea. If you see signs of dehydration, contact your baby's caregiver immediately. (See the next section for more info on dehydration and diarrhea causes, treatment, and prevention.)

Diarrhea Details

Diarrhea is a very common ailment among children; there are sixteen million cases per year in U.S. kids under five years old. So what, exactly, is diarrhea?

Diagnosis

It depends on your child. According to the American Academy of Pediatrics (AAP), if your child's poop suddenly becomes more loose, watery, and frequent than usual, it's diarrhea. (If your child has an occasional loose poop, it isn't considered diarrhea.) Naturally, you must know what's normal for your child before you can identify diarrhea; that's why it pays to pay attention to poop.

It can be tricky to diagnose diarrhea in breastfed babies because their poops are normally loose and frequent. Remember that breastfed newborns can have up to twelve bowel movements per day. If you suspect diarrhea in your breastfed baby, look for a foul odor and very watery poop.

Causes

Here's a list of the many possible causes of diarrhea in children:

- **Bacterial, parasitic, or viral infection in the digestive tract**: Children can contract infections like salmonellosis, shigellosis, gastroenteritis (rotavirus), or giardiasis by food contamination or hand-to-mouth transfer. Since all the organisms that cause these infections are spread via poop, diaper-wearing children in daycare are one group more susceptible to them. Another common route of transmission is swallowing contaminated water from swimming pools, lakes, rivers, streams, and shallow wells.
- **Bacterial or viral infection outside the digestive tract**: Infections that occur outside the digestive tract can also cause diarrhea. These include urinary tract infections, respiratory infections, and even ear infections.[1]
- **Medication**: Antibiotics often causes temporary lactose intolerance.
- **Sensitivity to nursing mom's diet**: Breastfed babies occasionally get diarrhea when mom eats a larger-than-usual amount of a certain food or eats a completely new food. Medications, herbal teas and supplements, and caffeine consumed by a nursing mom can have the same effect.

- **Food allergy or intolerance**: Diarrhea is a primary symptom of food allergy or intolerance. Cow's milk protein is a common irritant for both formula-fed and breastfed babies. Breastfed babies sometimes react to other nutrients in mom's diet. Once a baby is eating solids, the list of possible irritants expands greatly. (See page 133 for more on lactose intolerance and page 135 for more on allergies.)
- **Excessive juice, fruit, vegetables, sugar, or whole grains**: Children can develop diarrhea from drinking too much juice, especially juice with high sorbitol content, such as prune, pear, cherry, or apple juice. If your older child eats large quantities of fruit, vegetables, whole grains, or sugar at a single sitting, this can also bring on loose poops.

Treatment

In most cases diarrhea will resolve on its own in three to seven days. There's no effective treatment for viral diarrhea, which is the most common type. There are, however, several things you can do to keep your child nourished and hydrated and to prevent the problem from worsening. In this section I'll help you figure out what to do depending on your child's age and the severity of your child's diarrhea.

Troubleshooting
First, identify the type of diarrhea your child has:
- **Mild diarrhea**: If your child has just one or two loose poops, it's probably from something you or your child ate, and it's nothing to worry about. If your child has loose poops but isn't vomiting, has no fever, and is still active, you may not need to do anything but wait it out. Continue feeding on demand. If you're not sure how severe your child's diarrhea is, discuss it with your child's doctor.
- **Chronic diarrhea**: If your child's diarrhea lasts more than two weeks, it may be a sign of a more serious health problem. Call your child's doctor, who will probably recommend testing.
- **Toddler's diarrhea**: If your older baby or toddler acts normal, is still active, and shows no signs of dehydration but is having loose poops, it could be toddler's diarrhea. Does your child drink a lot of juice or eat a lot of high-fiber foods like fruits and veggies? If so, this could be the cause. Restrict juice to four to six ounces per day and give water when your toddler is thirsty, and slow down on the high-fiber foods. Toddler diarrhea can also be caused by a food intolerance. Keep track of your child's diet for a while to determine whether a particular food triggers loose poops.
- **Severe diarrhea**: If your child is having loose poops every one to two hours (or more often), this is considered severe diarrhea. If you're exclusively breastfeeding, nursing more often may be all you need to do—but depending on the cause, your baby's doctor may ask you to give an oral rehydration solution between feedings. If your baby is eating solid foods or drinking formula, your baby's doctor may ask you to withhold these for twenty-four hours and nurse more

Severe Diarrhea Feeding Guide

Age/Feeding Stage	Feeding Instructions[2]
Under six months and not eating solid foods	• Feed breast milk or formula and, if recommended, an oral rehydration solution. In most cases breastfeeding children don't need an oral rehydration solution.
Over six months or eating solids	• Feed breast milk or formula and, if recommended, an oral rehydration solution. In most cases breastfeeding children don't need an oral rehydration solution. • Offer solid foods already in the child's diet, emphasizing complex carbohydrates like rice, potatoes, peas, applesauce, pears, bananas, and wheat (toast, cereal, pasta). Chicken and egg yolks are good protein foods that may also help. Don't offer new foods. • Restrict high-sugar foods and drinks like soda, juice, Gatorade, and Jello as well as high-fat foods like fried foods, cheese, extra butter or margarine, bacon, sausage, and bologna.
Over eight months	• Follow instructions for children over six months. • Feed small amounts of yogurt to replenish "good" bacteria in your child's digestive tract.
Over twelve months	• Follow instructions for children over six months and over eight months. • Offer other fermented dairy foods like kefir to help replenish "good" bacteria in your child's digestive tract.

and/or feed an oral rehydration solution. (See the next section for more detailed instructions for severe diarrhea.)

What to Do for Severe Diarrhea

Following are feeding directions and tips to help you keep your child well-hydrated when he or she has severe diarrhea.

- Encourage fluid intake to prevent dehydration. (See the chart above for a guide to feeding according to your child's age and feeding stage.)

- If you suspect a reaction to food, keep a food diary—for yourself if you're exclusively breastfeeding and for you and your baby if you're breastfeeding along with solid foods—to track possible causes. You can also try removing highly allergic foods one at a time from your diets to see if eliminating a particular food helps.

- Also note whether your baby has just begun drinking formula or has recently switched formulas. Formula-fed babies may benefit from a temporary change to a lactose-free formula. Talk to your baby's doctor before switching.

- If your child's diarrhea is very severe and/or your child won't nurse, your child's doctor may ask you to feed your child only an oral rehydration solution for twenty-four hours. Pump your breasts to keep up your milk supply if necessary. Once your child is improving, resume breastfeeding or formula-feeding (along with oral rehydration solutions if recommended). Formula is sometimes given in half-strength at first. For babies eating solids, good foods to try first after a bad bout of diarrhea are applesauce, pears, bananas, rice, potatoes, toast, and cereal.

- Don't try to make a rehydration solution at home unless your baby's doctor instructs you and you have the proper instruments.

Oral Rehydration Solutions

If you've ever seen ads for Gatorade, you're probably familiar with the idea of replenishing the water, sodium, and potassium lost during extreme exercise or during a case of vomiting or diarrhea. But Gatorade is best left to the grownups in your family. When babies and children need rehydration solutions, they should have ones formulated just for them. Some widely available brands are Pedialyte, LiquiLytes, Rehydralyte, and Infalyte. These products are absorbed easily by and contain the right amount of sodium and potassium for babies and children.

- Don't feed your child salty broth or soup or boiled milk. Boiling milk concentrates it so that it's dangerously high in sodium and other minerals.
- Don't prevent your child from eating if he or she is hungry.
- If your child is younger than two years, don't give him or her an antidiarrheal medication. If your child is two years or older, consult your child's doctor before giving antidiarrheal meds.
- Be aware that antibiotics are effective against only specific bacteria or parasites. If your baby's doctor suspects a bacterial or parasitic infection, he or she will need to test a stool sample from your baby to prescribe the right antibiotic.

- About one in six children under the age of two years suffers from antibiotic-induced diarrhea. Children taking the drugs amoxicillin or clavulanate[3] are at even higher risk. (The drug clavulanate is combined with amoxicillin to make it more effective. Brand names of this drug combination include Augmentin and Timentin in the U.S. and Clavulin and Timentin in Canada.) If your child's diarrhea is antibiotic-induced, ask your child's doctor about probiotic therapy. Probiotics are "good" bacteria that reside in the digestive tract, where they improve intestinal function and promote good digestive health. Research has shown that probiotics prevent the growth of harmful organisms such as rotavirus.[4] Probiotic population in the digestive tract can be increased by eating foods containing probiotics. Breast milk naturally contains probiotics, as do fermented milk products like yogurt and kefir. Some foods, like acidophilus milk, are fortified with probiotics. Expect to see even more probiotic-fortified foods—possibly including infant formula—in the future. Several good clinical studies have shown that probiotics added to the diets of infants through formula could help reduce the risk of gastrointestinal infection,[5] colic, and irritability.[6] Stay tuned to see if larger studies confirm the benefits. So...how do you get probiotics into your sick kid? Here are a few tips:
  - If you're breastfeeding, eat foods that contain probiotics and/or take commercially prepared probiotic supplements. You'll find a wide variety of both at natural foods stores.

- If you're formula-feeding, ask your child's doctor about switching temporarily to a soy formula with added fiber, which has been shown to significantly reduce the duration of antibiotic-induced diarrhea in babies six months and older.[7] As of this book's publication, Isomil DF is the only such formula available. (It's also lactose-free and contains no cow's milk protein.)

- If your child is eight months or older and has already tried yogurt, offer yogurt. Make a fruit-and-yogurt smoothie if your child is more likely to drink yogurt than eat it. (See pages 303–304 for recipes.) Stonyfield Farms yogurt contains six different probiotics—the most of any yogurt on the market—and it's also organic.

- Ask your child's doctor if you should give your child a probiotic supplement.

- Call your baby's doctor if your baby shows signs of dehydration (see the next section) or has any of these symptoms:[8]
  - Fever lasting more than twenty-four hours
  - Change in behavior
  - Bloody poop
  - Severe abdominal pain
  - Swollen abdomen
  - Rash
  - Yellow skin (jaundice)
  - Vomit that's green, bloody, or looks like coffee grounds

Dehydration Alert

When your child is having more frequent, more watery poops, he or she may get dehydrated. Compounding the risk of dehydration are other symptoms like fever or vomiting. Dehydration can be very dangerous—even deadly—if it's not treated. That's why it's important to know the signs of dehydration. Check out the following list and call your baby's doctor immediately if you see any of these signs:[9]

- Decrease in urination
- No tears or fewer tears when your child cries
- High fever
- Dry mouth
- Weight loss
- Extreme thirst
- Listlessness (Your child is not active and seems to have no energy for movement.)
- Sunken eyes
- Cool, discolored hands and feet
- Wrinkled skin

If you think your child is moderately or severely dehydrated, take him or her to the emergency room right away.

Prevention

There are several things you can do to prevent diarrhea in children:

- Breastfeed as long as possible. Breast milk populates your baby's intestines with "good" bacteria that fight off disease-causing bacteria.

- Practice good personal hygiene, teach it to your child, and promote it with everyone who cares for your child. Most forms of infectious diarrhea are contracted by hand-to-mouth transmission of fecal matter.

- Never give your child raw or unpasteurized milk and avoid foods that could be contaminated with bacteria. (See page 195 for more food safety information.)

- Avoid unnecessary antibiotics.

- If your child drinks juice, limit him or her to four to six ounces per day.

Common Questions

Q: My two-week-old baby seems to poop all the time. Is this normal?

A: Yes. The gastrocolic reflex causes a poop after almost every feeding in breastfed infants. (Formula-fed infants have somewhat fewer poops.) As your baby gets older, this reflex will diminish. Your baby will begin to poop much less often between two and three months.

Q: Should I stop nursing if my baby has diarrhea?

A: Absolutely not! In fact, you'll probably want to nurse more often to prevent dehydration. Breast milk is the perfect food for a baby with diarrhea—and most other illnesses—because it's very digestible and it contains antibodies to fight illness. Breastfeeding is also comforting. You may need to change your nursing technique if you suspect lactose intolerance. (See page 133.) In rare cases your child's doctor may ask you to temporarily stop breastfeeding, but never do it on your own!

Q: When I started giving my breastfed baby formula, I noticed a big change in his poop. Is this normal? Should I switch formulas?

A: Yes, this is normal, and no, you probably shouldn't change formulas. Formula is a big change for your baby's system; because it's harder to digest than breast milk, it produces firmer poops. Unfortunately, the poops are also stinkier! Although switching formulas for this reason is very common, it's often unnecessary. Talk with your baby's doctor before switching formulas.

Q: My mother told me I should use low-iron formula or else my baby will get constipated. Is this true?

A: No. There are very few reasons why you should give your baby low-iron formula. The truth is: Babies need iron, and without it they could suffer from anemia, causing much greater problems than firm poops! Though iron in formula doesn't cause constipation, another ingredient might. Palm oil (or palmitic oil), a source of fat in some formulas, binds with calcium in the digestive tract. This results in firmer stools and less absorption of calcium and fat. You can avoid this problem simply by reading labels and avoiding formulas that contain palm oil.[10]

Q: Should I switch my baby to a different formula if he has diarrhea?

A: Not necessarily. You should always ask your baby's doctor before switching formulas. Sometimes diarrhea has nothing to do with formula. If, however, your baby's doctor determines that your baby has a milk allergy or temporary lactose intolerance (perhaps from illness or medication), you may be advised to switch to a lactose-free or soy formula temporarily.

Gas: What a Pain!

One thing parents often fret about is their babies' gas. Gas is common in young babies because of their immature digestive tracts. If gas doesn't seem to bother your baby, don't worry about it. However, if it does cause your baby pain, try to figure out the cause and treat it as best you can.

Following is a list of common causes of gas in babies, as well as simple remedies.

- **Swallowing air**: Babies may swallow too much air as a result of:
  - *Crying*: Be attuned to your baby's hunger and other needs to prevent meltdowns.
  - *Bottle-feeding*: Experiment with different bottles and nipples to find the one that gives your baby the least gas.
  - *Forceful letdown*: Rapid milk flow forces your baby to take large gulps of milk combined with air.

- **Inadequate burping**: See page 42 for info on burping while breastfeeding. See page 91 for info on burping while formula-feeding.

- **Positioning**: If your baby spends too much time horizontal during or after a feeding, he or she may have trouble getting rid of gas. Hold your baby at a forty-five-degree angle during a feeding and for thirty minutes afterward.

- **Sensitivity to mom's diet**: Your breastfed baby may have an intolerance to food, vitamins, or herbs you consume. If your baby's allergic to something in your diet, gas will be combined with additional symptoms. (See page 135 for more allergy info.) Changes in your diet may help—or they may not. (See the sidebar for my story.)

> **Tales from the Trenches: Trial and Error**
>
> My son Nicolas had terrible gas pains when he was a baby. They were so bad that he would sometimes stop nursing due to the pain. Every once in while he'd also have a large spit-up. After looking at possible causes with his pediatrician (and not coming up with anything), I put myself on a lactose-free diet. I also gave up all other foods that could be considered remotely gassy or spicy. I followed this bland diet for over a month to no avail. We finally chalked up Nicolas's gas to an immature digestive system and began giving him Mylicon drops. Thank goodness—it helped a lot.

- **Formula-feeding**: Formula-fed babies tend to have more gas than breastfed babies. Ask your baby's doctor if switching formulas might help.
- **Reaction to baby's diet**: If your baby's eating solids, drinking juice, or taking medications or vitamins, any of these could be the culprit. Be aware that babies have a hard time digesting some of the carbohydrates in juice. Don't offer juice until six months of age (if at all) and then in very limited amounts (no more than four to six ounces per day).

If you can't pinpoint a cause for your baby's gas or the preceding suggestions aren't working, here are a couple more gas-relief options:

- **Work it out**: Try gently massaging your baby's tummy and back, or bicycling your baby's legs.
- **Give simethicone drops**: This over-the-counter medication is safe for babies and is often recommended by doctors because it is not absorbed in baby's system but does break down gas bubbles. (Some widely available brands are Mylicon and Little Tummys.) Be aware that while clinical studies show simethicone reduces the amount of gas passed, it hasn't been shown to reduce crying time more than a placebo. Nonetheless, some parents have success with it.

Herbal treatments and teas aren't recommended for children because most have no clinical studies showing safety or effectiveness. Furthermore, they can be very dangerous to babies. Some herbs, such as star anise and peppermint oil, can be toxic. Finally, they add more substances to a baby's diet, which can aggravate digestive problems.

Spitting Up

Normal Spit-Up

Our next topic of discussion in the outbound department comes from the other end. Spitting up is another normal baby activity—that's why everyone who burps a baby sports a shoulder cloth!

Spitting up (also called gastroesophogeal reflux or GER) is what happens when your baby's stomach contents back up the esophagus (the tube that connects the mouth with the stomach) and out the mouth. Often your baby isn't even aware of spitting up; it just dribbles out. Spitting up usually peaks at about four months and goes away around one year.

Nearly all babies (both breastfed and formula-fed) have some GER, so spitting up is no cause for alarm. As long as your baby is gaining weight and isn't in pain, all is well. Your biggest problem is a little extra laundry. Here's what you can expect from a "happy spitter":

- Small amount of spit-up within an hour of feeding, as often as after each feeding
- An occasional big spit-up

Here are some tips to slow down spitting up:[11]

- Be sure to elicit a good burp during and after each feeding. Burp more often when your baby seems to be swallowing more air.

- If your baby spits up, don't try to feed your baby again until you see signs of hunger.

- Avoid exposing your baby to tobacco smoke.

- Avoid jostling your baby right after feedings.

- Avoid dressing your baby in tight diapers or waistbands.

- If you think breast milk oversupply or forceful letdown is contributing to spit-up, try the following:

  - Nurse your baby on just one breast for a two-hour period whenever your baby is hungry, then switch to the other breast for the next two hours, and so on. This may help your baby get a larger proportion of hindmilk.

  - Detach your baby from the breast when you feel letdown, and let your milk spray into a clean cloth. This will prevent the need for your baby to gulp to manage the milk flow and may reduce the amount of air your baby swallows.

- Avoid drinking excessive caffeine. Limit your intake to three to five hundred milligrams of caffeine per day—less if you think your baby is sensitive to it. (See page 23 for more on caffeine.)

- If you're bottle-feeding, don't coax your baby to finish the bottle if you're seeing signs of fullness. (See page 92.)

Gastroesophogeal Reflux Disease

If your baby's spitting up gets worse and more frequent over time, your baby may have gastroesophageal reflux disease (GERD). GERD is reflux with additional symptoms like poor weight gain, difficulty swallowing, pain, irritation of the esophagus, and respiratory disorders such as pneumonia. Here are some treatments that may help.

Tales from the Trenches: Peggy and Emma

Emma had trouble sleeping from birth. She slept very little at night and was fussy after being laid down. Doctors diagnosed her problem as colic. At first Peggy thought Emma wasn't getting enough hindmilk, so she began pumping after nursing and giving Emma the expressed milk also. It didn't help. Then Peggy thought it might be her diet, so she started a very bland, allergen-free diet. This didn't help either. Peggy, a registered nurse, suspected Emma might have reflux and elevated the head of Emma's bed. Still no luck. There was no rest for this weary family until Emma was about six weeks old. As Emma slept, Peggy noticed that she was choking and turning blue. An immediate trip to the doctor confirmed GERD, but Emma had the "silent" variety. She had painful acid reflux without ever spitting up, explaining why she was always fussy when she was laid down to sleep. Once she started taking medication, Emma slept much better. The moral of this story: Sometimes the problem isn't what you expect. If you're not convinced you've found the right answer, keep looking.

- **Positioning**:
  - Keep your baby upright for at least thirty minutes after meals and elevate the head of your baby's crib and changing table thirty degrees. Young infants who don't have good body control should be supported so they don't slump over.
  - Lying belly-down seems to help reflux the most. However, you should put your baby on his or her tummy only while awake and constantly monitored, since sleeping in this position increases the risk of sudden infant death syndrome (SIDS).[12]
  - Lay your baby on his or her left side.
  - Remember that lying on the back is the worst position for reflux. During diaper changing, roll your baby to the side instead of lifting up his or her legs. (Back sleeping is recommended for preventing SIDS; discuss any different sleeping positions with your baby's doctor.)
- **Tips for breastfed babies**:
  - Continue breastfeeding—breastfed infants usually spit up less than formula-fed babies.
  - If your baby is older when reflux begins, investigate whether the cause might be a new food in your baby's diet, a new food in your diet, or a food you've recently eaten in large quantities.
  - If you have forceful letdown or an abundant milk supply (common after a baby has gone through a growth spurt), this could cause your baby to gulp faster and swallow more air, which in turn causes spitting up. See page 48 for tips on managing this issue.
  - Don't thicken your milk with rice cereal (or anything else). Doctors sometimes recommend that formula-fed infants with GERD drink formula thickened with rice cereal, but breast milk won't thicken with rice cereal. Also, adding a thickener to breast milk introduces possible allergens and can decrease overall breast milk intake.
- **Tips for formula-fed babies**: Smaller amounts of formula given more often may be easier to digest. Ask your baby's doctor about switching formulas. He or she may recommend:
  - A rice starch-thickened formula (like Enfamil AR), which has been shown to decrease spit-up.

Why Do I Hear So Much about Babies with Reflux?

It's a chicken-and-egg case. No one knows which came first: more babies with reflux or more awareness of reflux. One thing's for sure: Reflux in babies is definitely on the radar of doctors and parents. In most cases (garden-variety GERD), babies outgrow it. For severe cases, doctors often recommend medication or, as a last resort, surgery to tighten the opening between the esophagus and the stomach. For more information about reflux in infants, see:
- http://www.kellymom.com/baby concerns/reflux.html#refluxsymptoms
- http://www.cdhnf.org/consumers.html
- http://www.infantrefluxdisease.com

- A soy formula (like Isomil DF), which has also been shown to decrease spit up.[13]
- A hypoallergenic formula if a milk allergy is the suspected cause of GERD.
- **Medication**: Your baby's doctor may prescribe a medication for reflux. Don't give your baby any medication, herbal preparations, or teas unless your baby's doctor advises you to do so.

Vomiting

Vomiting is forceful regurgitation that shoots out of a baby's mouth as opposed to dribbling out. Vomiting may be caused by viral or bacterial infections or by hypertrophic pyloric stenosis, an obstruction of the valve between the stomach and the small intestine. Vomiting always warrants a call to your baby's doctor so you can discuss accompanying symptoms and get advice on how to proceed. When your baby is vomiting, it's important to watch for signs of dehydration (pages 42 or 127) and get help if you see them. Following is a list of other vomiting and spit-up symptoms that should raise a red flag.[14]

- Vomiting with:
    - Blood
    - Green or yellow fluid
    - Poor weight gain
- Inconsolable or severe crying and irritability
- Persistent food refusal
- Difficulty eating
- Poor growth or failure to thrive
- Breathing problems:
    - Difficulty breathing
    - Repeated bouts of pneumonia
    - Apnea (temporary breathing stoppage)
    - Turning blue
    - Chronic cough
    - Wheezing

Lactose Intolerance

Lactose intolerance is malabsorption of lactose (milk sugar) due to a lack of the enzyme lactase. Common symptoms of lactose intolerance are bloating, gas, abdominal discomfort, and diarrhea.

Most adults are at least partially lactose intolerant. Research shows that certain populations are more prone to lactose intolerance than others. Groups who generally can digest lactose are northern Europeans, the Fulani and Tussi tribes of Africa, the Punjabi of India, Finns and Hungarians, and probably Mongols. The remainder of the world's people are lactose non-digesters. Since the world is now a melting pot, blending the genetics of different populations, our world population has varying degrees of lactose intolerance.[15]

There are a few different types of lactose intolerance. This section will describe them and provide tips for managing lactose intolerance.

Congenital Lactose Intolerance

Congenital lactose intolerance, also called primary lactase deficiency, is very rare. If your baby has this type of lactose intolerance, you'll know it immediately as soon as your baby drinks breast milk or cow's milk formula, which both contain lactose as their primary carbohydrate. Symptoms of congenital lactose intolerance are serious and can include vomiting, failure to thrive, and dehydration.

Primary Lactose Intolerance

Primary lactose intolerance is also sometimes called adult lactose intolerance (even though it starts in childhood). It occurs as the body gradually makes decreased amounts of lactase. Lactase decline can begin between ages three to seven years—or sooner in some populations. Primary lactose intolerance is genetic; some populations tend to have earlier and more extreme cases than others. Approximately 90 percent of Asians, 80 percent of African Americans, and 53 percent of Hispanics have it. People with primary lactose intolerance can often tolerate small amounts of lactose, especially with a meal.[16]

Temporary Lactose Intolerance

Temporary lactose intolerance is also called transient lactose intolerance or secondary lactase deficiency. If your baby appears to be doing fine on breast milk or cow's milk formula and then suddenly gets diarrhea, gas, or bloating, it could be temporary lactose intolerance.

Temporary lactose intolerance happens when anything damages the tips of the folds of the small intestine, where lactase is made. It can be caused by:

- Gastrointestinal infection
- Food allergy
- Food intolerance
- Antibiotic treatment
- Celiac disease (a condition that causes an immune response to gluten—found in wheat, barley, rye, or triticale—which can damage the small intestine)

Breastfed babies can also develop temporary lactose intolerance when they're getting too much foremilk (which is higher in lactose) and not enough hindmilk (which is higher in fat). If your baby has symptoms of lactose intolerance plus green frothy stools, but doesn't have any of the intestinal conditions described in the preceding bullets, your baby might just be getting more lactose than he or she can handle. This can happen if you're switching breasts before your baby self-detaches. This results in baby drinking milk that's lower in fat, and thus drinking more of it to get the calories he needs. A larger quantity of milk gives your baby a bigger load of lactose.

Managing Lactose Intolerance

To resolve foremilk/hindmilk imbalance, always let your baby self-detach before switching breasts.

If you're formula-feeding and your baby has any type of lactose intolerance, your baby's doctor may advise you to switch to a lactose-free cow's milk formula or a soy formula. If your baby is older than six months and has diarrhea, your baby's doctor may recommend a soy formula with added dietary fiber. (See page 127 for more information.)

If cow's milk and other dairy products are the norm for your family, there are ways for your child to enjoy dairy after weaning from breast milk or formula. Try small amounts of these foods first to see if your child tolerates them:

- Lactose-intolerant people can usually tolerate a cup of whole milk at a sitting. The fat in whole milk slows down its movement through the intestine, which gives bacteria and the small amounts of lactase in the intestine a chance to break down the lactose. (The same goes for whole-milk ice cream.)
- Chocolate milk and small amounts of plain milk with a meal are often better tolerated than a cup of plain milk alone.
- Cow's milk with the lactose already broken down is available at most supermarkets. (Lactaid is one popular brand.) You can also buy Lactaid drops to put in ordinary milk to break down the lactose for your child.
- Your child may enjoy these low-lactose dairy foods:
  - Yogurt
  - Acidophilus milk
  - Aged cheese like cheddar or Swiss

If you're concerned about your lactose-intolerant child's calcium intake, offer other calcium-fortified foods, such as soy milk, orange or apple juice, or bread.

Allergies

Allergy rates have exploded in the past two decades; they're reported ten times more often today than they were twenty years ago. Thirty percent of pediatrician office visits are related to allergies and 30 percent of school absences are related to asthma. So allergies are a hot topic—but what exactly are they?

What Is an Allergy?

According to the American Academy of Allergy, Asthma, and Immunology (AAAI), an allergy is an overreaction of the immune system. This reaction can be caused by something eaten, touched, or breathed in the environment. Because the digestive system is one of the routes by which children commonly get sensitized to allergens, allergies are an important (if not obvious) topic for this chapter. (For information on feeding children with food allergies, see page 163.)

So...what is an allergen? An allergen is a protein that causes the immune system of a person allergic to it to launch an immune response (or allergic reaction). An allergic person's body sees the allergen as an invader and releases antibodies to attack it. A non-allergic person's body perceives no threat and launches no reaction. Foods, drugs, chemicals, pet dander, insect venoms, and pollens can all be allergens.

An immune reaction involving immunoglobulin E (IgE) antibodies is called atopy. Atopic diseases are diseases that coincide with this IgE reaction. They include asthma, eczema, hay fever, allergic conjunctivitis, and hives. These diseases can be interrelated because they may be caused by the same allergen.

Why Does the Immune System Overreact?

A number of factors can increase a child's risk of developing allergies:

- **Genetics**: Infants can be genetically predisposed to allergies. Research shows that if both parents of a baby have an allergy, the baby has a 40 percent chance of developing the allergy. If both the baby's parents have the same allergy, the baby's risk goes up to 70 percent.[17]

- **Age**: Children seem especially prone to allergic sensitization during infancy. Sensitization means the child first meets up with a particular protein before the body is ready to deal with it, and the immune system reacts to it by producing antibodies. This is why babies (especially those at risk for allergies) shouldn't be fed anything besides breast milk or formula until six months, when their immune systems are more mature.

- **Other risks**:
  - Formula-feeding
  - Exposure to tobacco smoke, both prenatally and during childhood
  - Caregivers' ignorance about allergies
  - Premature introduction of highly allergenic foods
  - Environmental exposures: A large study at the University of Southern California showed that asthma diagnosis before five years of age was related to these exposures in the first year of life (listed in decreasing order of risk):[18] herbicides, pesticides, farm crops or farm animals, cockroaches, and wood or oil smoke, soot, or exhaust.

Allergy or Intolerance?

Food intolerance is often mistakenly labeled as allergy. One very common food intolerance is lactose intolerance, the inability to break down lactose due to lack of the digestive enzyme lactase. Like many food intolerances, it usually causes somewhat delayed symptoms like gas, bloating, and diarrhea that are mild at first.

A food allergy, unlike an intolerance, involves the immune system. The immune system thinks a new food is harmful to the body and makes antibodies against the food (sensitization). The next time the food is eaten, the antibodies recognize the food as an enemy and launch an immune response that can involve the respiratory system, skin, digestive system, and cardiovascular system. Food allergy symptoms typically occur within an hour of eating the offending food.[19]

See the chart below for a quick comparison of food allergy and food intolerance symptoms.

Food Allergy verses Food Intolerance

Anaphylaxis or Severe Allergic Reaction	Food Allergy	Food Intolerance
These symptoms require immediate medical attention. Warmth, itching, flushing of skin Severe sneezing Lightheadedness/loss of consciousness Shortness of breath/ difficulty breathing Vomitting/diarrhea	Hives Rash around mouth Eczema Asthma symptoms Swelling of eyes, lips, face Tingling of mouth or throat Sneezing, congestion, runny nose Nausea Vomiting Abdominal pain Diarrhea Gas or swelling of stomach Difficulty sleeping due to other symptoms	Diarrhea Bloating Gas Headache or migraine Abdominal discomfort Green, frothy poop (in breastfed babies)

Common Food Allergies

These eight foods are responsible for 90 percent of food allergies:

1. Milk
2. Eggs
3. Peanuts
4. Soy
5. Wheat
6. Tree nuts
7. Fish
8. Shellfish

The first allergy usually seen in babies is a milk allergy; it affects 2 to 7 percent of infants. If your baby is formula-fed, you'll find out if he or she has a milk allergy very quickly because cow's milk formula delivers a big, direct source of milk protein.

If you're breastfeeding, your baby may react to cow's milk or other allergenic foods in your diet because their protein molecules can pass through your milk to your baby's immature gut. (This is a fairly rare occurrence.) You don't need to stop breastfeeding—this would only raise your baby's risk of allergies—you simply need to remove the offending food from your diet.

How do you know if your child truly has an allergy? One common way to check for allergies is a skin prick test. Another is a blood test. The blood test is usually done on children because it's less traumatic, but it's also less sensitive and less specific. An allergist typically diagnoses allergies on the basis of one of these tests plus symptoms reported by a parent.[20]

Minimizing Allergies

If your child is at high risk for allergies, here are several ways you can delay, minimize, or prevent allergy development. To find out the most up-to-date advice in your area, go to http://www.worldallergy.org and click on global allergy links. And, ask an allergist about the current recommendations on allergy prevention.

- **Avoid peanuts while you're pregnant**: Research doesn't show that avoiding multiple allergens during pregnancy reduces the risk of allergic disease in your child, and it can be difficult to avoid all the common allergens and still get the nutrients you need for pregnancy.[21] However, research does show a correlation between eating a lot of peanuts during pregnancy and a younger age of peanut allergy onset in high-risk infants.

- **Breastfeed your baby**: All experts agree that breastfeeding is very important for those at high risk for allergies. Exclusive breastfeeding provides direct protection against allergies by limiting early exposure to antigens and provides indirect protection by limiting absorption of allergens in the digestive tract.[22] Research shows that it can reduce or postpone asthma and allergies. Also, taking probiotics while breastfeeding can reduce the risk of atopic disease in infants.[23] (See page 126 for more on probiotics.)

- **Avoid allergenic foods while you're breastfeeding**: Stay away from cow's milk, eggs, fish, peanuts, and tree nuts until your baby weans. This has been shown to reduce the risk of eczema, asthma, and respiratory allergic symptoms.[24] Test eating beef and chicken cautiously, because they have been known to cross-react with milk and eggs.[25] (You can try this strategy, but be aware that as of this book's printing, it's not currently recommended by the American Academy of Allergy, Asthma and Immunology [AAAAI][26] or the Australian Society of Clinical Immunology [ASCI].[27])

- **Examine the fats in your diet**: Preliminary data show that increasing omega-3 fats in the maternal diet may offer breastfed babies some protection from allergies.[28]

- **If breastfeeding isn't possible, use a hypoallergenic formula**: The AAAAI and ASCI recommend that if you need to introduce formula to your allergy-prone infant before six months, you should use an hypoallergenic (extensively hydrolyzed) formula like Alimentum or Nutramigen. Although expensive, research shows they can help prevent allergies. In one study, using hypoallergenic formula prevented the development of allergy during the first eighteen months of life in high-risk infants.[29]

- **Avoid peanuts, period**: Even if you aren't breastfeeding, peanut protein on your clothes and skin could sensitize your baby to peanuts.

- **Follow these suggestions from the AAP**:[30]
  - Don't introduce solid foods until your baby is six months old.
  - Delay introducing dairy products until one year.
  - Delay introducing eggs until two years.
  - Delay introducing peanuts, nuts, and fish until three years.

If your child is *not* at high risk for allergies, follow the timetable described in Chapter 8.

Colic

Your new baby, who was so pleasant just one week ago, is suddenly showing a "dark" side. Crying for hours every afternoon or evening, your baby is driving your family to the edge.

Sound familiar? You're the proud parents of a colicky baby. You're not alone; up to 28 percent of infants have colic in the first few months of life.

What Is Colic?

Colic sounds like a clinical term for a specific disorder, but actually it's just a catchall name for a poorly understood—though common—problem. Doctors define colic as three hours of inconsolable crying per day. Unfortunately, the cause of colic is unknown. Over the years, many people have pointed fingers at allergies and gas. These could be the causes of a few cases, but most cases are unexplained.

One factor associated with colic is stress during pregnancy. General stress and physical discomfort during pregnancy and/or negative experiences during childbirth seem to increase the risk of colic. Most experts think colic is mainly a symptom of adjustment to life outside the uterus. Some babies have a tough time getting used to their new environment and are very sensitive, so they cry. It's the only way they have to express their frustration. Then a cycle begins. Baby cries, swallows air, and then cries some more because of the discomfort. Parents get tense, baby feels the tension, and the crying continues to escalate. Pretty soon everyone's crying.

> **Tales from the Trenches: Grandpa Lee's Advice**
>
> Lee, a five-time grandpa from Hartsville, Ohio, recommends laying your baby skin-to-skin on your chest. He thinks the warmth of your skin passed on to your baby's skin helps. Clinical researchers agree with Lee: Skin-to-skin contact, also called kangaroo care, does help babies deal with pain. Kangaroo care during heel sticks has been shown to reduce signs of pain like crying time and accelerated heart rate by 82 percent.[31]

What Can You Do?

First, make sure your baby's crying isn't a symptom of illness. Check for signs of illness, such as decreased appetite, not wanting to be held, diarrhea or other abnormal poop, vomiting, or fever.

Next, try these feeding changes to see if they help:

- Try feeding your baby smaller quantities more often.
- Be sure to burp your baby during and after a feeding.
- Keep your baby upright for a while after feeding.
- Feed your baby in a quiet, dim room to help you both relax.
- If you're nursing, change your diet. Following are some changes that might be worth a try.
    - Eliminate dairy and nuts from your diet. You can also try removing eggs, wheat, soy, and fish from your diet. While this is a drastic step, a small study showed that 74 percent of colicky babies whose moms followed this allergen-free diet showed fewer hours of crying time.[32] Be warned that this diet may be challenging to stick with. Also, know that you'll need to take a calcium supplement and make sure you eat other high-quality proteins.
    - Eliminate or reduce your caffeine intake.
    - Make sure your baby has a good latch to prevent air swallowing.
    - Record everything you eat, including quantities and times. Keep a separate record of your baby's colicky times. After a week or two, compare the records and see if any connections emerge. Remember that food intolerance symptoms can appear from one to three days after you've eaten the offending food. See lactose overload, below.
    - Add probiotics (especially lactobacillus acidophilus) to your diet via yogurt or a supplement. "Good" bacteria has been shown to improve colic.[33]
- Another possible breastfeeding-related cause of colic is lactose overload resulting from foremilk/hindmilk imbalance. See page 135 for more information on this problem and tips for solving it.
- If you're formula-feeding and you think your baby's colic might be aggravated by cow's milk, ask your doctor about switching to a soy formula, a lactose-free formula, or a hypoallergenic formula.
- Don't introduce your baby to juice until at least six months (if ever). Colicky babies are more likely to have trouble absorbing the natural sugar in juice. They tend to experience gas, fussiness, and sleep disturbance after drinking juices such as apple juice and pear juice.[34] Babies don't really need juice anyway— especially in large amounts. It's a calorie-dense, low-nutrient food that's bad for teeth. Eating whole fruit is a much better way to get the hundreds of antioxdants and nutrients in fruit.[35]

After making any necessary feeding changes, try the following colic-soothing tips.

- Rock your baby.
- Dance with your baby.

- Wear your baby in a sling or front carrier.
- Place your baby in a baby swing or infant seat that rocks.
- Find a noise that soothes your baby, such as soft music, a fan, or a vacuum cleaner.
- Take your baby for a car ride.
- Put your baby in a baby seat on top of the washer or dryer while it's running, making sure that your baby's seat won't shimmy off and fall on the floor.
- Place your baby in a bouncy seat that vibrates.
- Lay a warm water bottle on your baby's tummy.
- Rub your baby's tummy in a circular motion.
- Take a warm bath with your baby to relax you both.

Coping with Colic

As you cope with colic, keep these important points in mind: You haven't done anything wrong to cause your baby's colic. Neither has your baby. Your baby needs extra attention and cuddling—don't worry that you will spoil him, because it simply isn't possible to spoil a baby.

> **Tales from the Trenches: Michael, Theresa, and Baby Addie**
>
> Colic ran in Theresa's family—she and her dad both had it—so she wasn't surprised when her daughter Addie became colicky at two weeks. She said, "I truly believed I had a child who'd never smile. She had only three modes: eating, sleeping, or screaming."
>
> When asked what worked, Theresa replied, "Nothing worked all the time. The two things that worked best were buckling her in her car seat then gently swinging the seat back and forth, and walking outside with her. We'd take turns eating dinner and walking Addie. She'd finally fall asleep on Mike's shoulder around 8:30.
>
> Theresa's advice to other parents: "There is a light at the end of the tunnel. Your baby's colic will go away eventually."
>
> In the meantime, get support from family and friends so you can take time away from your baby. Talk with other moms, too; you're sure to find someone who survived a colicky baby, and that will help.

As important as it is to try to console your baby, it's also important to take a break when you feel frustrated. The emotions triggered by colic can bring parents to tears and worse. Shaken baby syndrome often results from tension and frustration generated by a baby's crying or irritability.[36] *Never shake your baby*—shaking can cause severe brain injury, blindness, or even death. Here are some ways to care for yourself:

- Take turns with your partner so you both can get a break from the constant crying.
- Don't forget to eat well. Lack of sleep combined with a poor diet generally leads to sickness. Try some of the one-handed snacks listed on page 66.
- Accept help from anyone who offers. If no one offers, *ask*.
- If you feel your emotions spinning out of control, leave your baby in a safe place (even if he or she is crying) so you can go to a quiet room for a brief rest.

Finally, remember that colic won't last forever. It usually goes away by the time a baby is three months old.

Chapter 7

Nutrition 101 for Babies and Toddlers

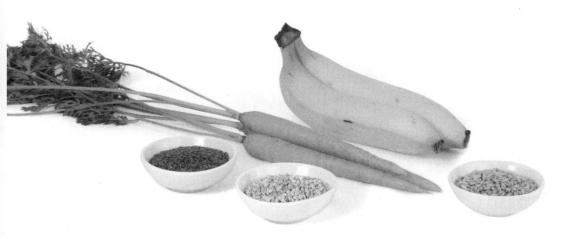

*Children are survivors. If your intentions are good,
it's hard to screw them up too badly.*

—Lise, mom of Benjamin

Joanna never gave a thought to what she ate—until she got pregnant and then had a daughter of her own to feed. She realized that her eating habits would become her daughter's, and she knew that probably wasn't great news for her baby. So she began researching what kind of nutrition her baby did need. She found out babies have far different needs than adults and that early eating habits tend to stick—for better or worse.

This chapter will tell you everything you need to know about your young child's nutrient needs by answering these questions:

- Is your child growing properly?
- What nutrients does your baby need and why?
- How much food do babies and toddlers really need?
- What about special diets and supplements? How do you feed a child with food allergies?
- Does food affect children's behavior?
- What can you do to protect your child's teeth?

Is Your Child Growing Properly?

Luckily there's an easy way to find out! Babies and toddlers have frequent checkups with their doctors. At these visits, your baby's height, weight, and head circumference are checked and charted. For children over two years, doctors may also calculate body mass index (BMI), a calculation that considers height and weight and is plotted by age. BMI is a good indicator of underweight, overweight, and risk for overweight.

It's normal for kids to change percentiles on growth charts until about eighteen months; after that they usually settle into their own unique growth curves. If your baby shows a dramatic change in growth, such as dropping from the fiftieth to the fifth percentile, this may signal a feeding, developmental, or other health problem, and your child's doctor will want to look into it.

Growth Charts

Types of Growth Chart

Following I've listed the different growth charts U.S. doctors use for children of different ages. These charts are provided by the Centers for Disease Control and Prevention (CDC).

- Infants, birth to thirty-six months:
  - Weight for age
  - Length for age
  - Weight for length
  - Head circumference for age

- Preschoolers, two to five years
  - Weight for stature
- Children and adolescents, two to twenty years:
  - Weight for age
  - Stature for age
  - Body mass index for age

You can download all of these charts by visiting http://www.cdc.gov/nchs/about/major/nhanes/growthcharts/clinical_charts.htm.

What the Growth Charts Mean

Health professionals use growth charts to identify changes in growth pattern, which helps them screen for feeding, developmental, or health problems. The charts have curved lines with percentile rankings that show how your child's size compares to other kids of the same age and gender. For example, if your child's height falls at the sixtieth percentile, it means that 40 percent of children the same age and gender are taller and 60 percent are shorter.

Your child's doctor considers parental stature and gestational age at birth when evaluating growth measurements. Although one measurement can be used as a screening tool, multiple measurements are needed to evaluate a growth pattern.

- **Weight for age** reflects body weight compared with other children your child's age. This measurement is used to detect changes in health or nutritional status, not to classify children as underweight or overweight.

- **Length for age or stature for age** describes linear growth in relation to age. Babies and toddlers under two years old are measured lying down for length. Children over two years old are measured standing up for stature. This growth measurement indicates relative shortness or tallness. Your baby's family history plays into this measurement.

- **Weight for length or weight for stature** looks at weight in relation to height.

- **Head circumference for age** reflects brain size. It provides critical information during infancy.

- **Body mass index (BMI) for age** estimates body fat and is calculated using height and weight for children over two years. When plotted on the graph, your child's BMI falls into one of four areas: underweight, healthy weight, at risk for overweight, or overweight. (See chapter 17 for more information.)

Be aware that some populations can't be accurately charted on the CDC growth charts because they aren't fully represented in the data used to create these charts:

- **Exclusively breastfed infants**: The CDC charts use data from breastfed and formula-fed infants to plot the growth curves. However, it's important to note that the growth pattern of exclusively breastfed infants is different from that of formula-fed infants. Breastfed babies generally grow the same or faster than formula-fed babies the first three months and slower than formula-fed babies the next nine months. Between six and eight months, growth in breastfed infants may slow down to the point that they may drop in growth percentiles on the CDC growth charts.[1] This may lead doctors to a faulty conclusion that a baby is not growing adequately. A doctor may then advise a formula supplement. This is *not necessary* if your baby is achieving what is considered normal, healthy growth for a breastfed baby! That's why it's best to use a growth chart that is specifically for *breastfed infants*. The CDC currently has no growth charts for exclusively breastfed infants, but the World Health Organization (WHO) does. Visit http://www.who.int/childgrowth/standards/en to learn about and download the charts.

- **Premature infants**: Premature infants can be plotted on the CDC charts, but the gestation-adjusted or "corrected" age must be used. For example, if your baby is now three months old but was born four weeks premature, he or she would be plotted at an age of two months on the growth chart. Your doctor might also use an alternative chart. (You can find growth charts for premature infants at www.kidsgrowth.com.) Corrected age is used for premature infants until two or three years, or sooner if the child catches up with normal height and weight for his or her age.

- **Very low birth weight (VLBW) infants**: The CDC charts do not use data from VLBW babies. So when a VLBW baby's growth is plotted on these charts, the baby's gestation-adjusted age should be used, and the growth pattern should be evaluated with caution.

Keeping Growth Charts in Perspective

Babies come in all shapes and sizes. Your baby's place on the growth charts isn't particularly important; what matters is a consistent and smooth growth pattern.

My kids, who both weighed seven pounds at birth, started on the fiftieth percentile for weight. But within a few months, they both dropped to the fifth percentile. My husband and I didn't worry; the doctor explained that they were just finding their normal growth curve. Because we're both petite, it was expected for our kids to hover between the fifth and tenth percentiles.

Remember: It's important to compare your baby to *your baby*, not to others, and to respect your baby's natural growth curve. Trying to change it is flirting with disaster and can lead only to misery for the whole family!

Health professionals may show concern if your baby is at either extreme on the growth charts. Several things would warrant a closer look at health, diet, and genetics: a drastic upward or downward change in growth pattern, short stature for age, relatively high or low weight for length, or a BMI above the eighty-fifth percentile.

Normal Growth

Height, Weight, and Head Circumference

Now you know how your baby's growth is charted, but what kind of growth should you expect? In a word: lots. During the first year, your baby will grow at a phenomenal rate. Expect your child to grow about ten inches (twenty-five centimeters) in length and to triple his or her birth weight! Read on for a more detailed breakdown of normal growth during the first two years.

Your baby is born with excess body fluid and will lose it during the first few days after birth. This loss may be up to 10 percent of your baby's body weight. However, if breastfeeding is going well, weight loss should not be more than 7 percent. So if your baby weighs 7 pounds (3.17 kilograms) at birth, expect a loss of 8 to 11 ounces (225 to 310 grams) during the first five days. Your baby should gain back the loss over the following five days. By day ten, your baby should be back at his or her birth weight.

From week one to week four, your baby will gain about 0.7 ounce (20 grams) per day! Your baby will grow taller before your very eyes, too—at a rate of 1 to 1.5 inches (2.5 to 3.7 centimeters) during this first month. Your baby's brain is also growing tremendously. The skull grows faster during the first four months of life than at any other time. At the end of the first month, your baby's head circumference will increase by about 1 inch (2.5 centimeters).[2]

From month two to month three, your baby will continue growing with the same phenomenal speed. Expect your baby to gain 1.5 to 2 pounds (0.7 to 0.9 kilograms) and grow 1 to 1.5 inches (2.5 to 3.7 centimeters) in height each month.[3] At about two months your baby will look decidedly round. That's normal. (I distinctly remember my kids at this age, looking like tadpoles with their round bellies!) You may also notice that your baby's head looks big for his or her body. That's a good sign; your baby's brain and head are growing so rapidly—about 0.5 inch (1.25 centimeters) per month—that the rest of the body hasn't caught up yet.

From month three to month six, your baby will, on average, gain 1 to 1.25 pounds (0.45 to 0.56 kilograms) per month and grow an average of 0.75 inch (1.9 centimeters) per month. Most babies will double their birth weight by the end of the sixth month.

From month six to month twelve, your baby's weight gain will slow down to about 1 pound (0.45 kilograms) a month, and your baby's height will increase an average of 0.75 inch (1.9 centimeters) per month. For the next six months, as your baby gets more mobile, he or she will thin out a bit. By the end of the first year, your baby will have tripled his or her birth weight and increased in length by 50 percent!

Don't be worried if you notice that at the end of the first year, your child's growth slows down even more. Your child will gain only 3 to 5 pounds (1.4 to 2.3 kilograms) and grow only about 5 inches (12.5 centimeters) during the entire second

Growth Spurts

Growth spurts tend to happen at about these times:[4]

- Seven to ten days
- Two to three weeks
- Four to six weeks
- Three months
- Six months
- Nine months

Take a lesson from Kitee on breastfeeding through a growth spurt…. Kitee was about to give up; when her baby, Ethan, wanted to nurse every hour, she was sure she wasn't making enough milk. Quite the contrary: Ethan was ensuring that she *would* make enough.

Breasts make whatever amount of milk is demanded of them. Ethan was nursing more often to tell Kitee's breasts to ramp up their milk production. It was exhausting for Kitee to nurse every hour, but in a few days her supply caught up with Ethan's demand.

Kitee experienced a typical "breastfeeding marathon." It typically lasts from a few days to a week. When you find yourself in this situation, let everything else go, nurse like crazy, and don't supplement with formula. Most importantly, don't worry—you can make all the milk your baby needs!

year! Your child's head growth will also slow down, increasing in circumference by only 1 inch (2.5 centimeters) during the second year. By the age of two, your child's head will reach 90 percent of its adult size. Your child will start looking less like a baby and more like a toddler as arms and legs lengthen, muscles build, and baby fat starts coming off. Your child's face will start to look less round and more angular.

During the preschool years, children grow an average of 2.5 inches (6.2 centimeters) per year and gain about 4 pounds (1.8 kilograms) per year. You'll continue to see changes in your child's body proportions as legs and trunk lengthen. As your child's body fat decreases and muscles grow stronger, your child will have a leaner, stronger look. Children start to show more variety in shape and size at this age; continue to honor your child's normal growth pattern without comparing it too closely to his playmates'. Your child will continue to grow at this slow and steady pace until puberty.

Other Kinds of Growth

In addition to the growth you can see—height, weight, head size, hair, skin, fingernails, and so on—there's also a fantastic amount of development you can't see happening inside your child's body during the first few years.

It's beyond the scope of this book to describe every detail of your baby's growth, but here's a quick list of the cool stuff happening to your baby's body:

- Your child's vision is getting sharper; focus, depth perception, and color discrimination are all improving.

- Your child's permanent teeth are developing beneath the baby teeth that keep popping up.

- Your child's immune system continues to develop throughout the first two years. That's why breastfeeding is so important!

- Your child's bones are lengthening and strengthening. Your child's height growth is a result of bone growth. The first two years, when you have the most control over your child's diet, is the perfect time for your child to bank as much calcium in his or her bones as possible.

- Your child's muscles are strengthening.

- Your child's coordination is improving.

Naturally Nutrient-Rich Foods

If you find yourself nodding off while reading the informative (but boring) nutrient charts on pages 149–151, here's a shortcut to great nutrition: If you serve your child a variety of naturally nutrient-rich foods, he or she will have a great diet!

What are naturally nutrient-rich foods? They're foods that are minimally processed and inherently rich in vitamins, minerals, or antioxidants that a body needs to thrive. They are *not* foods that are highly enriched or fortified. Here are some examples of naturally nutrient-rich foods:
- Fruits
- Vegetables
- Legumes (beans and peas)
- Nuts
- Whole grains
- Milk, cheese, and yogurt
- Soymilk and tofu
- Eggs
- Seafood
- Lean beef, lamb, and wild game
- Chicken and turkey (especially the dark meat)

Nutrients and the Jobs They Do

When you look at the nutrients listed in the following charts, you'll see that every vitamin and mineral contributes somehow to your baby's growth. During the first six months, your baby will get virtually all the necessary nutrients from breast milk or formula. By the end of the first year, your baby will get some of these nutrients from other foods, and the ratio of food nutrients to milk nutrients will grow as your baby becomes a toddler. That's why it's important to get in the habit of providing your child a balanced diet with plenty of variety early on.

Energy Nutrients

Nutrient	Function	Baby/Toddler Foods
Fat	Energy, growth (especially of brain), building hormones	Breast milk or formula, whole milk,* vegetable oil, avocado, egg yolk*
Protein	Building tissues, blood, skin, organs, muscles, bone, antibodies, and hormones	Breast milk or formula, whole milk,* meats, egg yolk*
Carbohydrate	Energy	Breast milk or formula, whole milk,* grains,* fruits, vegetables

*These foods should be restricted during a child's first year, longer for those at high risk for food allergies. See page 136 for more information.

Fat-Soluble Vitamins

Nutrient	Function	Baby/Toddler Foods
Vitamin A, beta carotene (vitamin A precursor found in non-animal foods)	Healthy skin and immune system, vision	Breast milk or formula, whole milk,* spinach, carrots, broccoli, sweet potato, winter squash, mango, cantaloupe, watermelon
Vitamin D	Building bones and teeth	Sunshine, formula, fortified whole milk,* vitamin supplements†
Vitamin E	Protecting muscles, cardio-vascular system, and nerve cells from damage	Colostrum, breast milk or formula, vegetable oils (especially corn oil), wheat germ,* nuts,* and seeds*
Vitamin K	Promoting blood clotting	Breast milk or formula, green leafy vegetables (spinach, lettuce), cauliflower

*These foods should be restricted during a child's first year, longer for those at high risk for food allergies. See page 136 for more information.
†See page 154 for more information.

Water-Soluble Vitamins

Nutrient	Function	Baby/Toddler Food
Vitamin C	Maintaining collagen, promoting iron absorption, healing wounds	Breast milk or formula, citrus fruit and juices,* berries, melon, tomatoes,* peppers, broccoli, kale, turnip greens, collards, potatoes
Vitamin B$_1$ (thiamine)	Producing energy, maintaining appetite and muscle tone	Breast milk or formula, meat (especially pork and chicken), eggs,* milk,* dried peas and beans, nuts,* whole-grain or enriched breads and cereals*
Vitamin B$_2$ (riboflavin)	Producing energy, promoting healthy skin and good vision	Breast milk or formula, whole milk,* cheese,* eggs,* fish,* dark green leafy vegetables, enriched grains and cereals*
Niacin	Promoting normal appetite, metabolizing carbohydrate	Breast milk or formula, meat, poultry, fish,* dried beans and peas, nuts,* whole-grain or enriched cereals or breads*
Vitamin B$_6$	Building and breaking down carbohydrate, fat, and protein; making red blood cells	Breast milk or formula, meat, poultry, fish,* sweet potatoes, vegetables, whole grains,* fortified cereal*
Vitamin B$_{12}$	Processing carbohydrate, fat, and protein; building nerve cell covering (myelin sheath), dividing cells	Breast milk or formula, animal foods only (meats, fish,* poultry, eggs,* milk*)
Folic acid (folacin, folate)	Making red blood cells, building new cells	Breast milk or formula, dark green leafy vegetables, meats, poultry, fish,* eggs,* whole grain cereals*
Choline	Building cell membranes, transmitting nerve signals, supporting memory center of developing brain	Breast milk or formula, eggs*, fish (especially salmon),* meat, wheat germ,* broccoli

*These foods should be restricted during a child's first year, longer for those at high risk for food allergies. See page 136 for more information.

Minerals

Nutrient	Function	Baby/Toddler Food
Calcium	Building bone and teeth, clotting blood, contracting and relaxing muscles, regulating blood pressure	Breast milk or formula, dairy products,* kale, broccoli, collards, turnips, dried beans and peas, almonds,* molasses
Chromium	Working with insulin in carbohydrate, protein, and fat metabolism	Breast milk or formula, brewer's yeast, meat, cheese,* whole-grain cereals*
Copper	Making blood cells, healing wounds, making nerve coverings	Breast milk or formula, shellfish,* meats, nuts,* legumes, whole-grain cereals*
Fluoride	Promoting healthy bones and teeth	Fluoride supplements, fluoridated water
Iodine	Regulating metabolism as part of thyroid hormones	Breast milk or formula, ocean fish* and shellfish,* iodized salt, food grown in iodine rich soil
Iron	Part of hemoglobin in red blood cells, enzyme involved in energy metabolism	Breast milk or formula, red meat, poultry, egg yolk,* enriched and whole-grain breads* and cereals,* dark green vegetables, legumes, dark molasses, prunes
Magnesium	Making protein, helping muscles and nerves work	Breast milk or formula, whole-grain cereals,* nuts,* legumes, meat, milk,* green leafy vegetables
Manganese	Metabolizing carbohydrate and protein, forming bone	Breast milk or formula, legumes, nuts,* whole-grain cereals*
Phosphorus	Building strong bones and teeth; metabolizing fat, protein, and carbohydrate; forming cell membranes and enzymes	Breast milk or formula, breads,* cereal,* lima beans, meat, poultry, fish,* milk,* cheese,* yogurt*
Selenium	Protecting muscles, cardiovascular system, and nerve cells from damage	Breast milk or formula, meat, seafood,* cereal foods
Zinc	Promoting growth and development, maintaining health of eyes, reproductive system, muscles, and skin	Colostrum, formula, shellfish,* fish,* meats, whole grains,* wheat germ,* yeast, legumes

*These foods should be restricted during a child's first year, longer for those at high risk for food allergies. See page 136 for more information.

Appetite

There's only one thing that parents worry about more than their child's growth, and it's their child's appetite! Many things can change your baby's or toddler's appetite.

Appetite Decrease

An appetite decrease can last from a few hours to a few days. If your baby has a chronic health condition or is taking medications that blunt hunger or upset digestion, you may struggle with long-term low-appetite issues. (In this case, it may be helpful to discuss feeding strategies with a dietitian or your baby's doctor.) Here's a list of several possible reasons for a decreased appetite.

- Illness
- Teething
- Distraction
- Medication

- Anemia
- Normal growth slowdown after one year
- Fatigue
- Very large meal eaten earlier in the day

As your child grows and settles into an eating rhythm, you'll begin to know what's normal and when to worry about an appetite decrease. That's what happened to us. When our son Robert was a toddler, he loved eating a big breakfast and a moderate lunch, but when it came to dinner, he just wasn't very interested. (In fact, breakfast continues to be his favorite meal!) So we made sure he had very healthy foods on his plate the first half of the day and we learned not to worry when he picked at his dinner. Nicolas, on the other hand, ate all his meals with equal interest. We also learned that he wouldn't eat dinner if he went "past hunger," which happened sometimes if our dinner was delayed.

Appetite Increase

Your child's appetite will probably increase— and then some—after an appetite decrease ends. Children have a way of catching up on their eating when they need to. Your child's appetite will also increase during a growth spurt. In fact, it may be hard to get enough food into your kid! You may worry that you aren't producing enough milk or that your baby's formula is somehow inadequate. Neither case is true; your baby is simply ravenous because he or she needs a lot of fuel right now.

The bottom line on appetite: As a parent, it's your job to trust that your child's appetite will ebb and flow when it needs to.

Fad Diets = Bad Diets

You may be wondering if a special diet might help your child's health or weight. First, remember that your child should never be put on any special diet (especially for weight control) without the advice of your child's doctor. Diets that restrict or overemphasize one food group inevitably end up harming children. So use caution with the following diets or any diet or lifestyle program that seems restrictive or unbalanced.

Low-Carb

You may have improved your health following Atkins, South Beach, or another low-carb diet. Perhaps you're wondering whether your diet would also be good for your child. Is it?

No. A low-carb diet doesn't provide the fiber, vitamins, minerals, or carbohydrates a kid needs for growth and development. Most experts agree that kids need ample fruits, vegetables, and grains to function well. And we're not just talking about growing, we're also talking about thinking.

When a diet lacks sufficient carbs, the body draws its energy from ketones, a byproduct of breaking down body fat. According to Bruce Rengers, assistant professor of nutrition and dietetics at the Saint Louis University Doisy School of Allied Health Professions, "Ketones have a dulling effect on the brain. Low-carb diets work by fooling the body to think it's starving. If you're putting kids into a starvation situation, they don't grow as well and they are not as likely to do well in school."

Low-Fat

With skyrocketing childhood obesity making headlines, you may wonder if your child should eat a low-fat diet right from the start. No! Babies need about 50 percent of their calories from fat. The AAP recommends that children between one and two years continue to have a moderate-fat diet. Not until your child turns two should you switch her to low-fat milk and modify her calories from fat to between 30 and 35 percent.[5] Why? The brain is growing quickly during the first two years, and one of its main building blocks is fat.

The type of fat babies and toddlers eat is important, too. While most of the fat in the diet will still come from breast milk or formula (or whole cow's milk after one year for most babies), the majority of other fat should be unsaturated—from vegetable and marine sources like canola oil, olive oil, avocado, fish, and nut butters. (Delay fish and nuts if your family has a history of food allergies.) You can control the saturated fat in your child's diet by choosing lean meats and low-fat cheese. Also, limit your child's intake of trans fats (found in many processed foods like shortening, margarine, fried foods, crackers, and cookies) and provide more fats from natural sources.

Supplements

In the United States 60 percent of the population takes some kind of dietary supplement. In 2002, Americans spent nearly nineteen billion dollars on supplements; 25 percent of that on herbal supplements. Using vitamin and mineral supplements as well as herbs is part of a growing system of healthcare called complementary and alternative medicine (CAM). CAM also includes Chinese and ayurvedic medicine, mind-body interactions, manipulative methods (chiropractic and osteopathic adjustments), and energy therapies.

Should Your Baby Take a Supplement?

You may wonder if your baby should also take a supplement. That depends on your baby's age and health, what your baby eats, and even the amount of sunshine your baby gets. The following vitamins are ones that some babies need. If your baby was premature or has any chronic health conditions, he or she may have different vitamin requirements than the typical full-term baby. Ask your baby's doctor about the need for supplements.

Vitamin D

If your baby is exclusively or partially breastfed (less than seventeen ounces of formula a day) the AAP and the National Academy of Sciences (NAS) recommend that your baby take a supplement of 200 IU of vitamin D per day.[6] Don't be alarmed when you see that many infant vitamin D supplements actually contain 400 IU; this is still way below the Tolerable Upper Intake Level set by the NAS.[7]

Vitamin B_{12}

If your baby is exclusively breastfed and your diet doesn't contain a reliable source of vitamin B_{12} (you eat no animal products), your baby should take a supplement to meet the dietary reference intake (DRI) for B_{12} (0.4 micrograms for babies birth to six months and 0.5 micrograms for babies seven to twelve months). To increase *your* dietary intake of vitamin B_{12}, see page 158.

Fluoride

Fluoride is associated with tooth and bone mineralization, but it's best known for its role in cavity prevention when applied topically to the teeth. Children from six months to sixteen years old should take a fluoride supplement if:

- They drink ready-to-feed formula that's not mixed with water.
- They drink (or have formula prepared with) only bottled or filtered water that doesn't contain fluoride.
- They use tap water that has fluoride content of less than 0.3 parts per million (ppm)[8]. Contact your city's water department to find out the level of fluoride in your neighborhood.

Be aware that bottled water for infants can contain more fluoride than the AAP recommends; discuss its use with your baby's doctor.

Iron

Iron should be given only to infants who need it—that is, infants who are diagnosed with anemia. When iron supplements were given to breastfed infants who had normal hemoglobin levels, it had negative effects: decreased growth in length and head circumference.[9]

Probiotics

Your baby's doctor may recommend a probiotic supplement if your baby is taking an antibiotic or if your doctor thinks your baby's digestive or immune system could benefit from it. See page 126 for more about probiotics.

Herbs

It's certainly likely that some herbal products are safe for babies, but there's very little research to show it. On the other hand, we know that some botanicals—especially those containing pennyroyal oil—can cause serious damage. Case in point: Infants given yerba buena, an herbal tea common in Mexico, were admitted to the hospital with liver failure.[10] Homegrown herbs can be particularly risky because it's sometimes difficult to distinguish what's safe and what's dangerous. Why take a chance?

Should Your Toddler Take a Supplement?

Once your baby weans from breast milk or formula and is getting most calories from table foods and conventional milk, things change a lot. Cow's milk (and milk alternatives) are nutritious, but they aren't nearly as nutrient-packed as breast milk or formula. Plus, you may find, as I did, that when you switch from baby foods to table foods, your baby's former favorites take a hit! Toddlers' sudden lack of interest in food may be caused by a combination of a decrease in appetite, the transition to adult food, and blossoming independence.

If your baby is a picky eater, it can't hurt to provide a multivitamin supplement. Children between the ages of one and two years are notorious for not eating their fruits and vegetables. In fact, a large study of toddlers found that 18 to 23 percent of them ate no vegetables on a given day and 33 percent ate no fruit![12]

Here are some reasons your child might need a daily multivitamin:

- Your child is a very picky eater.
- Your child eats limited amounts of one or more food groups.
- Your child has chronic health problems.
- Your child takes medications that affect his appetite or nutrient absorption.

Herbs: Proceed with Caution

There are about four hundred different herbal supplements on the market; sixty million Americans are using them. Even though herbs are widely used, you should use extreme caution if you choose to administer herbal products to children. Here's why:[11]

- Most herbal medicines haven't been subjected to rigorous clinical trials.
- Herbal product ingredients aren't standardized, so research on their effectiveness is difficult.
- There's no governmental regulation on the manufacture, purity, concentration, or labeling claims of herbal remedies and dietary supplements.
- The active ingredients in herbs can interact with other herbs or medications.
- Some herbs contain contaminants like lead and mercury.
- An analysis of imported traditional Chinese medicines by the California Health Department found that half had high levels of contaminants.
- Infants and young children are more vulnerable to the adverse effects of herbs.

- Your child gets very little unprotected exposure to sunshine and drinks less than a pint of milk per day. (In this case, your child may need a multivitamin containing vitamin D.)

- You're raising your child vegan. Your toddler will need a reliable source of vitamin B$_{12}$ (to meet the DRI of 0.9 micrograms for children one to three years) and possibly others:

  - If your child gets very little unprotected sunlight exposure (especially if your child has dark skin), he or she might need more vitamin D.

  - If your child's diet contains limited amounts of iron- and zinc-rich foods, he or she might need more iron and/or zinc.

  - If your child drinks only bottled water without added fluoride, or if your water supply is low in fluoride, ask your doctor about a fluoride supplement.

Too Much of a Good Thing

A recent study in the *Journal of the American Dietetic Association* uncovered an interesting fact: Many infants and toddlers are getting too much vitamin A and zinc. Nearly all toddlers who took a vitamin supplement exceeded the recommended intake, and 15 percent of toddlers who didn't take a vitamin supplement did, too. A substantial number of infants and toddlers (who did and didn't take vitamins) had too much zinc.

It just goes to show that many children are getting more than enough of these vitamins without supplements. So many foods are now fortified that kids are getting multiple vitamin doses. It's easy to go overboard. Pay attention to the number of fortified foods your child eats and also how much of each nutrient is in each food. For example, if your child eats several servings of a cereal that contains 100 percent of the recommended intake for most vitamins, and eats other fortified foods as well, *and* takes a multivitamin your child can easily overdose on vitamins. Getting excess water-soluble vitamins isn't usually a problem, but overdoing it on some minerals and fat-soluble vitamins (like vitamin A) can be.[13]

Choosing a Vitamin Supplement

Vitamin supplements for infants come in drops. One brand that's very widely available is Tri-Vi-Sol, which contains vitamins A, D, and C. You can also buy a version of Tri-Vi-Sol with iron. Poly-Vi-Sol, made by the same company, contains nine vitamins and comes with or without iron. Some other infant vitamin brands are Baby Plex, Just D, Infant Care, and Kindermins.

Once your child can chew well—generally between two and three years old, you can introduce chewable vitamins. Earlier than that can pose a choking hazard. The selection of supplements is not as simple as you'd probably like! Like vitamins for adults, children's vitamins come in endless variety. In general, those with close to 100 percent of the dietary reference intake (DRI) for each of the vitamins they contain are best.

If a little bit is good, is a lot better? No! Some vitamins in excess can be toxic—especially iron and vitamin A— so please follow the dosage guidelines on the label of your child's vitamins. Also, make sure all vitamin bottles have childproof caps and that you always close them properly. Because children's vitamins look and taste so appealing, kids equate them with candy. Let your child know that vitamins are medicine and that he or she should take vitamins only when a parent supplies them.

So you've found a vitamin supplement your child likes. Now you don't have to worry about what your kid eats. Right? Wrong! Food contains many nutrients, antioxidants, phytochemicals, and essential fats that supplements don't contain, so you still need to encourage your child to eat the healthiest diet possible! A vitamin supplement can take the pressure off a bit, but it's no reason to relax your standards.

Vegetarian Eating

It's not easy being green sometimes. Whether you've chosen a vegetarian lifestyle for your child or your child has chosen it by refusing to eat meat, this section will help you ensure that your child gets all the nutrients he or she needs.

Nutritional Concerns for Lacto-Ovo Vegetarian Kids

Children who are lacto-ovo vegetarians don't have as many nutrient concerns as vegan children because they do consume dairy products and eggs. Dairy and eggs contain all the vitamin B_{12} and vitamin D a child needs. The minerals that might be in short supply include iron and zinc, since meats are one good source of iron and zinc for kids. Omega-3 fats could also be in short supply since the best source is cold-water fish. See the sections about iron, zinc, and fat on the following pages for more information.

Nutrition Concerns for Vegan Kids

A well-planned vegan diet can be just as healthy—or even healthier—than a meat-eater's diet, but it can be hard to get enough of certain nutrients without eating animal foods. Also, because a vegan diet is very high in fiber, its sheer bulk can prevent a child from getting sufficient calories. On the following pages I've listed some nutrients of concern for vegan children.

Iron

Iron is important for red blood cells and for cognitive development. Severe iron deficiency can affect a child's cognitive development ten years later! Here are some tips for increasing iron in your vegan child's diet:

- You may hear that breast milk is low in iron. That's true, but the iron in breast milk is highly bioavailable. If you're breastfeeding, your milk is your baby's best source of iron.
- If your baby drinks formula, make sure it's iron-fortified.
- Once your baby starts eating solid foods, make sure he or she eats iron-rich foods several times a day. Iron-rich vegan foods include fortified cereals, tofu, soybeans, blackstrap molasses, garbanzo beans, lentils, tahini, sea vegetables, and some soy convenience foods. According to the WHO, breastfed infants have difficulty meeting iron needs unless fortified foods (such as cereal) are used.

- Vitamin C enhances iron absorption, so serve vitamin C–rich fruits and vegetables with iron-rich foods to enhance iron absorption. Some foods high in vitamin C are fortified fruit juices, melon, broccoli, berries, and green leafy vegetables.

Zinc

Your child's body needs zinc for growth and development, including brain development, and also to maintain the immune system. The best vegan sources of zinc are whole grains, wheat germ, fortified cereals, adzuki beans, hyacinth beans, other legumes, tempeh, textured vegetable protein (TVP), nuts, and seeds.

Vitamin D

Vitamin D is necessary for calcium regulation, which affects bone mineralization. Vitamin D deficiency can cause rickets, a disease characterized by bowed legs and curvatures of other bones. The best source of vitamin D is sunlight. For your child to naturally produce enough vitamin D, he or she must be exposed (with no sunscreen) to thirty minutes of sunshine a week wearing only a diaper, or two hours per week fully clothed without a hat.[14]

Dark skin, sunscreen use, and living at far northern or southern latitudes can all make it hard to get enough sunlight to produce adequate vitamin D. If your child has dark skin, it may take him or her six times the sun exposure a light-skinned person needs to make the same amount of vitamin D. If, for example, you live in northern Canada, your child likely won't receive enough sunshine throughout the year to produce the vitamin D he or she needs. Finally, sunscreen (widely used to reduce the risk of skin cancer) blocks the ultraviolet light necessary to produce vitamin D. For these reasons, many children need dietary sources of vitamin D.

Because breast milk is low in vitamin D and formula is fortified with vitamin D, the AAP recommends a vitamin D supplement for all exclusively breastfed infants (and any other infants who drink less than seventeen ounces of formula a day). For babies and toddlers eating solid foods, vegan sources of vitamin D include fortified cereals and fortified soy and rice milks. Be sure to check food labels, because vitamin D levels vary among brands.

Vitamin B_{12}

Vitamin B_{12} is critical for development of the nervous system; a deficiency can cause irreversible nerve damage. Be aware that high levels of folic acid in the diet can mask the symptoms of B_{12} deficiency, which is a potential problem with vegans, who generally have a high folate intake. Many foods are reported to contain vitamin B_{12} (tempeh, sea vegetables, and algae), but most contain either no active vitamin B_{12} or very little. The only reliable vegan sources of vitamin B_{12} are nutritional yeast grown on a vitamin B_{12}–rich medium (Red Star brand T6635), fortified cereals, fortified meat analogues (such as veggie burgers), fortified soymilk, and other fortified foods.

Fat

Your child's brain and eye development continue past the first year, and certain fats are important for this growth. The essential dietary fats alpha-linolenic acid (ALA) and linoleic acid (LA) are converted into longer-chain fats necessary for growth. However, current research suggests that infants and vegetarian breastfeeding moms don't convert ALA very efficiently into docosahexaenoic acid (DHA), a long-chain omega-3 fat needed for infant brain and eye tissue.

If your vegan baby is formula-fed, you can choose a follow-up formula containing DHA and ARA. The DHA and ARA in formula are from vegetarian sources; 70 percent of the world's infant formula supply as well as some other food products and supplements contain Life's DHA, which is made from microalgae. (For more information about this type of DHA, visit http://www.martek.com.)

If your vegan baby is breastfed, consider the following recommendations based on the latest research.

- Take a daily supplement containing 300 milligrams of DHA, as recommended by an expert panel of scientists.[15]

- Get most fats from whole foods such as nuts, flaxseed and other seeds, olives, avocado, and soy foods.

- For oils, choose those rich in monounsaturated fat, such as olive, canola, high oleic sunflower and safflower oils, and nut oils. Omega-3–rich flaxseed oil can also be used but shouldn't be heated.

- If you eat eggs, choose those enriched with omega-3 fatty acids. These eggs contain 60 to 150 milligrams of DHA per egg.

- To avoid consuming too much omega-6 fat (LA), don't use these oils as primary cooking oils: safflower oil, grapeseed oil, sunflower oil, corn oil, cottonseed oil, and soybean oil. Also, be aware that omega-6 oils are often found in processed foods.

- Don't drown yourself in omega-3 fats. Too much ALA can hamper the conversion of LA, the other essential fatty acid, to ARA, the other long-chain fatty acid.[16]

- Limit your trans fat intake. Trans fats can hamper the conversion of ALA to DHA. Trans fats are found in hydrogenated oils like shortening and stick margarine, as well as in foods containing hydrogenated oils, such as bakery goods, crackers, cookies, and fried foods. Look for trans fat content on your food labels.

- Try to eat a good diet overall; this helps in the metabolism of essential fats. Insufficient energy or protein reduces the activity of the enzymes that convert ALA and LA into DHA and ARA. So can deficiencies of vitamin B_6, biotin, calcium, copper, magnesium, and zinc.[17]

Raising Your Child Vegan: Step by Step

Raising a healthy vegan child takes a bit of planning and care, especially as your child begins eating solid foods. Following is a description of the progression from liquid to solid foods for vegan babies and toddlers.

The First Six Months

While your baby is on an all-liquid diet, he or she will get all the necessary nutrients as long as:

- Your baby drinks only breast milk or iron-fortified formula.
- If you're breastfeeding, you follow the supplement guidelines on page 154.

Do *not* feed your baby soymilk, rice milk, or homemade formula. These drinks don't have the right proportion of nutrients that a young infant needs.

A Day in the Diet of a Vegan Ten-Month-Old

Breakfast
- Breast milk or formula
- Rice, oat, or barley cereal
- Chopped apricots

Mid-morning
- Soy cheese
- Crackers
- White grape juice

Lunch
- Breast milk or formula
- Creamy Split Peas (page 267)
- Soft, cubed carrot and avocado
- Applesauce fortified with vitamin C
- Teething cracker

Mid-afternoon
- Half slice of toast
- Soy yogurt
- Banana slices

Dinner
- Breast milk or formula
- Soy burger chunks
- Whole-Grain Risotto with Sweet Potato (page 299)

Bedtime
- Breast milk or formula
- Ready-to-eat cereal with blueberries

Six to Twelve Months

Once your vegan baby begins eating solid foods, it gets a bit more challenging to keep the right balance in his or her diet. At the usual time for introducing meats (seven to nine months), you'll want to introduce vegan counterparts: puréed legumes, tofu, and soy yogurt. (If your baby is at high risk for allergies, hold off on soy until one year.) As your baby gets skilled at eating finger foods (ten to eleven months), you can introduce other vegan foods like well-cooked black beans, chickpeas with the hulls slipped off, pintos and other beans, soy crumbles, soy burgers, and Quorn patties cut into baby-safe nibbles.

Iron and zinc, nutrients usually supplied by meat, may be in shorter supply in a vegan diet. To make sure your baby gets enough of these minerals, follow the tips on page 157. And because a vegan diet can be very bulky, making your baby feel full before he or she has eaten enough calories, make sure you provide calorie-dense foods like vegetable oils, avocados, puréed olives, and dates.

Of course, you'll also need to continue breastfeeding or formula-feeding. For more information on providing essential fats via breast milk or formula, see page 159.

Milk Alternatives for Vegan Toddlers: Nutrient Comparison

Nutrients in 16 Ounces (500 Milliliters) and Percent of DRI for One- to Three-Year-Olds

Nutrient	DRI	Silk Soymilk	Similac Isomil Advance 2 Soy Formula	Baby's Only Organic Soy Toddler Formula
Vitamin B$_{12}$	0.9 mcg	6 mcg (660%)	1.44 mcg (160%)	1.44 mcg (160%)
Iron	7 mg	2.16 mg (30%)	6 mg (86%)	5.76 mg (82%)
Zinc	3 mg	1.2 mg (40%)	2.4 mg (80%)	3.2 mg (106%)
Calcium	500 mg	600 mg (120%)	432 mg (86%)	432 mg (86%)
Vitamin D	200 IU	240 IU (120%)	192 IU (96%)	192 IU (96%)

Nutrient-Rich Vegan Foods

Food	Amount	Calcium	Protein	Vitamin B$_{12}$	Vitamin D	Zinc	Iron
DRI for one- to three-year-olds		500 mg	13 g	0.9 mcg	200 IU	3 mg	7 mg
Calcium-fortified juice	1 cup	350 mg	2 g	0	0	0	0
Rice Dream enriched rice milk	1 cup	300 mg	1 g	1.5 mcg	100 IU	0	0
Fortified soymilk	1 cup	300 mg	7 g	3 mcg	120 IU	0.6 mg	1.08 mg
Silk kid's pack	6.5 ounces	350 mg	4 g	2.4 mcg	100 IU	0.6 mg	1.08 mg
Silk Live! cultured soy smoothie	10 ounces	350 mg	7 g	1.5 mcg	100 IU	1.5 mg	1.8 mg
Cultured soy yogurt plain	8 ounces	300 mg	5 g	0	0	0	0.72 mg
White Wave soft tofu	⅛ block	100 mg	11 g	0	0	0	1.2 mg
White Wave firm tofu	⅛ block	100 mg	10 g	0	0	0	0
MorningStar Farms vegan burger	1 burger	20 mg	13 g	0	0	0	2.7 mg
Refried beans	½ cup	44 mg	7 g	0	0	1.47 mg	2.09 mg
Tahini (ground roasted sesame seeds)	2 tablespoons	128 mg	5 g	0	0	1.39 mg	2.69 mg

Check labels; nutrient content sometimes changes.

Twelve Months and Older

At one year your child should be on the way to eating like you do, with three meals a day plus a few snacks. Your child should be eating the same kinds of foods you do, too.

Just like other toddlers, vegan toddlers can be picky. And just like other parents, you may wonder if your child is getting enough calories and nutrients to grow properly. A unique challenge your family faces, though, is the bulkiness of a vegan diet. Try to see that your child doesn't get too full on high-fiber foods before getting the calories he or she needs. Continue offering healthy sources of concentrated calories and protein like avocados, nut and seed butters (mixed with fruit and only if your child isn't allergy-prone), soy cheese and other soy products, some refined grains, fruit juices, and peeled fruits and vegetables. Also be sure to include omega-3 fats like flaxseed oil, ground flaxseed, and canola and soybean oil (often found in mayonnaise and salad dressings).

Be sure to keep up with well-child appointments to assess your toddler's growth. It's also probably a good idea to give your toddler a vitamin-mineral supplement. (See pages 155–157 for more information.)

If your baby weans between the first and second year, you can offer either full-fat soymilk or soy formula made for older babies (follow-up formula). Both are fortified with vitamin B_{12}, zinc, and iron, which can bolster your toddler's diet (especially if you've got a picky eater on your hands). Each choice has its advantages.

Soymilk has more calcium per serving than a soy follow-up formula but less iron. Soymilk contains three times the vitamin B_{12} a one- to three-year-old needs. This may seem like a lot, but don't worry: the NIH hasn't set an upper limit for B_{12} intake because research hasn't revealed any problems with excess. Soymilk is, of course, available in organic and non-organic versions.

If you go with soy follow-up formula, you can choose one with DHA and ARA, which contribute to brain building that continues into your child's second year. There's one brand of organic soy follow-up formula available: Baby's Only Organic Soy Toddler Formula. (For more information, visit http://www.naturesone.com.)

Coping with a Food Allergy

A diagnosis of food allergy—especially a life-threatening one—is the beginning of a journey that's often emotionally and physically exhausting. Coping with a food allergy is very scary and time-consuming at first, but over time, as you gain experience and knowledge about your child's allergy, it will come to seem normal. This section isn't a food allergy bible, but it *will* help you start this journey on the right foot.

Letting the World Know

The first thing you should do when you find out your child has a food allergy is make sure everyone else knows, too.

Start by getting your child a MedicAlert bracelet. This internationally known organization provides members with a well-known emblem signifying a potentially dangerous health condition. Enrollment provides access to a toll-free phone number emergency professionals can call to get critical treatment information about your child.

Next, explain the situation to your family and friends, your child's daycare and/or school staff, and the parents of your child's classmates and friends. Everyone who spends time with your child needs to know what to do if your child has an allergic reaction. Providing an EpiPen Jr at all locations where your child might spend time is another smart move.

Finally, give your child some tools to spread the word. As soon as your child can talk, teach him or her to say, "No peanuts—they make me sick," or, "I'm allergic to milk." Consider some of the following products your child can wear to help spread the word.

- Catchy t-shirts (http://www.cafepress.com/buy/allergy)

- Allergy-identifying adhesive labels (http://www.labelitorloseit.com/allergy.htm and http://www.mypreciouskid.com/allergy-labels.html)

- Embroidered canvas allergy awareness patches that can be sewn or ironed onto backpacks, diaper bags, and so on (http://www.jeeto.com/patchcollection.html)

Feeding an Allergic Kid

Label Reading

One of the most important things you must learn to do is diligently read food labels—*every label, every time*—because ingredients often change.

As of 2006, the Food Allergen Labeling and Consumer Protection Act of 2004 (FALCPA) requires manufacturers to state in plain language if their products have any ingredients that contain the protein of the eight major allergens: milk, eggs, fish, crustacean shellfish, tree nuts, peanuts, wheat, or soybeans. Food labels can state this information in two ways:

- The allergenic food can be included parenthetically in the list of ingredients. For example, the list might say, "casein (milk), lecithin (soy), enriched flour (wheat)."

- The label can include a statement listing all allergenic foods adjacent to or at the end of the ingredient list. For example, the statement might say, "Contains milk, soy and wheat."

FALPCA doesn't apply to:

- Highly refined oils derived from the top eight allergens, such as highly refined peanut oil

- Raw agricultural products like fresh fruits and vegetables

- Ingredients added to a food unintentionally, such as by contact with machinery used to grow, transport, or process an allergenic food. You may see allergy advisory statements about cross-contamination, but be aware that they're voluntary, not required—which means that cross-contamination can also occur without an advisory statement.

- Food that doesn't fall under Food and Drug Administration (FDA) jurisdiction, such as meat, poultry, and egg products
- Foods that aren't prepackaged, such as food bought at a restaurant, deli counter, or food kiosk

Here are some tips for label reading and food buying:

- Buy only foods for which you can identify every ingredient.
- Keep checking labels for foods you've deemed safe. Manufacturers sometimes change ingredients in a product.
- Keep up with product recalls and mislabeling at http://www.foodallergy.org/alerts.html. At this website you can also sign up for free e-mailed allergy alerts.
- Avoid buying foods in bulk. Bulk foods are often cross-contaminated.
- Be aware that deli foods may also be cross-contaminated due to shared machinery.
- If you have doubts about an ingredient, call the manufacturer's toll-free phone number.

Allergen-Free Convenience Foods

Even though your child has food allergies, as time goes on he or she will want to eat what other kids are eating: chicken nuggets, fish sticks, and the like. For occasional convenience food purchases, check out the following brands:

- Ian's Natural Foods, a company that makes kid-friendly, antibiotic- and hormone-free frozen food, has a line of frozen foods that are also wheat- and gluten-free. For more information, visit http://www.iansnaturalfoods.com.
- Kinnikkinnick Foods has cookies, crackers, muffins, and baking mixes that are wheat- and dairy-free. I've tried them, and they're tasty! For more info, visit http://www.kinnikkinnick.com.
- Amy's Kitchen also offers foods that are dairy- and gluten-free. For more information, visit http://www.amyskitchen.com.

Check Out the Asian Aisle

If your child has a wheat allergy, check out the Asian aisle at your grocery store. Many Asian foods are based on rice or other starches instead of wheat. Here are a few examples:

- Rice noodles
- Rice flour
- Bean threads (made from mung beans and potato starch)
- Spring roll wrappers (made from tapioca starch)

As with all foods, read the labels of Asian foods carefully. Since these foods are often imported, you may need to contact their distributors to double-check ingredients or ask about cross-contamination.

Storing Food at Home

The best way to keep your child safe from allergenic foods at home is to avoid bringing them in the house! However, that's not always practical for the rest of the family. Other strategies include:

- Having a shelf or cabinet that contains only non-allergenic foods
- Labeling all foods that are off-limits with a special red allergy label (This is especially useful if you have a nanny or babysitter in your home.)
- Labeling a shelf in the refrigerator either "safe" or "off limits" for your child

Cooking at Home

Doing your own cooking and baking gives you the most control over your allergic child's diet. If you find yourself cooking different meals for different family members, you may benefit from bulk cooking and freezing of non-allergenic dishes. The most important thing to keep in mind is avoiding cross-contamination of non-allergenic foods with allergenic foods. Here are some cooking and preparation tips:

- If you prepare separate meals for your allergic child, cook the non-allergenic food first and then cover it.
- Be careful not to cross-contaminate foods with utensils, pans, or cutting boards.
- Be aware that baking sheets and muffin pans often retain food remnants. Your best bet is to use separate pans dedicated to cooking only for your allergic child.
- Make sure to clean countertops well between preparing non-allergenic and allergenic foods.
- Use separate utensils for serving allergenic and non-allergenic foods.
- Don't reuse frying oil used for allergenic foods.
- Plastic or metal utensils may be better than wooden ones to prevent cross-contamination.

> **Non-allergenic Organic Baby Food**
>
> Bobo Baby baby food is great for a baby with allergies or who is at high risk for allergies. These products contain none of the top eight allergens and are also organic, vegetarian, and kosher. The food comes in twenty-five–milliliter (about one-ounce) frozen portions. For more information, see http://www.bobobaby.com.

Eating Away from Home

Eating away from home can be tough with a food allergy. Keep it simple. Order whole, unprocessed foods—like baked potatoes or steamed vegetables without sauce—when possible. Make sure foods that you order aren't cooked with allergenic foods or cooked in the same pan. Keep in mind that foods cooked in a deep-fryer or wok or on a grill can be cross-contaminated easily. If you take your child out to eat with you, it may be easier and safer to bring food from home and have the restaurant heat it up in a microwave.

When you're eating at a friend's or relative's house or at daycare, it's a bit easier because people who know you are generally understanding. Still, they may not understand just how little of an allergenic food it takes to cause a reaction. It may be best to bring something safe for your child to eat or to offer to bring a dish for everyone that your child can also eat. At large get-togethers where there are many people, have your child wear an allergy T-shirt that says, "No peanuts for me—I'm allergic!" (or whatever). It's a friendly reminder that's impossible to miss.

To protect your baby from unintentional exposure to allergens while eating away from home, look into table toppers, disposable adhesive placemats your child can use at daycare or when eating out. (For more information, visit http://www.tabletopper.com.) Dietary cards are another handy product especially useful when you're traveling. These personalized cards alert servers and cooks about food intolerances or allergies. They're available in several languages. (For more info, visit http://www.dietarycard.com.)

More Resources

The information I've presented here is really just to get you started. Following are more resources to educate yourself further.

Websites

The Internet is home to many great resources for allergy information. Here are some of the best:

- http://www.foodallergy.org
- http://www.niaid.nih.gov/factsheets/food.htm
- http://www.nal.usda.gov/fnic/etext/000004.html
- http://www.anaphylaxis.ca
- http://www.foodallergyconnection.org

Books

Below is a list of written resources for families with allergies. Here are some great books for adults:

- *The Parent's Guide to Food Allergies* by Marianne Barber
- *Was It Something You Ate?* by John Emsley and Peter Fell
- *Caring for Your Child with Severe Food Allergies* by Lisa Cipriano Collins
- *Food Allergies: Tips from the Nutrition Experts* by the American Dietetic Association
- *The Food Allergy News Cookbook* by the Food Allergy Network
- *Food Allergy: Adverse Reactions to Foods and Food Additives* by Dean Metcalfe, Hugh Sampson, and Ronald Simon

And here are some helpful books for children:

- *Allie the Allergic Elephant* by Nicole Smith
- *Taking Food Allergies to School* by Ellen Weiner

- *No Nuts for Me!* by Aaron Zevy and Susan Tebbutt
- *A Preschooler's Guide to Peanut Allergy* by Lauri Habkirk

Food and Hyperactivity

Parents, health professionals, and researchers have been debating for decades whether sugar, artificial sweeteners, and food colorings cause hyperactivity. Here are the facts:

- Activity levels in children vary. A two-year-old is usually more active and has a much shorter attention span than a ten-year-old. It's easy to mistake this natural difference for a food reaction.

- There's little evidence to support the claim that refined sugar has a significant effect on behavior.[18] However, refined sugar—the kind found in table sugar, corn syrup, sweet beverages, and sweet foods—*can* affect a child's activity, especially when eaten on an empty stomach. Simple sugars enter the bloodstream quickly, which leads to rapid increase in blood sugar, which in turn could trigger an adrenaline release to make a child more active. Parents also need to realize that high sugar events like birthday parties and Halloween are also very exciting to kids, and a high level of activity is normal at these events.

- Giving your child a fiber-rich diet can help keep adrenaline levels steady. Provide plenty of whole-grain cereals and breads as well as fruits and vegetables to mitigate the effects of any sugar your child may eat.

- Some studies have shown a relationship between hyperactivity and some artificial colorings; others don't.

- Some experts believe that the change in behavior sometimes seen when a child follows a new special diet is due to the changed dynamics among family members. A special diet is a way of giving extra positive attention to the child.

Dental Health

Regardless of the true impact of sugar on children's activity levels, one thing's for sure: Sugar definitely affects children's dental health. Before I explain how to keep your kid's teeth healthy, let's discuss how those pearly whites develop.

Teething

Teething is one of those developmental milestones that brings both triumph and tribulation. In other words, you're excited that your child will soon be able to sink her teeth into family foods, but you don't treasure the fussiness, drooling, and fever that sometimes accompany teething.

The timing of first tooth emergence varies, but it's usually between four and seven months. Don't be alarmed if your baby's first tooth is late—it happens, and it's no big deal. Candi's daughter Cara was close to a year when she got her first teeth. It didn't bother Cara a bit—she was able to gum most of the same foods as her peers!

The first teeth to emerge are usually the two bottom front teeth (central incisors), followed four to eight weeks later by the four upper front teeth (central and lateral incisors). About a month later, the two lower lateral incisors should appear. The first molars come in next, followed by the canine or eye teeth. With this teething schedule, it's no wonder you feel like your baby's on drool overdrive—with a fussy attitude to match—for months!

Drooling is often the first teething symptom a parent recognizes, but there are others, too. The most common teething symptoms are:

- Biting
- Drooling
- Gum rubbing
- Irritability
- Sucking
- Sleep awakenings
- Ear rubbing
- Facial rash
- Reduced appetite for solids
- Slightly elevated temperature (not over 101°F or 38.3°C)

The topic of teething has spawned lots of myth and misunderstanding through the ages. Debates on how infant teething affects health go back at least five thousand years! Everyone—from ancient Hindu scholars to those old Greeks Aristotle and Homer to modern doctors and parents—has a mixed-up idea or two about teething.

Kristina's son, Marco, was fussy and had diarrhea. Kristina thought he was teething, but actually he'd picked up a virus at daycare. Kristina's not alone in misinterpreting symptoms of other conditions as signs of teething. In a study just twenty years ago, fifty parents reported infant teething as a reason for hospital admission. In forty-eight of those cases, medical evaluation found other causes for the babies' symptoms. These causes ranged from upper respiratory tract infections to bacterial meningitis![19] In a more recent survey of Florida doctors, 35 percent believed diarrhea to be a symptom of teething.[20]

To help you find your way through the fog of folklore surrounding teething, here are a few research-backed facts:[21]

- Teething symptoms usually occur within eight days of a tooth eruption, from four days before a tooth emerges to three days afterward.
- Babies are more likely to suffer a mild fever or wakefulness on the day before or the day of a tooth eruption.
- Babies are more likely to have a reduced appetite for solids and ear rubbing on the day a tooth emerges beyond the gum.
- There's a slight association between teething and loose poops. Increased saliva production is one explanation. A change in diet is another. (For example, if your child refuses solids, you're more likely to offer more liquids, which can result in looser poops.)
- In one study, 35 percent of the participating babies had no teething symptoms.

If you're lucky, your child may not have any teething symptoms. But chances are, you'll see a few—and it pays to know how to help your baby. Expect your baby's gums around new and emerging teeth to swell and feel tender. Your baby will want to chew on something to relieve the pain. Here's how you can help:

- Gently rub your baby's gums with your clean finger.

- Let your baby chew on something safe, such as your finger or a firm teething ring. Make sure whatever you give your baby is intended for teething; hard objects can do more harm than good. Also make sure your baby's teething objects aren't choking hazards.

- If your older baby has already had similar foods, offer a teething biscuit or a frozen bagel. Some babies enjoy chewing on these.

- Be aware that teething rings containing liquid may get too hard when frozen. Either chill them in the refrigerator or freeze them not-quite-solid.

- If your baby is miserable, a teething gel rubbed onto the gums might help. However, it'll provide only temporary relief, since saliva will soon wash it away. Over-the-counter infant pain relievers such as acetaminophen or ibuprofen may provide longer-lasting relief.

- If your baby has fever over 101°F or 38.3°C, if your baby seems particularly miserable, or if your baby has diarrhea, call your baby's doctor. These symptoms may be signs of a problem more serious than teething.

Tooth Care

How Do Cavities Happen?

It's a simple equation: Sugar or starch + bacteria in the mouth + time = acid that destroys tooth enamel and makes a small hole or cavity. How do you prevent cavities? That's simple, too: If you remove any part of the equation, no cavities can occur. Let's look at the parts more closely.

Sugar and Starch

Sugars and cooked starches (collectively called fermentable carbohydrates) are the only foods that can cause cavities.

Sugar is the number one cavity-causing ingredient. Sticky sugars—caramel, gum, dried fruit, toffee, taffy, and other chewy or sticky sweets—are especially bad. Because they stick to teeth, they provide an ongoing snack for bacteria. You also need to watch out for sweet drinks. Bacteria use added sugars in beverages, like sucrose, very effi-

> **Most Cariogenic Beverages**
>
> A recent study in the journal *General Dentistry* showed that the following beverages are the worst culprits for destroying tooth enamel. The drinks are listed in order from most to least offending:[24]
> - Lemonade
> - Energy drinks
> - Sports drinks
> - Fitness water
> - Sweetend iced tea
> - Cola

ciently. Sweet drinks like soda, lemonade, and sports drinks also contain acid, which contributes to cavity-making. Recent research shows that even cough syrups can cause cavities because they're both sweet and acidic.[22]

Starchy foods like bread, potato chips, and pretzels are also cavity-causing. Research shows that some starchy foods linger on the teeth longer than some types of candy. Five minutes after eating, there are more food particles left in the mouth from plain donuts, potato chips, cookies, or saltine crackers than from caramel, milk chocolate, or milk chocolate–caramel bars.[23]

Bacteria

The lead cavity-causing bacteria is Mutans streptococci. This bacteria converts the sugar in the mouth into acid.

Chances are, this bacteria gets into your baby's mouth courtesy of you! Mothers are the prime suspects in the transfer of salivary bacteria to babies' mouths via shared utensils, food, and even kisses.[25] If you have active or untreated cavities, or if you eat a lot of sugar, you're at higher risk of transferring bacteria to your baby. The best ways to reduce bacteria in your mouth are eating a healthy diet and practicing proper dental care.

Some people are more prone to cavities than others because they tend to have more cavity-causing bacteria than others. This tendency has a genetic component: If mom and/or dad has more bacteria, their child probably will, too.

Time

After bacteria converts sugar or starch in the mouth into acid, it takes twenty to forty minutes for saliva to neutralize or wash away the acid. So the more often you eat sugar or starch and the longer it stays on your teeth, the more acid bacteria can produce.

Dental Hygiene

See a tooth? See a dentist.

A consumer poll done by the Academy of General Dentistry showed that 70 percent of parents wait until their child is three years old to see a dentist.[26] This is way too late! By this age, about 25 percent of kids will already have cavities. Even waiting until age two is too late—at this age, one out of every ten kids already has a cavity.

The best time to visit a dentist is within six months of your baby's first tooth appearing. This first visit is simple, educational, and friendly. The dentist usually discusses hygiene techniques and takes a quick look at your baby's teeth while your baby sits on your lap.

Between dentist visits, keep an eye out for cavities: A white, chalky spot or lesion on the tooth close to the gum line precedes a cavity. This is where bacterial acid has removed calcium from the enamel. A lesion can be reversed with fluoride treatment, so see a dentist fast! Active cavities are usually golden brown.

Of course, it's also important to keep your child's teeth clean. Wipe a baby's teeth with clean gauze once or twice a day. Introduce a soft toothbrush with plain water at about one year.

Once your child is a bit older—between one and two years—you should start brushing his or her teeth with a soft brush and fluoride toothpaste. Use no more than a pea-size amount—kids sometimes swallow toothpaste while brushing, and a fluoride overdose can be harmful. Make brushing fun—you're establishing a habit that will make or break your child's future smile!

When your child wants to start brushing independently, let him or her. But be sure to follow up with a brushing of your own. Kids often just brush the teeth they can see and ignore the rest. Flossing isn't necessary until there are touching teeth.

Don't let your baby or toddler fall asleep with a bottle of anything except water. When children fall asleep drinking breast milk, formula, cow's milk, juice, or other beverages, the liquid tends to pool and cause cavities. Ditto for letting a toddler walk around all day with a bottle or sippy cup of juice, soda, or any sweet drink—every sip bathes the teeth with sugar. Finally, if your child is taking a sweet and/or acidic medication like cough syrup, be sure to brush your child's teeth after each dose.

Cavity-Preventing Foods

Here's a bit of good news: Some foods can actually prevent cavities from forming:
- Cheese
- Vegetables
- Xylitol (a low-calorie sweetener)

Also, eating a protein food along with a starchy food can decrease the starch's cavity-causing ability.

Part 2

Adding
Solids

CULVER PUBLIC LIBRARY

Chapter 8

Starting Solids

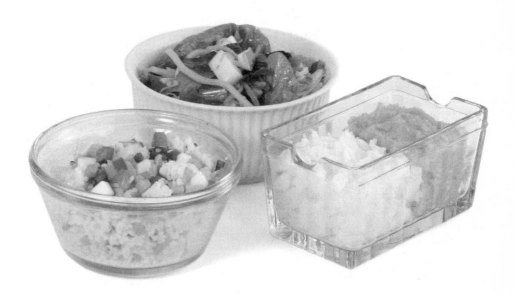

*"There's nothing to worry about" is a
typical example of the kind of easy-for-you-to-say
remarks that pediatricians like to make.*

—Dave Barry, writer and humorist

Not So Fast!

There's no rush to start solids, but don't be surprised if you get pressured to do so by well-meaning grandparents or friends who think your baby needs them. You might also be tempted to push solids after hearing that solid foods will help your baby sleep longer at night.

Be aware that research shows starting solid foods does *not* help babies sleep through the night. And on the flip side, starting solids too soon *does* increase your child's risk of allergies—especially if your child has a family history of allergies.

Confused about Feeding Advice?

If you're confused about contradictory feeding recommendations in this book and elsewhere, don't worry: It's not you.

Experts like to disagree. The AAP itself offers two different guidelines for when to introduce solids! You'll also see varying advice on how long to wait between introducing new foods. La Leche League and the AAP disagree about cosleeping and pacifier use. Even Bridget, the author of this book, and Christine, the editor (both well-educated moms) don't agree on every issue. And disagreement certainly isn't limited to experts; friends with opposing philosophies and relatives from different generations often debate child feeding and other parenting issues.

How do you cope with so much contradictory advice? Realize that if there's expert debate on an issue, it probably means there isn't enough evidence to make a concrete rule. Also, remember that a lot of child feeding advice is a matter of custom, not science. Gather all the evidence-based info you can and use common sense to apply it to your family's needs.

Large proteins found in solid foods can sometimes get through the lining of the immature intestinal wall. When this happens, your baby's immune system produces antibodies to the proteins, resulting in an allergic reaction. Finally, pushing solids before your baby is ready can make feeding unpleasant and start a negative feeding relationship between you.

When to Start

Allergies can cause lifelong problems, and your relationship with your child is too precious to tamper with, so I suggest you wait as long as possible to introduce solid foods—preferably around six months.

If you're breastfeeding, be confident that your breast milk supplies all the nutrients your child needs for the first six months. The American Academy of Pediatrics (AAP) recommends that breastfed infants be introduced to an iron-rich supplemental food beginning at about six months.

If you think your baby really might need solids before six months or isn't ready at six months, discuss it with your baby's doctor. It's also possible that your baby's doctor may suggest starting solids before six months. In either case, know that the AAP Committee on Nutrition says it's okay to begin earlier than six months if your baby is showing all the signs of readiness—but that you should *never* introduce solids before four months. The AAP also notes that some babies may not be ready for solids until eight months.[1]

Signs of Readiness

Certain developmental signs show your baby is ready to try solid foods. (See the following list.) If your baby is around six months old (or even a bit younger) and showing all these signs, you can feel confident that you're offering solids at the right time.

- Your baby seems to be nursing or drinking formula around the clock but still isn't satisfied. (This can also happen during growth spurts before four months; don't confuse these two situations.)
- Your baby sits well with minimal or no support.
- Your baby shows good head control.
- Your baby shows interest in food by trying to take food off your plate or trying to grab your fork.
- Your baby turns his or her head when done feeding.
- Your baby has lost the tongue-thrust reflex.
- Your baby opens his or her mouth upon seeing a spoon approaching.

Gearing Up

All you really need at first is a rubber-tipped infant spoon and a small plastic bowl you can hold in one hand. (Why plastic? Just in case. Baby tableware often ends up on the floor.) You might fasten a small bib around your baby's neck just to look official.

Once your little one gets in the groove of solids, you'll probably want more supplies. Here's a list of popular baby feeding items:

- **Plate with compartments**: Consider getting one with a suction cup on the bottom, which can't be thrown!
- **Several spoons**: You'll want a spoon for you and a spoon for your baby to hold. Spoons with curved handles prevent your baby from pushing the spoon too far into his or her mouth.
- **Highchair**: You can use anything from an heirloom chair to a brand-new one with features like a one-hand tray release, a reclining seat, and so on. If you do use an heirloom chair, make sure it has a waist and crotch belt that prevents your baby from sliding out. Also, be aware that wooden chairs are harder to clean.
- **Travel feeding chair**: If your favorite restaurant doesn't stock highchairs, or your best friend is childless (and therefore gearless) but likes to invite your family for dinner, you'll find a travel feeding chair very handy. Many models fold up or collapse very small and are easy to tote with you.
- **Bibs**: You'll need a drawer full of them! For easy on and off, you may find Velcro closures convenient. For some foods, you'll almost want body armor! We had a long-sleeved bib for my son Nicolas when he ate watermelon. Without it, his arms and clothes would be soaked with melon juice and pulp!
- **Floor mat**: Some parents use an inexpensive plastic tablecloth; it can be hosed off if needed or tossed if it's beyond saving. At our house, we didn't bother with

a mat because we had a four-legged cleaning crew. (Our dogs loved having a baby in the house!) If you have a dog, you may want to keep it out of the kitchen until cleanup time.

Introducing Solid Foods: A Road Map

Timing Your Baby's First Meals

There's no specific time of day when babies accept new foods better. In the beginning, it's best to feed your baby solids when you're both in a sunny mood, well rested, and not sick. Babies don't do well with new experiences when they're already grumpy! Remember that you're creating more than a great picture for your baby's scrapbook; you're setting the foundation for future good eating habits. Relax and make it pleasant!

Most experts recommend starting with a small amount of breast milk or formula, then trying the new food, then finishing up with more breast milk or formula. This way your baby is hungry when you offer solids—but not too hungry. Remember that until your baby is one year old, solid foods are an addition to—not a replacement for—breast milk or formula.

Division of Responsibility

Do you ever find yourself pleading, "Just one more bite"? It may make *you* feel better if your child is a plate cleaner, but it's not healthy for your child.

Take a load off, Mom and Dad! You're responsible *only* for offering your child nutritious food when he or she is hungry. Your child is responsible for deciding whether to eat it and how much to eat.

Children have very good appetite control (unlike adults, who are often forced to eat by the clock). If left to their own devices, they'll eat when hungry and stop when full. If you try to force eating when your child is ready to stop, you may override your child's innate ability to eat exactly what his or her body needs. And if you mix emotions into meals, your child may learn to eat to make you happy—which isn't healthy physically or emotionally.

New Foods Protocol

During the next few months your baby will be trying many new foods. There's a certain protocol for introducing new foods; this protocol gives your baby a chance to get used to each new food and gives you a chance to assess your baby's reactions. Remember the following tips as you add foods to your baby's repertoire.

- Introduce only single-ingredient foods at first. For example, introduce carrots, wait a while, then introduce potatoes, wait a while, and so on. When you're sure there is no allergic reaction to either food, you can serve them mixed together.

- Wait three[2] to seven[3] days between introducing new foods to watch for signs of allergy: diarrhea, rash, or vomiting. (Experts disagree on how long you should wait. The standard recommendation is three to five days; waiting a bit longer is wise if you have allergies in your family.) Waiting also helps your baby get used to a new food before trying another one.

- Many parents offer a new food once and if their baby spits it out, it's ceremoniously crossed off the list of foods their baby will eat. Don't do this! It can take ten to fifteen tries for a baby to accept a new food. Why give up on the eighth try when your baby would have loved a food on the ninth?

Progression of Foods and Textures

Have you ever wondered why parenting books have different age ranges for introducing various foods and textures, or overlap ages in their feeding advice? It's because babies develop the skills they need to eat and show readiness to progress at different rates. The following charts combine developmental milestones with feeding skills to help you figure out how and when to introduce various foods and textures. Please use them as guides only—they're not written in stone!

Development and Feeding: 0 to 6 Months

Developmental Stage	Newborn	Young Infant	Sitter (Supported)
Approximate age	*0 to 1 month*	*1 to 4 months*	*About 6 months*
General development	Sleeps a lot; has little or no head control; keeps hands in tight fists; may turn head side to side when lying down	Pushes up on arms when lying on belly; opens and shuts hands; tries to bring hand to mouth; reaches for objects; may turn head side to side when lying down	Sits with support; brings hands and objects to mouth; turns head side to side
Feeding skills development	Roots reflexively; learns to coordinate sucking, swallowing, and breathing	Moves tongue forward and back to suck	Loses tongue-thrust reflex; moves food from front to back of mouth with tongue; closes mouth around spoon
Hunger signs	Early signs: rooting, lip smacking, sucking fingers; late sign: crying	Cries or fusses; smiles and looks at caregiver when eating	Cries or fusses; appears happy while eating
Fullness signs	Stops sucking; spits out nipple or falls asleep	Stops sucking; spits out nipple or falls asleep	Closes mouth; turns head side to side
Foods	Breast milk or formula only	Breast milk or formula only	Rice cereal or pureed meats
Textures	Liquids	Liquids	Semi-liquid at first, progressing to puréed, adding more texture as needed
Poop	After almost every feeding	Frequency slows down	More solid

Development and Feeding: 6 to 18 Months

Developmental Stage	Sitter (Independent)	Crawler	Stander/Walker	Walker/Runner
Approximate age	*6 to 8 months*	*8 to 10 months*	*10 to 12 months*	*12 to 18 months*
General development	Sits without help; is teething; sits well in highchair; may crawl	Is teething; crawls	Pulls up to standing; takes first steps	Walks; runs; says short phrases
Feeding skills development	Picks up food; holds food in hand; tries to hold cup	Transfers objects hand to hand; turns objects upside down; moves jaw in chewing motion	Picks up small objects with thumb and index finger (pincer grasp); wants to self-feed with spoon; bites through firmer textures; drinks through straw	Spoon-feeds self with finesse; upends cup on purpose; follows simple instructions
Hunger signs	Moves head toward spoon; points to food	Eagerly anticipates food; fusses if food doesn't come fast enough; reaches for food	Uses words or sounds to ask for food; fusses if food doesn't come fast enough	Uses words and phrases to express hunger
Fullness signs	Closes mouth and keeps it closed; pushes food away; slows down eating	Shakes head; pushes food away	Shakes head; says *no*	Uses words and phrases to express fullness: *all done, get down*; plays with food; throws plate or spoon
Foods	Barley and oat cereals, whole grain cereals, then vegetables and fruits, then egg yolk* at 7 months	Meats and other protein foods like legumes and soy,* combination foods, small amounts of yogurt* and cheese,* wheat cereal,* non-citrus juices, and finger foods	Diet similar to rest of family, with a few exceptions	Can add whole milk,* egg white,* citrus, and tomato, peanut and other nut butters* (mixed with mashed fruit to prevent choking)
Textures	Thin puréed, thicker puréed, soft mashed	Thicker puréed, ground, soft mashed with small lumps, crunchy foods that dissolve easily (cereal Os, teething biscuits)	Soft to moderate textures, lumpy foods, and bite-size table foods	Bite-size table food, finely chopped or ground meats
Poop	Stronger smelling, more varied in color	Sometimes contains seeds; diarrhea possible from excess juice	Sometimes contains undigested food like corn or tomato skin	Texture and frequency will reflect dietary habits

*If your baby has a family history of allergies, these foods should be introduced later: wheat and soy after one year; eggs after two years; peanuts, other nuts, and fish after three years.

Your Baby's First Food

During the second half of your baby's first year, the iron naturally stored in his or her body before birth gets used up. That's why your baby needs an iron-rich food around six months, when he or she starts eating solids. Most parents offer a fortified single-grain cereal; a few offer meat. Though meat is higher in iron and zinc than cereal, parents usually try cereal first—probably because it looks a lot more appetizing! However, you'll find that home-puréed meats like the ones in this book are very tasty and look more appealing than jarred meats, too.

There are three groups of infants who might benefit most from meat as a first food as opposed to cereal: breastfed infants, premature infants, and low birth weight infants. A recent study at the University of Colorado showed that a significant number of breastfed infants had marginal zinc and iron status. Introducing meat instead of cereal greatly increased zinc intake and appeared to increase head growth.[4] Research has shown breastfed babies to be equally accepting of meat and cereal as a first food. Though cereal looks better to adults, babies don't seem to prefer it.

Premature and low birth weight infants are prone to have less insulin sensitivity (also called insulin resistance)—this means the body needs to produce more of it to process glucose. Insulin resistance is a well-recognized abnormality that can eventually lead to adult-onset chronic disease like type 2 diabetes and coronary heart disease. A higher carbohydrate diet increases the body's need to produce insulin; it's possible that starting your infant with a high-protein food (meat) instead of a high-carbohydrate food (cereal) could, in the short term, temper insulin production.[5]

If you're starting with a grain, experts recommend trying rice cereal first, because it's the grain least likely to cause an allergic reaction in your baby.

Textures: Go with the Flow

It's pretty amazing: In twelve short months, your baby goes from only drinking liquids to eating almost everything the rest of the family eats. How will you know when your baby is ready to go from liquid to semi-solid to lumpy foods? You need to let your baby's development and cues guide you. Trust your parental instinct; it's usually right.

Cereal in a Bottle: Just Say No!

The first texture a baby eats is really a thickened liquid. So, why not just put the cereal in a bottle? There are a few good reasons why you shouldn't (unless your baby's doctor recommends it):

- Learning to eat from a spoon is an important developmental step that your baby won't learn if he or she drinks cereal. If your baby rejects spoon-feeding, this means that your baby isn't ready for solid foods—not that you should force the issue by using a different method.
- Babies who don't have a good suck-swallow reflex may inhale small particles of cereal into their lungs.
- If you feed cereal in a bottle, it may encourage your baby to eat more than he or she needs. Right now your baby is pretty good at matching the volume of breast milk or formula he drinks to his or her appetite. Cereal in a bottle increases the calories without increasing the volume of liquid, so your baby is tricked into eating more calories.

To adults, eating is second nature. You put the food in, you chew it up, and you swallow it. What could be simpler? It's not that simple for our children. From birth, babies are developing the many skills they need to eat like us. Eating involves many different processes: opening the mouth to let food in, coordinating breathing and swallowing, moving the tongue back and forth and side to side, holding the head up, chewing in a rotary motion, and putting food into the mouth.

Learning to eat is also a matter of losing certain reflexes. When babies are rid of their tongue-thrust reflex, they do a better job of keeping food in their mouth and moving food to the back of the mouth for swallowing. When babies lose their plantar grasp and develop the pincer grasp, picking up objects and self-feeding become much easier.

Here's a guide to the textures your baby will learn to eat, in the order he or she should try them:

- **Semi-liquid**: like thick milk
- **Thin purée**: like even thicker milk
- **Purée**: smooth food with no lumps
- **Mashed**: thick purée with some lumps
- **Chopped**: finely cut pieces of food, like meat
- **Cubed**: small pieces of soft food that can be picked up between thumb and finger

If at any time your baby seems uncomfortable with a new texture, go back a step. Your baby may spit out the food, make a funny face, or gag. If he doesn't gag, you can try another time or two to see if your baby just needs to get used to the new texture. If your baby still doesn't like it by the third try, wait a few days or a week.

Sample Menus for Babies of All Ages

The following chart suggests daily menus to help you plan a balanced and appropriate diet for your baby at various ages. Bear in mind, though, that there's no wrong or right time of day to give your baby different types of foods. You and your baby will find a way that works for you—and it may vary from day to day. Also keep in mind that babies and toddlers eat much smaller servings than adults!

Daily Intake

Every baby is different, but the following guide gives you an idea of how much of each food your baby might eat daily at various ages.

- **At the end of seven months**:
    - Up to ½ cup (125 milliliters) of dry cereal mixed with breast milk or formula
    - Up to 1 cup (250 milliliters) of fruits and vegetables (8 ounces total)
- **Eight to nine months**:
    - ¼ to ½ cup (60 to 125 milliliters) of dry cereal mixed with breast milk or formula

Sample Menus for Babies of All Ages

Meal	About 6 months	6 to 7 months	7 to 8 months	8 to 10 months	10 to 12 months	12 to 18 months	18 to 24 months
Rise and shine	Breast milk or formula	Breast milk or formula	Breast milk or formula	Breast milk or formula	Breast milk or formula		
Breakfast	Breast milk or formula, rice cereal	Breast milk or formula, oat or barley cereal	Breast milk or formula, cereal or egg yolk,* fruit	Cereal or egg yolk,* grain, fruit	Cereal or egg yolk,* grain, fruit	Whole milk,* cereal or egg,* grain, citrus fruit	Whole milk,* cereal or egg,* grain, citrus fruit
Snack	Breast milk or formula	Breast milk or formula	Breast milk or formula	Dairy,* fruit or veggie	Dairy,* fruit or veggie	Dairy,* fruit or grain	Dairy,* fruit or grain
Lunch	Breast milk or formula	Breast milk or formula, veggie	Breast milk or formula, fruit, veggie	Breast milk or formula, veggie, grain, protein	Breast milk or formula, veggie, grain, protein	Whole milk,* veggie, grain, protein	Whole milk,* veggie, 1 or 2 grains, fruit, protein
Snack	Breast milk or formula	Breast milk or formula	Breast milk or formula, fruit	Breast milk or formula, finger food, fruit or juice	Breast milk or formula, finger food, fruit or juice	Finger food, fruit or juice	Finger food, fruit or juice
Dinner	Breast milk or formula, rice cereal	Breast milk or formula, oat or barley cereal, fruit	Breast milk or formula, cereal, 1 or 2 veggies	Protein, 1 or 2 veggies, grain	Protein, 1 or 2 veggies, grain	Whole milk,* protein, grain, 2 veggies	Whole milk,* protein, grain, 2 veggies
Bedtime	Breast milk or formula	Breast milk or formula	Breast milk or formula	Breast milk or formula	Breast milk or formula		

*If your baby is at risk for allergies (or in the case of wheat, also a gluten intolerance), put this food off until later.

- 2 to 3 4-ounce (120-gram) jars of baby fruits and vegetables or 1 to 1½ cups (250 to 375 milliliters) puréed
- 1 to 2 ounces (30 to 60 grams) of puréed high-protein food (beef, lamb, pork, poultry, beans, or tofu)
- Up to 1 egg yolk per day
- 2 to 3 grain servings

- **Ten to twelve months**:
    - ½ cup (125 milliliters) of dry infant cereal or regular iron-fortified cereal
    - 1½ cups (375 milliliters) of fruit and vegetables
    - 1 to 2 ounces of chopped or puréed high-protein food (beef, lamb, pork, poultry, beans, or tofu)
    - Up to 1 egg yolk per day
    - 4 grain servings
    - 1 to 2 servings of yogurt or cheese (optional)

Guide to Commercial Baby Foods

If you visit the baby food aisle at your grocery store, many choices will meet you. Here's a summary of the different types of commercial baby foods you'll find.

- **Jarred baby foods**:
    - *Stage one/first foods–about six months*: These are puréed, strained single-ingredient foods that come in small 2.5-ounce portions, perfect for the beginning eater.
    - *Stage two/second foods–six to eight months*: These are also puréed but come in larger four-ounce jars and are often combinations of foods.
    - *Stage three/third foods–eight to ten months*: These come in six-ounce jars and offer more combinations that often include wheat and dairy. The texture is also thicker. The flavors are more complex, with three or more ingredients plus spices.
    - *Toddler foods–twelve months and older*: These have different names depending on the brand, but they're all diced foods and combination dinners with many ingredients, including salt.
- **Shelf-stable foods**: These microwaveable dinners and entrées are perfect for sending to daycare with an older baby or toddler.
- **Finger foods**:
    - *Diced fruits and veggies*: are available for older babies and toddlers. These soft, easy-to-grab foods are healthy and handy for older babies and toddlers.
    - *Cereal Os*: Earth's Best has a line of organic cereals that make great finger foods. Cheerios is a low-sugar, whole-grain mainstay that many parents can't do without! (You might also want to check out Oatios, a popular organic alternative.)

- *Gerber Fruit Puffs and Veggie Puffs*: These are puffed-up pieces of real fruits and veggies with no added ingredients. I think these taste delicious!
- *Meat sticks*: If your toddler doesn't like meat, these are alternatives. They are soft sausages that contain salt, but much less than conventional sausages. (Note: These are a choking hazard if not cut into smaller pieces.)
- *Crackers*: There's a large variety of teething crackers and other toddler-friendly crackers available.

Many parents choose to buy organic baby foods. For some, organics are a lifestyle choice for the whole family. Others are concerned about their baby's vulnerability to pesticide residues found in regular baby food. I think organic foods are a pretty good idea; I've used a combination of regular and organic foods for my family. But organics do tend to be pricey, so an all-organic diet is hard for most people to afford. (See pages 210–212 for other ways to reduce the pesticides in your child's diet.)

Earth's Best and Gerber Tender Harvest are organic baby food brands widely available in the United States. Earth's Best has the most variety and also uses only whole grains in their baby foods. Healthy Times has a line of organic jarred food as well as cereals, crackers, and cookies. Happy Baby Organic is a frozen baby food. All these brands are available at natural food grocers in the U.S. Heinz Organic, Earth's Best, Sweet Pea, and Bobo Baby are organic brands widely available in Canada. Around the world (especially in the United Kingdom) many other brands are available. Hipp (http://www.hipp.co.uk) is available all over Europe. If you live in a small town where organic brands aren't available, you can buy these products online: Earth's Best (http://www.earthsbest.com) and Healthy Times (http://www.healthytimes.com).

No GMOs

According to Greenpeace, Earth's Best, Heinz, and Baby Times foods are free of genetically modified organisms.

Beechnut offers a line of foods with added DHA and ARA called First Advantage. (See page 79 for more information on DHA and ARA.) The source of its DHA and ARA is egg yolk. According to Beechnut, one to two jars per day provides the same amount of DHA and ARA that a breastfed baby would get. If you're breastfeeding and you're vegan or you don't have a consistent source of DHA in your diet, First Advantage may be a good choice. If your baby drinks a formula with DHA and ARA, you don't need this type of baby food.

Breast Milk or Formula: Still the Main Dish

When you begin adding solids to your baby's diet, it should correspond with your baby's increased need for calories. Your baby should still drink about the same amount of breast milk or formula because those liquids are still the main source of important nutrients for your baby's growth and development.

As your baby gets older, more of his or her calories will come from food. For example, from six to eight months, complementary foods typically provide only about 130 calories a day. Their contribution increases to 300 calories per day at nine to eleven months and to 550 calories per day at twelve to twenty-three months. Between nine and twelve months, solids begin replacing some of the calories from breast milk or formula. So as your baby begins eating three meals a day, he or she may gradually reduce liquid feedings. This may translate to drinking six to eight ounces less formula, or perhaps one less breastfeeding session. However, your baby should not drink less than twenty ounces of formula or breast milk on a regular basis.

Chapter 9

Making Baby Food: The Basics

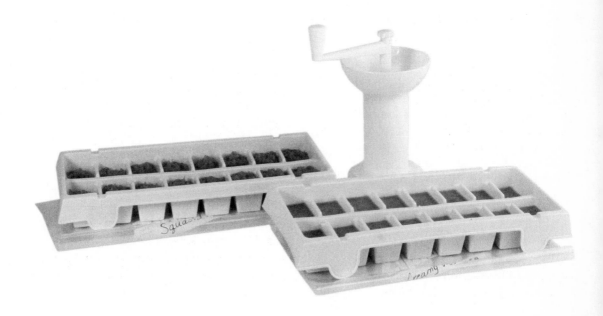

*I always wondered why babies
spend so much time sucking their thumbs.
Then I tasted baby food.*
—Robert Orben

This chapter describes the tools you'll need and the basic information you should know before you start making your own baby food. See chapters 11–15 for recipes.

Debbie made all of her son Parker's food with a blender starting when he was five and a half months old. "I thought it was the healthy way to go, being so much fresher. It's also a lot less expensive than jarred baby food," she explained. "It definitely takes more time than opening a jar. But the way I did it, in large quantities once a week, made it very simple."

Like Debbie, you may decide to make some or all of your baby's food for these reasons:

- You can better control what's in your baby's food.
- It's cheaper.
- It's better for the environment.
- You can use organic produce and natural meats and poultry.
- You can provide more variety than commercial baby foods do.
- You can make foods that fit with your culture.
- You can help your child get used to flavors and spices your family normally eats.

You may have grand intentions regarding baby food, but life can get in the way of great goals. You don't have to make *all* your baby's food if you just can't swing it. Anything you can make from scratch will benefit your baby. You can just make extra quantities of family foods here and there, pop them in the blender, and then freeze them in ice cube trays. For example, if your family loves broccoli but you can't find it in baby food jars and want your baby to get familiar with this food that appears often on your dinner table, make an extra pot whenever you cook broccoli. Purée it and store it and you have a month's supply!

One-Stop Shop

KidCo makes a complete line of baby food preparation and storage tools, from manual and electric baby food mills to freezer trays to covered microwavable feeding dishes. You can buy the tools individually or all in one kit. For more information, visit http://www.kidco.com.

Tools of the Trade

As with most endeavors, you can make baby food with simple tools that rely on elbow grease or fancy tools that rely on technology (and deeper pockets). The tools you need depend on how much food you plan to make and how much you want to spend. This section explains the basic jobs you'll need to do and the various tools that can help you do them.

Cooking

There are several ways you can cook your baby's food. Whichever way you choose, the key to retaining nutrients is to cook as little as possible in as little water as possible. (See page 191 for more information.) Any pot or pan will do, but here's some equipment that you might find especially useful.

- **Steamer**: A steamer can be anything from a metal colander or steamer basket over a pot of water to a stand-alone electric steamer to a microwave steamer. They all do the same thing—cook food using steam so no vitamins are lost in cooking water.

- **Microwave and microwave-safe containers**: A microwave cooks food quickly and also steams great! I often use a glass microwave plate and plastic wrap to cook vegetables—it takes only a few drops of water in the plate to steam them.

- **Crock-Pot**: This is a handy tool if you and your partner both work outside the home and you don't have much kitchen time. In the morning, put large chunks of food in the Crock-Pot with a squirt of water and set the pot on low heat. When you get home, toss the cooked food in a blender with the cooking water. Voilà—baby's dinner (and lots of extra for freezing) is ready in minutes! The Crock-Pot works great for batches of beans, roasts, and other foods that take a while to cook—steam your veggies later.

> ### Tales from the Trenches: Janet and Ellicea
>
> Ellicea ate only seven jars of baby food her first year. Her mom, Janet, made her first foods in a blender and froze them in ice cube trays. "We were eating organic and natural foods, and I wanted to give my daughter the same," she explained. As Ellicea got older, Janet varied the texture of her foods by blending the food less or pulsing it. Ellicea's favorite meals were garbanzo beans and mixed broccoli and carrots—she didn't take to eating meat until after her first year.

Puréeing and Chopping

Manual Tools

The following tools are great for low-budget baby food making. Some of these tools are also handy when you're out and about, because they don't need electricity.

- **Fork**: When your baby is just starting solids, a fork works well for bananas, avocados, and other very soft foods. Later, you can use it when your baby needs thicker textures.

- **Baby food mill**: This small plastic device has a handle at the top, which you turn to push the food through the mill. It works well for making small amounts of food. (For example, it's great for making your baby's food from what's on the dinner table.) Some models come with a carrying case, which makes it convenient for traveling or eating out.

- **Small food mill**: This mill is a little bigger than a baby food mill and allows you to make larger amounts. It has a fine disc for puréeing and removing seeds. It's made of stainless steel, so it's very durable.

- **Large food mill**: Large food mills (also stainless steel) can hold up to four quarts and come with fine, medium, and coarse discs. The different discs let you make different textures as your baby grows.

- **Potato ricer**: This tool looks like a giant garlic press. You push the food through, and it comes out looking like long grains of rice. It's good for when your baby is ready for thicker textures.

- **Purée sieve**: This tool is similar to a food mill. It has a very fine mesh screen to finely purée foods.
- **Strainer**: If you use a food mill without a screen to remove seeds, and you like to make fruit purée using fruits with seeds, like strawberries or blackberries, you'll need a fine-mesh strainer.
- **Food chopper**: A manual food chopper is a great tool for dicing finger foods for your baby, and it's hard to over-chop with one.

Electric Tools

- **Baby food processor**: This small food processor makes 3.5 ounces at a time. It's perfect for single servings of food puréed from your dinner table.
- **Blender**: Chances are you already have a blender, and it's perfect for making big batches of puréed baby foods or for grinding up dry, whole-grain cereals. (However, it's not convenient if you just want to make a few small portions.)
- **Hand blender**: This tool is great when you want to purée food as you cook. You can use it right in the pan, which makes cleanup a lot easier. It also works well for making soups, sauces, and smoothies. Some come with a whisk attachment for whipping, too. (I used the Braun hand blender for most of the recipes in this book and absolutely loved it—it puréed foods in seconds!)
- **Mini food chopper**: This tool is good for more coarsely chopped food, especially meat.
- **Food processor**: Many kitchens today are already equipped with food processors. Like a blender, this tool is best when you are making a big batch of baby food. A processor is a little more versatile than a blender, as it allows a wider range of textures. It's especially good for chopping meats. You can use a food processor for making fine whole-grain cereals. As your baby gets older and starts eating nuts, you can use a food processor to make your own nut butters.
- **Electric food mill**: For those who can't easily turn the crank on a manual mill, electric ones are available.
- **Hand mixer**: You know that big mixer on your counter—the one you don't have time to use anymore? Well, you can buy a variety of attachments to use for making your own baby food (or you may already have them tucked away and just didn't know what to use them for).

> **Tales from the Trenches: Sallee and Shelby**
>
> Sallee makes her daughter Shelby's baby food. Like many parents, she's concerned about pesticides in food. She has a history of food allergies, too. She feels she can better control what's in Shelby's food if she buys organic and makes it herself.

Storing

Now you've got a chopper, a steamer, and a blender. You're all ready to cook and purée, but what will you put your baby's food in once you've made it? Here are some suggestions:

- **Ice cube trays**: If you don't already have these, they're cheap—and they make perfect baby-size portions.
- **Baby food storage trays**: These are one step better than ice cube trays because each tray has a lid to protect the food from freezer odors and freezer burn. Because of the lids, the trays stack easily. Each compartment holds one ounce.
- **Baby cubes**: These cubes are individual one-ounce containers with attached lids that can go from the freezer to the microwave. They fit in a tray and can also be stacked.
- **Food storage containers**: We all have these in our cabinets, but most are too big for baby food. If you do use these, use ones that are smaller than three inches high—any deeper and food will take too long to cool safely. Particularly useful are ones that can go from freezer to microwave.
- **Cookie sheet**: An alternative to the cube method of freezing baby food is the "plop" method. Simply plop one- to two-tablespoon portions on a cookie sheet and freeze.
- **Small freezer zipper bags**: Freezer bags are perfect for storing frozen cubes or plops of baby food, as well as single portions of finger foods like chicken pieces or chopped veggies.

Tales from the Trenches:
Ana and Michael and Grandma

"When my mom saw me opening up jars of baby food for Michael, she was disgusted," said Ana. "When I was a baby in Spain, she boiled potatoes, a tiny bit of garlic, and a little olive oil for me. For Michael she puréed a week's supply. When he could eat more texture, she would combine the potatoes with chicken and carrots. Whenever she cooked dinner, she would keep some food separate and cook it longer until it was soft enough for Michael. Thanks to my mom, my kids are not picky eaters. They love my mom's cooking!"

Healthy Baby Food How-To

Cooking to Keep the Vitamins

Many parents make their own baby food because they think it will be fresher. Maybe it will, maybe it won't—it depends on how fresh your food is to begin with and how quickly you prepare it. Jarred baby food is generally processed soon after picking. To make sure your homemade baby food is at least that fresh, follow these tips:

- If you're going to prepare baby food from fresh produce, try to buy it no sooner than the day before you plan to prepare it. Buying from a farmer's market or food co-op can help guarantee freshness. And of course, picking fruits and veggies from your own garden or a you-pick farm is the freshest option of all.
- Keep bananas, avocados, tomatoes, and other soft fruits at room temperature until they reach peak ripeness.
- Don't wash produce until you're ready to prepare it.

- Chop foods before you cook them; they'll cook quicker and will retain more nutrients.
- Cook as little as necessary. Steaming or cooking in the microwave with a tablespoon of water preserves the most vitamins.

Keeping Things Clean and Safe

Your baby or toddler's immune system is still immature, so he or she is more vulnerable to food-borne illness and other contaminants than adults or older kids are. Use the following precautions when making your baby's food. For more information about food safety, see Chapter 10.

- Wash produce well, using a produce rinse like Fit to help remove pesticides. Some foods, like grapes, spinach, and strawberries, come clean better when soaked in water for a few minutes. You'll be shocked at the dirt you find at the bottom of the bowl.
- Wash your hands in warm soapy water before preparing food and after using the bathroom, changing diapers, blowing your nose, and handling pets. For best results, wet your hands, apply soap, rub your hands together for twenty seconds, then rinse thoroughly. (That's roughly one verse of "Happy Birthday to You.")

- Keep food prep utensils and cutting boards used for raw meats, poultry, and fish separate from those that'll be used for raw fruit or vegetables.
- Wash cutting boards, knives, utensils, and countertops with hot soapy water after preparing each food item and before going on to the next one.
- Blenders can be hard to clean; they have lots of nooks and crannies to hide food. Take your blender apart after each use and wash each part separately, using a brush if necessary. (A bottle brush is ideal for scrubbing tall blender pitchers.) Thoroughly dry the parts (or let them air-dry) before putting them back together.
- Use plastic or other non-porous cutting boards. Wash cutting boards in a dishwasher or in hot soapy water after use.
- When you're cooking meat, test doneness with a food thermometer. That way you don't have to guess whether it's cooked to the right temperature.

Tales from the Trenches: Neat versus Clean

I'm not really a neat cook, but I'm meticulously clean. What's the difference?

I tend to use a lot of utensils, bowls, and so on, and unfortunately I never really learned to clean as I go—except when it comes to germs. When I break an egg or touch raw meat, I wash my hands immediately! When I spill fish juice or raw egg on the counter, I wipe it up with a paper towel and follow it up with an anti-bacterial wipe. Yeah, I really do use a different cutting board for raw meat and produce. And when I drop lettuce in the sink while washing it, it goes in the trash.

Some people accuse me of being a little over-the-top on this topic. But I figure you just can't be too careful about food safety—especially when it comes to your children, who are extra vulnerable.

Now, if only I could translate that meticulousness into neatness!

Homemade Baby Food Storage Guide[1]

Food	Refrigerator (40°F or 4°C)	Freezer (0°F or -18°C)
Cooked fruits and veggies	1 to 2 days	6 to 8 months
Cooked meat, poultry, fish, and eggs	24 hours	1 to 2 months
Frozen fruits and veggies that are thawed	2 days	Do not refreeze.
Cooked meat, poultry, or fish that has been thawed	24 hours	Do not refreeze.

- Store raw meat, poultry, and seafood on the bottom shelf of your refrigerator to minimize drips onto other food.
- Never place cooked food on a plate that previously held raw meat, poultry, or seafood.
- Make sure storage containers are clean.
- Consider using paper towels to clean kitchen surfaces. If you use cloths, wash them often in the hot cycle of your washing machine. If you use sponges, wash them in the dishwasher and replace them often.
- Avoid leaving any raw meat, poultry, or fish at room temperature.
- Refrigerate cooked foods after a brief cooling period.
- Follow the guide above when storing homemade baby food in your refrigerator or freezer.

Making Different Textures

Following is a description of the various baby food textures you should make for your child as he or she learns to eat solid foods. The exact timing of this progression isn't important, and your baby should guide it. It *is* very important, though, that you do progress the texture in your baby's food as he or she masters each step.

- **Thin purée**: Your baby's first food will be a very smooth purée. To purée food, you should use a blender, food processor, or food mill. You'll need to add some liquid to thin the purée. Use reserved cooking liquid, breast milk, or formula. Like your baby's first cereal or meat meal, his or her first vegetable or fruit meal should be a thick liquid.
- **Thick purée**: Once your baby gets used to a thin purée and is skilled at closing his or her mouth around a spoon, you can make thicker purées by adding less liquid. Let your baby be your guide—if the thick purée seems to be gagging your child, then add a bit more liquid.
- **Mashed**: This texture is the consistency of mashed potatoes. For thick purées and mashed food, you can use a fork or potato masher.
- **Chunky**: When your baby has a few teeth (or is very good at gumming) and is developmentally able to go through the motions of chewing, it's a good time to introduce chunkier foods. Stews and casseroles are great for this stage; sauce

mixed with chunks helps the chunks go down. You'll still need to cut up large chunks of food into smaller pieces.

- **Diced family fare**: Finally, your baby has graduated to eating everything the family eats—cut into pieces he or she can easily chew and swallow. (You'll need to continue to finely chop some meats until your baby has his or her molars.) It's inevitable at this point that your baby will be eating foods with salt. To prevent sodium overload, cook with a minimum of salt (and don't serve too many high-sodium convenience foods).

Chapter 10

Food Safety for Babies and Toddlers

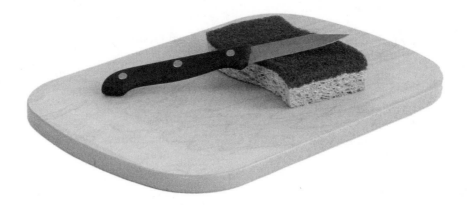

Let your food be your medicine, and your medicine be your food.
—Hippocrates

Food-Borne Illness

Food-borne illness is increasing all over the world. The U.S. Centers for Disease Control and Prevention (CDC) estimates 76 million Americans suffer from food-borne illnesses each year, accounting for 325,000 hospitalizations and more than 5,000 deaths.[1] In Canada there are an estimated 11 to 13 million food-borne illnesses annually,[2] and in Australia there are an estimated 4 million cases each year.[3]

Babies and young children are more vulnerable than adults because their immature immune systems can't fight off infection as well. Every year, at least 800,000 children under ten years old in the U.S. get sick from food poisoning.

The Clean-Kitchen Quiz[4]

What comes to mind when you think of a clean kitchen? Shiny waxed floors? Gleaming stainless steel sinks? Spotless counters and neat cupboards? These things can help, but a truly clean kitchen—one that ensures safe food—doesn't just look great; it also uses safe food practices. Preventing food-borne illness at home depends on proper food storage, handling, and cooking.

To see how clean your kitchen is, take the following quiz. For each question, choose the answer that best describes the practice in your household. Then read on to learn how you can make all the meals and snacks from your kitchen as safe as possible.

Questions

1. **The temperature of our refrigerator is:**
   a. 50°F (10°C)
   b. 40°F (5°C)
   c. A mystery

2. **The last time we had stew or another cooked food with meat, chicken, or fish in it left over, we:**
   a. Cooled the food to room temperature, then put it in the refrigerator
   b. Put the food in the refrigerator immediately after it was served
   c. Left the food at room temperature overnight or longer

3. **The last time we sanitized our kitchen sink drain, disposal, and connecting pipe was:**
   a. Last night
   b. Several weeks ago
   c. Never

4. **When we use a cutting board to cut raw meat, poultry, or fish and then want to use it for another food, we:**
   a. Reuse it as is
   b. Wipe it with a damp cloth
   c. Wash it with soap and hot water
   d. Wash it with soap and hot water then sanitize it

5. **The last time we had hamburgers at home, I ate mine:**
   a. Rare (140°F/60°C)
   b. Medium (160°F/71°C)
   c. Well-done (170°F/77°C)

6. **The last time there was cookie dough in our house, the dough was:**
   a. Made with raw eggs, and I sampled some
   b. Made with raw eggs and refrigerated, and I sampled some
   c. Store-bought, and I sampled some
   d. Not sampled until baked

7. **We clean our kitchen counters and other food preparation surfaces with:**
   a. Water
   b. Hot water and soap
   c. Hot water and soap, then a bleach solution
   d. Hot water and soap, then a commercial sanitizing agent

8. **When we wash dishes at our house, they're:**
   a. Washed and dried in an automatic dishwasher
   b. Left to soak in the sink for several hours, then washed with soap in the same water
   c. Washed right away with hot water and soap, then air-dried
   d. Washed right away with hot water and soap, then immediately towel-dried

9. **The last time I handled raw meat, poultry, or fish, I cleaned my hands afterward by:**
   a. Wiping them on a towel
   b. Rinsing them under hot, cold, or warm tap water
   c. Washing them with soap and warm water

10. **We defrost meat, poultry, and fish by:**
   a. Setting them on the counter
   b. Placing them in the refrigerator
   c. Microwaving them

11. **When we buy fresh seafood, we:**
   a. Buy only fish that's refrigerated or well-iced
   b. Take it home immediately and put it in the refrigerator
   c. Sometimes buy it straight out of a local fisher's creel

12. **I realize people should be especially careful not to eat raw seafood if they have:**
   a. Diabetes
   b. Human immunodeficiency virus (HIV) infection
   c. Cancer
   d. Liver disease

Answers and Explanations

1. **Refrigerators should stay at 40°F (5°C) or less, so if you chose answer b, give yourself two points.** If you didn't, you're not alone. According to Robert Buchanan, senior science advisor and director of science in the Food and Drug Administration's (FDA's) Center for Food Safety and Applied Nutrition (CFSAN), many people overlook the importance of maintaining an appropriate refrigerator temperature. "According to surveys, in many households the refrigerator temperature is above 50°F (10°C)," he said. His advice: Measure the temperature with a thermometer and adjust the control dial if necessary. A temperature of 40°F (5°C) or less is important because it slows the growth of most bacteria. It won't kill bacteria, but it will keep them from multiplying, and the fewer there are, the less likely you are to get sick. Freezing at 0°F (-18°C) or less stops bacterial growth (although it won't kill bacteria already present).

2. **You should refrigerate hot foods promptly; give yourself two points if you picked answer b.** Refrigerate hot foods as soon as possible within two hours after cooking. But don't keep the food if it's been sitting out for more than two hours (one hour if the temperature is over 90°F [32°C]). Don't taste-test it, either. Even a small amount of contaminated food can make you sick. Date leftovers so you can use them within a safe time. Generally, leftover cooked food is safe when refrigerated for three to five days. If in doubt, throw it out, says FDA microbiologist Kelly Bunning: "It's not worth a food-borne illness for the small amount of food usually involved."

3. **Your kitchen sink's drain needs occasional sanitizing. If answer a best describes your practice, give yourself two points. Give yourself one point if you chose answer b.** According to John Guzewich, CFSAN's director of emergency coordination and response, people often overlook their kitchen sink drain, disposal, and connecting pipe, where food particles get trapped and combine with moisture to create an ideal environment for bacterial growth. You should sanitize this apparatus periodically by pouring a solution of one teaspoon (five milliliters) of chlorine bleach in one quart (about one liter) of water (or a commercial kitchen cleaning agent) down the sink.

4. **Cutting boards are major cross-contamination culprits. If you chose answer d, give yourself two points.**
   If you picked answer a, you're violating an important food safety rule: Never let raw meat, poultry, or fish come in contact with other foods. Answers b and c aren't good either. Washing with a damp cloth won't remove bacteria. And washing only with soap and water may not do the job. To prevent cross-contamination from a cutting board, the FDA advises these practices:

   - Use smooth cutting boards made of hard maple or a non-porous material like plastic that are free of cracks and crevices. Hard, smooth boards are easier to clean. Avoid boards made of soft, porous materials.

   - Wash cutting boards with hot water, soap, and a scrub brush to remove food particles. Then sanitize the boards by running them through an automatic dishwasher or rinsing them in a solution of one teaspoon (five milliliters) of chlorine bleach in one quart (about one liter) of water.

- Always wash and sanitize cutting boards after using them for raw foods and before using them for ready-to-eat foods. Consider dedicating one cutting board to foods that will be cooked and another to ready-to-eat foods. For those into gadgets, check out Rachael Ray's Clean-Cut Cutting Board. It features a sturdy wood base with six color-coded plastic cutting mats to be used for different types of foods to prevent cross-contamination. (You may not need all six, but the different colors are a good reminder to not cross-contaminate.) You might also consider using disposable cutting sheets, for especially messy prep or when you don't have time to clean up properly.

5. **Eating rare ground beef is never a good idea. Give yourself two points if you picked answer b or c.** Ground beef isn't safe to eat unless you cook it to an internal temperature of 160°F (71°C). Using a food thermometer is crucial, the U.S. Department of Agriculture (USDA) says, because one out of every four burgers turns brown before it has reached a safe internal temperature. Research also shows that some ground meat patties cooked to 160°F or higher may remain

Safe Cooking Temps for Meat, Eggs, and Seafood

- Ground beef, veal, pork, and lamb: 160°F (71°C)
- Poultry (whole, ground, and pieces): 165°F (74°C)
- Egg dishes: 160°F (71°C)
- Fish and seafood: 145°F (63°C)
- Ground or flaked fish, as in a fish cake: at least 155°F (68°C)
- Stuffed fish: 165°F (74°C)
- Sauces and custards: 160°F (71°C)
- Casseroles and leftovers: 165°F (74°C)

Seafood Cooking Tips

Cooking seafood is a bit tricky. It's easy to overcook, and sometimes it's too thin to check the temperature easily. Here are a few tips to help you determine whether seafood is safely cooked:

- When microwaving seafood, rotate the dish several times to ensure even cooking. Follow recommended standing times. After the standing time, check the seafood in several spots with a meat thermometer to be sure it has reached the proper internal temperature.

- For fish, slip the point of a sharp knife into the flesh and pull it aside. The edges should be opaque and the center slightly translucent, with flakes beginning to separate. Let the fish stand three to four minutes to finish cooking.
- Use the ten-minute rule: Measure fish at its thickest point and cook it for ten minutes per inch of thickness. Bake it at 450°F (232°C), broil it two to four inches from heat, or grill it four to six inches above heat. Turn it once halfway during cooking time. Add five minutes to cooking time if fish is in foil or in a sauce. Double the cooking time if you begin with frozen fish.[5]
- For shrimp, lobster, and scallops, check color. Shrimp and lobster turn red and their flesh becomes pearly opaque. Scallops turn milky white or opaque and firm.
- For clams, mussels, and oysters, watch for the point at which their shells open; this means they're done. Boil three to five minutes longer. Throw out those that stay closed.

pink inside. Thus the color of cooked ground beef alone isn't a reliable indicator of its safety. When you're eating out, order your hamburger well-done to be on the safe side.

6. **Eggs can contain salmonella bacteria, so you should always cook foods that contain raw egg. If you answered a or b, you're risking salmonellosis.** Cooking eggs or egg-containing foods to an internal temperature of at least 160°F (71°C) kills any salmonella bacteria that might be in the eggs. Refrigerating won't. So answer d—eating the baked product only—will earn you two points. Commercial cookie dough is usually made with pasteurized eggs (eggs that have been heated enough to kill bacteria) and may also contain an acidifying agent that kills bacteria. But the best practice, even when using products containing pasteurized eggs, is to eat the foods only as they're intended to be eaten. So answer c won't earn you any points. Consider using pasteurized eggs for homemade recipes that aren't cooked, such as eggnog or Caesar salad dressing. Here are two more tips to ensure egg safety:

   • Buy only refrigerated eggs, and keep them refrigerated until you're ready to cook and serve them.

   • When you're frying, poaching, or boiling eggs, cook until both the yolk and white are firm; when you're scrambling eggs, cook until there's no visible liquid egg.

7. **Water alone may get rid of visible dirt, but not bacteria. Answers c and d will earn you two points each; answer b, one point.** According to CFSAN director John Guzewich, bleach and commercial kitchen cleaning agents are the best sanitizers—provided they're diluted according to product directions. Hot water and soap does a good job, too, but may not kill all strains of bacteria. Also, be sure to launder dishcloths often in hot water. Wet kitchen cloths can harbor bacteria and spread it around.

8. **Prompt dishwashing and air-drying is your best bet. Answers a and c are worth two points each.** There are potential problems with b and d. When you let dishes sit in water for a long time, it creates a bacteria soup. Automatic dishwashers avoid this problem and also wash and dry dishes very effectively by using high water pressure and heat. When you're washing dishes by hand, it's best to wash them all within two hours. Also, it's best to air-dry them so you don't handle them (and spread bacteria) while they're wet.

9. **Raw meat, poultry, and fish can contain dangerous bacteria, so when you handle them, you need to make sure you don't spread it. The only correct practice is answer c. Give yourself two points if you picked it.** Wash your hands with warm water and soap for at least twenty seconds before and after handling food—especially raw meat, poultry, and fish. If you have an infection or cut on your hands, wear rubber or plastic gloves. Wash gloved hands just as often as bare hands.

10. **Leaving raw meat, poultry, or fish at room temperature is a recipe for disaster. Give yourself two points if you picked b or c.** Food safety experts recommend

thawing these foods in a refrigerator or microwave, or putting the food in a watertight plastic bag submerged in cold water and changing the water every thirty minutes. Gradual defrosting overnight in the refrigerator is best because it helps maintain quality. When microwaving, follow package directions. Leave about two inches (about five centimeters) between the food and the inside surface of the microwave to let heat circulate. Smaller items defrost more evenly than larger ones. Foods defrosted in the microwave oven should be cooked immediately after thawing. Do not thaw meat, poultry, or fish on the counter or in the sink without cold water; bacteria can multiply rapidly at room temperature. You should also marinate food in the refrigerator, not on the counter. Discard the marinade after use because it contains raw juices, which may harbor bacteria. If you want to use the marinade as a dip or sauce, set aside a portion before adding raw food.

Tips for Choosing Safe Seafood

- Don't buy cooked seafood displayed in the same case as raw fish. Or at least make sure the raw fish is on a level lower than the cooked fish, so the raw fish juices don't flow onto the cooked items and contaminate them.
- Don't buy frozen seafood if the packages are open, torn, or crushed on the edges. If the package cover is transparent, look for signs of frost or ice crystals. This could mean that the fish has been stored for a long time or has been thawed and refrozen.
- If you plan to use seafood within two days after purchase, store it in the coldest part of your refrigerator, usually under the freezer compartment or in a special meat keeper. Avoid packing it in tightly with other items; let air circulate freely around the package. Otherwise, wrap it tightly in moisture-proof freezer paper or foil to protect it from air leaks and store it in the freezer.
- Discard shellfish if they die during storage or if their shells crack or break. Live shellfish close up when the shell is tapped.

11. **Fresh seafood should always be sold cold. Answers a and b are both correct; Give yourself two points for either.** When you're buying fresh seafood, buy only from reputable dealers who keep their products refrigerated or properly iced. Be wary of vendors selling fish out of a canvas bag or out of the back of a truck. Once you buy the seafood, immediately put it on ice, in your refrigerator, or in your freezer.

12. **Various diseases make eating raw seafood especially dangerous. Give yourself two points for knowing one or more of these risky conditions.** People with the following diseases and conditions need to be especially careful to avoid raw seafood because their diseases or the medicines they take may put them at risk for serious illness or death from contaminated seafood.

- Liver disease from any cause
- Hemochromatosis (an iron disorder)
- Diabetes
- Stomach problems, including previous stomach surgery and low stomach acid (for example, from antacid use)

- Cancer
- Immune disorders, including HIV
- Long-term steroid use, as for asthma and arthritis

What's Your Clean-Kitchen Rating?

24 points: Bacteria doesn't stand much of a chance in your kitchen. Feel confident about the food you make and eat in your home.

12 to 23 points: Take a closer look at food safety practices in your home. You're violating some key rules.

11 points or fewer: Your current practices are putting you in danger of food-borne illness. Correct your family's food handling, storage, and cooking techniques right away.

Food-Borne Illness Prevention Primer

Common Bacteria Affecting Kids

The following bacteria are common causes of food-borne illness in children.

- **Salmonella** infects about 1.4 million people and causes six hundred deaths each year; an antibiotic-resistant strain is now the second most common type of salmonella found in the U.S. Salmonella is more likely to sicken children under five years; it infects thirteen times more children than adults. According to the CDC, reptiles, including turtles, are a common carrier of salmonella and are not recommended as pets for small children, nor should they be in the same house as an infant.[6] Salmonella is most often associated with eating raw or undercooked eggs, poultry, and beef, or by foods and objects that have been cross-contaminated with infected foods. Fruit at room temperature that comes in contact with salmonella is the perfect carrier—especially when it's not washed before eating.

- **Campylobacter** is the leading cause of bacterial diarrhea in children. It can be caused by handling raw poultry, eating undercooked poultry, or drinking non-chlorinated water or unpasteurized milk. Cattle and poultry waste are often the source of the bacteria that causes this illness, but it can also be spread by cat and dog poop.

- **Yersinia** most often causes illness in children less than a year old—often from eating raw and undercooked pork products. The preparation of raw pork intestines (chitterlings) may be particularly risky, especially if an infant's caretaker prepares chitterlings and doesn't adequately wash his or her hands before handling the infant or the infant's toys, food, or pacifier.

Fight Bac!

Clean: Wash hands and surfaces often.

Separate: Don't cross-contaminate.

Cook: To proper temperatures.

Chill: Refrigerate promptly.

- **E. coli 0157:H7**: There are hundreds of mostly harmless strains of E. coli; this dangerous strain was discovered in the United States in 1982. E. coli lives in the intestines of healthy cattle, deer, goats, and sheep; the organism can be mixed into meat when it is ground. Undercooked ground beef has been the most common cause of infection. Illness with E. coli 0157:H7 has also been caused by eating sprouts, lettuce, spinach, unpasteurized milk and juice, and by swimming in or drinking sewage-contaminated water.

The Basics

Here are some basic tips to help you protect your family from food-borne illness:[7]

<aside>

Off-Limits for Baby

Several foods pose a particular danger of food-borne illness to babies:

- **Honey**: Don't let your child have any until one year. Honey may contain botulism spores that affect babies, but not older children.
- **Unpasteurized soft cheeses**: To make sure a cheese is safe, look for the term *pasteurized milk* on the label.
- **Raw sprouts**: See page 204.
- **Undercooked hamburger**: No one in your family should be eating this!
- **Deli meats**: Don't give these to your baby or toddler unless you've heated them to steaming.

</aside>

- Wash your hands carefully before preparing food. Remove jewelry and use a nail brush.
- Wash your hands, utensils, and kitchen surfaces with hot soapy water after they touch raw meat or poultry. (See page 200 for more info.)
- Cook beef, poultry, and eggs thoroughly. (See page 199.)
- Eat cooked food promptly and refrigerate leftovers within two hours after cooking. (See page 198.)
- Wash all fruits and vegetables thoroughly—even those you plan to peel or cook.
- Drink only pasteurized milk and juice and clean drinking water.
- Wash your hands carefully for twenty seconds after using the bathroom, changing a diaper, blowing your nose (or someone else's), or cleaning up animal poop.

Here are some tips especially for parents:

- Wash your hands before every nursing session.
- Dry, cracked hands (a common result of frequent hand-washing) provide a perfect route for bacteria and viruses to enter your body. Keep your hands hydrated with lotion. A dispenser next to the sink will remind you.
- When you express breast milk for your baby, follow the storage guidelines on page 114. Offer only small amounts at a time to avoid waste.
- If your baby is formula-fed, follow the formula feeding and storage guidelines on page 89.

Sprout Safety

If you're into health, you know that sprouts are *really* good for you. Broccoli sprouts, for example, have twenty times the cancer-fighting substance sulforaphane glucosinolate than mature broccoli has.

If you're a sprout eater, you're probably discouraged to hear that sprouts are one of the many foods associated with E. coli and that they're not recommended for high-risk groups. The good news is that almost all cases of bacteria in sprouts can be traced back to the seed. Not all seeds used for sprouts are grown just for food production.

Picture this: Healthy, grass-fed beef are grazing (and pooping) in the alfalfa field. When alfalfa season is over and the field goes to seed, the seeds are harvested and sold for various purposes—including for growing sprouts. Those contaminated with E. coli from cow poop will go on to grow into contaminated sprouts. Not a pretty picture.

Growing sprouts from seeds that are produced for food production prevents this problem. Buying sprouts (or seeds, if you sprout your own) from a company that uses organic seeds and rigorous growing conditions substantially decreases your risk of food-borne illness from sprouts.

Brassica Protection Products is a company created by scientists at Johns Hopkins University School of Medicine to ensure that food products made from plants (including sprouts) are produced under strict food safety standards. For more information about Brassica sprouts, see http://www.broccosprouts.com. Another source for organic seed that is tested for bacteria is http://www.sproutpeople.com.

- It's difficult, but wash your child's hands as often as you can. Use an alcohol hand sanitizer when soap and water aren't available. Babies and toddlers touch a lot of dirty things like dog toys and the floor and then put their hands in their mouths—whether they're eating or not!

- Look for more tips on preventing food borne illness in Chapters 11 through 16.

Produce Safety

From 1990 to 2003, more cases of food poisoning resulted from eating produce than from any other food! In late 2006, there were several large outbreaks of E. coli and salmonella from produce. Since you should be eating lots of fruits and veggies, it's important to handle produce safely. Here's how:[8]

Check

- Make sure the fresh fruits and vegetables you buy aren't bruised or damaged.

- Make sure fresh cut fruits and vegetables like packaged salads and melons are refrigerated at the store before you buy them. Don't let your child eat a sample of fresh produce at the store unless it's on ice.

Clean

- Starting with clean hands, rinse fresh produce under running tap water, including those with skins and rinds you don't plan to eat. Wash produce just before eating.

- Scrub firm-skinned produce like cantaloupe with a clean produce brush.

- Dry rinsed produce with a clean cloth towel or paper towel.

- Never use detergent or bleach to wash fresh produce; these products aren't meant for human consumption. Special produce washes like Fit are okay to use.

Separate

- When you're shopping, separate fresh produce from household chemicals and raw foods in your cart and in your bags.
- Keep fresh produce away from raw meat, poultry, and seafood in your refrigerator, too.
- Use a clean cutting board for preparing produce that will be eaten raw.

Cook

- Cook or throw away produce that has touched raw meat, poultry, seafood, or their juices.

Chill

- Refrigerate all cut, peeled, or cooked fresh produce within two hours.

Throw Away

- Throw away fresh produce that hasn't been refrigerated within two hours of cutting, peeling, or cooking.
- Cut out and throw away bruised or damaged portions of fruits and vegetables when preparing to cook them or before eating them raw.
- Throw away any produce that won't be cooked after touching raw meat, poultry, or seafood.
- If in doubt, throw it out!

Cold Food Storage Guide

Copy this chart and stick it on your fridge to remind you how long you can safely keep refrigerated or frozen food. (Recommended freezer storage times aim to preserve a food's taste and nutrient content; they're more for food quality than food safety.)

Food Safety Resources by Phone

FDA/CFSAN Information Line
888-SAFEFOOD (888-723-3366)
Recorded messages are available twenty-four hours a day. Information specialists are available Monday through Friday from 10:00 A.M. to 4:00 P.M. Eastern time.

USDA Meat and Poultry Hotline
888-MPHOTLINE (888-674-6854)
Recorded messages in English and Spanish are available twenty-four hours a day. Food safety specialists are Monday through Friday from 10:00 A.M. to 4:00 P.M. Eastern time.

Cold Food Storage Guide

Food	Refrigerator (40°F or 4°C)	Freezer (0°F or -18°C)
Eggs		
Fresh in shell	3 to 5 weeks	Don't freeze
Raw yolks or whites	2 to 4 days	1 year
Hard-boiled	1 week	Don't freeze well
Ground Meat and Stew Meat		
Hamburger or stew meat	1 to 2 days	3 to 4 months
Ground turkey, veal, pork, lamb, and mixtures	1 to 2 days	3 to 4 months
Fresh Beef, Veal, Lamb, and Pork		
Steaks	3 to 5 days	6 to 12 months
Chops	3 to 5 days	4 to 6 months
Roasts	3 to 5 days	4 to 12 months
Stuffed, uncooked pork chops, lamb chops, or chicken breast	1 day	Doesn't freeze well
Soups and Stews		
Any kind	3 to 4 days	2 to 3 months
Meat Leftovers		
Cooked meat and casseroles	3 to 4 days	2 to 3 months
Gravy and meat broth	1 to 2 days	2 to 3 months
Fresh Poultry		
Whole chicken or turkey	1 to 2 days	1 year
Chicken or turkey pieces	1 to 2 days	3 to 4 months
Cooked Poultry		
Pieces or casseroles	3 to 4 days	4 to 6 months
Pieces covered with broth or gravy	1 to 2 days	6 months
Chicken nuggets or patties	1 to 2 days	6 months
Commercial	2 months	Doesn't freeze well
Fish		
Lean fish (cod, flounder, sole, haddock)	1 to 2 days	6 months
Fatty fish (salmon, mackerel)	1 to 2 days	2 to 3 months
Raw shellfish	1 to 2 days	3 to 6 months
Cooked shellfish	3 to 4 days	3 months
Dairy Products		
Hard cheeses (Cheddar, Swiss)	6 months unopened, 3 to 4 weeks opened	6 months
Cottage cheese	1 week	Doesn't freeze well
Milk	7 days	3 months
Yogurt	7 to 14 days	1 to 2 months

Continued on the next page

Food	Refrigerator (40°F or 4°C)	Freezer (0°F or -18°C)
Prepared Foods		
Egg, chicken, ham, tuna or macaroni salad	3 to 5 days	Doesn't freeze well
Hot dogs, opened package	1 week	1 to 2 months
Luncheon meats, opened package	3 to 5 days	1 to 2 months
Cooked, sliced ham	3 to 4 days	1 to 2 months

Modified from Cold Food Storage Chart, USDA/FDA Center for Food Safety and Applied Nutrition, May 2002.

Environmental Contaminants

Many chemicals found in small amounts in the environment can be harmful to children. Some examples are heavy metals like lead and mercury, persistent organic pollutants, and pesticides. This section will focus on how children are exposed to some of the most common environmental contaminants via diet and how to reduce your child's dietary exposure.

Lead

You can't see or smell lead. However, it does taste sweet, which attracts children to eat leaded paint chips and paint dust. Children's bodies also absorb more lead. According to the Environmental Protection Agency (EPA), "It only takes lead dust equal to two grains of sugar a day on a child's fingertip transferred to the mouth, for perhaps a month, to cause that child's nerve velocity to decrease, making the child slower both physically and mentally."[9] Lead exposure can cause nervous system and kidney damage; learning disabilities; attention deficit disorder; speech, language and behavior problems; poor muscle coordination; decreased muscle and bone growth; and hearing damage.[10]

Why Children Need Protection from Environmental Contaminants

Since World War II, at least seventy-five thousand new synthetic chemicals have been released, but few have been tested for safety to children. Babies and children are very vulnerable to the effects of chemicals because:
- Pound for pound, they breathe more air, drink more water, and eat more food than adults.
- They're growing, and hormone-like chemicals can disrupt normal growth.
- They spend a lot of time on the floor, where contaminated dust may settle.
- They put everything in their mouths; it's a natural part of their learning process.

Lead is a naturally occurring element found in soil and rock; it's also used in manufacturing, in ceramic glazes, solders, and storage batteries. In the past it was added to paint and gasoline and was used in plumbing pipes. Here's where lead is typically found today:

- In leaded paint in homes built before 1978 and on old toys and furniture
- In drinking water if pipes or solder contains lead

- In food and liquid stored in lead crystal decanters and lead-glazed pottery
- In soil containing lead, especially near lead or copper smelters and other industries that release lead
- In folk remedies that contain lead (sometimes called greta or azarcon)

How to Reduce Your Child's Dietary Exposure

- Wash your child's hands, bottles, and cups often.
- Make sure your child eats healthy foods rich in calcium and iron. Well-nourished children absorb less lead.
- If you suspect your water supply contains excess lead:
  - Use only cold water for drinking and cooking.
  - Run water for fifteen to thirty seconds before drinking it, especially if you haven't used your water for a few hours.
- Don't store acidic foods like fruit juices in ceramic or leaded crystal containers.
- Don't use ceramic dishes that say "for decorative purposes only." Remember that lead glazes are still used on some imported pottery.
- Use pottery for serving, storing, or cooking food only if it's labeled "lead-free."
- Don't store beverages in lead crystal containers for extended periods.

Mercury

Much of the mercury load in the environment is from the actions of humans. Solid waste incineration and fossil fuel combustion contributes 87 percent of mercury emissions. Fertilizers, fungicides, and disposal of mercury-laden waste like batteries and thermometers in landfills contribute to mercury found in soil. Mercury also enters water or soil from natural deposits, volcanic activity, and bacterial activity. Mercury makes it to the food chain via water.

Mercury is a potent neurotoxin and can damage the developing nervous systems of fetuses and babies. It's also a possible carcinogen. Babies and children can be exposed to mercury through food (usually fish that's high in mercury) and through breast milk (depending on the mother's lifetime exposure to mercury and current dietary intake of mercury).

How to Reduce Your Child's Dietary Exposure

Fish is the main source of dietary mercury exposure. The FDA and EPA advise breastfeeding women, infants, and children as follows:[11]

- Fish and shellfish are an important part of a healthy diet for breastfeeding women and young children. A well-balanced diet that includes a variety of fish and shellfish contributes to heart health and proper growth and development.
- Avoid shark, swordfish, tilefish (also called golden bass or golden snapper), and king mackerel, which are highest in mercury. (See the following page for more info on the mercury content of various fish.)

Mercury Content of Seafood

Fish at the top of the food chain (usually large predatory fish) accumulate the most mercury. Preparation and cooking don't affect mercury content much because the mercury is bound to proteins in fish. The following list, modified from guidelines developed by Charles Santerre at Purdue University, groups fish by mercury content.

High Mercury Content[12]

Children under six years and women of childbearing age should avoid these fish:
- Chilean sea bass
- Grouper
- King Mackerel
- Marlin
- Orange roughy
- Shark
- Spanish mackerel (Gulf of Mexico)
- Swordfish
- Tilefish (golden bass or golden snapper, Gulf of Mexico)
- Tuna (fresh or frozen)
- Tuna (canned albacore or white)
- Walleye (Great Lakes, Canada)

Moderate Mercury Content[13]

Limit your family's consumption of these fish to four ounces per week:
- Bass (saltwater, black or striped)
- Bluefish
- Buffalo fish
- Halibut
- Lobster (Northern)
- Sablefish
- Scorpion fish
- Sea trout (weakfish)
- Snapper
- White croaker (Pacific)

Low Mercury Content[14]

Limit your family's consumption of these fish to eight ounces per week:
- Carp
- Mahi Mahi
- Monkfish
- Perch (freshwater)
- Skate
- Sheephead
- Spanish mackerel (South Atlantic)
- Tilefish (Atlantic)

Lowest Mercury Content

It's safe to eat as much as twelve ounces per week of these fish:
- Anchovy
- Butterfish
- Catfish (farm-raised)
- Clams
- Cod
- Crab (blue, king, and snow)
- Crawfish
- Croaker (Atlantic)
- Flatfish (flounder, plaice, sole)
- Haddock
- Hake
- Herring
- Jacksmelt
- Lobster (spiny)
- Mackerel (Atlantic jack or Pacific chub)
- Mullet
- Ocean perch
- Oysters
- Pickerel
- Pollock
- Rainbow trout (farm-raised)
- Salmon
- Sardine
- Scallops
- Shad (American)
- Shrimp
- Squid
- Tilapia
- Whitefish
- Whiting

If you don't recognize all the fish names on this list, check out the FDA's Regulatory Fish Encyclopedia at http://www.cfsan.fda.gov/~frf/rfe0.html.

- Limit fish consumption to twelve ounces per week.
- If you fish recreationally, pay attention to local fish advisories. If there are no local fish advisories posted, limit consumption of recreationally caught fish to six ounces per week and don't eat any other fish that week. (To find fish advisories for rivers and lakes in your area, visit http://www.epa.gov.)

To calculate the amount of canned tuna you or your child can safely eat based on body weight, go to the Environmental Working Group site: http://www.ewg.com. To calculate the amount of mercury in your diet from seafood (based on EPA safe levels), use the National Resources Defense Council mercury calculator at http://www.nrdc.org/health/effects/mercury/calculator/calc.asp.

Persistent Organic Pollutants

Persistent organic pollutants (POPs) are chemicals that linger in the environment for a very long time and travel thousands of miles from where they were used. Some examples of POPS are polychlorinated biphenyls (PCBs), dioxins, and pesticides like dichlorodiphenyltrichloroethane (DDT), chlordane, and dieldrin. Animals (including people) store POPS in fatty tissue, and POPs accumulate over time up the food chain. Some POPS may harm the immune and reproductive systems and may be carcinogenic. Children, who may be exposed to POPs through breast milk, formula, food, and water, are at particular risk from POPs.

Resources on Organic Foods and Pesticides

- http://www.theorganicpages.com: This website provides easy access to organic suppliers of food, ingredients, and other products
- http://www.ams.usda.gov/NOP/indexIE.htm: This is the U.S. National Organic Program website.
- http://www.localharvest.org: This website helps you find organics by locating local farmer's markets, community-supported agriculture, and food co-ops.
- http://www.foodnews.org: This website provides a report card on pesticides in produce.
- http://www.eatwild.com: This website offers sources for grass-fed meat and dairy products.

How to Reduce Your Child's Dietary Exposure

- Choose lean meats and poultry; serve fish from the low-mercury list. Cut off any skin and fat before cooking, since many chemicals are stored in fat.
- Consider buying organic meats, poultry, and eggs, as well as produce.
- Remove skin and fatty layer from fish before cooking it.
- Choose low-fat or skim milk once your child is older than two years.
- To avoid pesticides, consider buying organic produce or growing your own. Also consider buying or making organic baby food. (For more information on avoiding pesticides, see the next section.)
- Make sure your drinking water is as pure as possible. (See page 86 for more info.)

Avoiding Pesticides

One way to reduce your pesticide load is to know which produce has the most—and least—and choose accordingly. If price were no object, we'd all probably fill our pantries and fridges with nothing but organic foods. But most of us need to pick and choose the organic foods we buy, because they cost from 50 to 100 percent more than conventional foods.

To help in that task, the Environmental Working Group (EWG), a nonprofit environmental research organization, has developed the Shopper's Guide to Pesticides in Produce. EWG developed the guide by using the pesticide data from the FDA and USDA collected between 2000 and 2004.[15] (It can be downloaded at http://www.ewg.org) Below is a list of the worst and best produce available in the U.S. compiled from the EWG guide:

The Twelve Cleanest Fruits and Veggies

These are the fruits and vegetables with the lowest pesticide ranking, listed in ascending order (lower pesticides first):

- Onions
- Avocado
- Sweet corn (frozen)
- Pineapples
- Mango
- Asparagus
- Sweet peas (frozen)
- Kiwi fruit
- Bananas
- Cabbage
- Broccoli
- Papaya

The Twelve Dirtiest Fruits and Veggies

These are the fruits and veggies with the highest pesticide load. It's best if you can buy these organic or limit how often your child eats them. They're listed in descending order (most pesticides first).

- Peaches
- Apples
- Sweet bell peppers
- Celery
- Nectarines
- Strawberries
- Cherries
- Pears
- Grapes (imported)
- Spinach
- Lettuce
- Potatoes

Here are some more tips for avoiding pesticides:[16]

- Wash all fruits and vegetables thoroughly. Some foods, such as grapes, are best soaked for several minutes. Produce washes may remove waxes and pesticides more easily.
- Peel apples, peaches, nectarines, and pears before eating them and remove the outer leaves of lettuce; this will get rid of much of the pesticide residues.

- In the summertime, buy your produce at a local farmer's market. These foods are mostly grown close to home so they have fewer post-harvest pesticides.
- Grow your own produce. Plant some fruit trees or a vegetable garden. Strawberries and tomatoes can be grown in containers on a patio. You'll know where your fruit comes from and what chemicals (if any) are on them, and you can pick and eat your fruit at the peak of ripeness. Alternatively, find an organic you-pick farm.

Other Contaminants

Microwave-Safe Packaging

Microwave cooking in containers and with wraps not safe for the microwave can result in melting and migrating of some plastic into food. Never microwave food using foam takeout containers, used margarine tubs, foam meat trays, or used microwave food packaging. Always use glass, ceramic, or plastic containers labeled "microwave safe." For covering cooking containers in the microwave, use microwave-safe plastic wrap, wax paper, parchment paper, or paper towels. (When you use microwave-safe plastic wrap, the wrap should not touch your food.) Never use plastic storage bags, grocery bags, newspapers, or aluminum foil in the microwave.[17]

Insects, Rodents, and Dirt

Avoid storing food in cupboards under a sink or cupboards that have pipes passing through them. Food stored in these places can attract insects and rodents through openings that are difficult to seal adequately. And regardless of where you store them, wash the tops of cans with soap and water before opening.

Choking Hazards

Children under five years are more prone to choking on small objects (including food) than adults and older kids. Why? Babies and toddlers put everything in their mouths, and their airways are smaller and more easily blocked by small round objects. Here are some tips to prevent your child from choking:

- Always supervise your child's eating. It's best not to let your child eat when you can't watch him or her closely (for example, in the car). If your child must eat in such a situation, provide food he or she is unlikely to choke on, such as very soft food, very small food, and food that crumbles or dissolves quickly in the mouth.
- Make sure your child is seated when eating. Kids are more likely to choke if they eat while walking or running.
- Encourage your child to take small bites of food.
- Discourage talking with food in the mouth.

- Don't give your child hard candy. Of all children treated for choking in 2001, 60 percent choked on food and 25 percent of children under five choked on hard candy or gum. Here are some other foods to avoid until your child is four years old:[18]
  - Round foods like hot dogs, whole olives, and whole grapes
  - Nuts and seeds
  - Chunks of peanut butter
  - Hard, gooey, or sticky candy
  - Raisins
  - Chewing gum
  - Large and/or round pieces of hard raw vegetables, such as carrots and celery. Grate, finely chop, or lightly steam these veggies first.
  - Popcorn and pretzels
  - Large chunks of meat or cheese
- Keep an eye on older siblings, who may accidentally give your child foods he or she could choke on.
- Know what to do if your child does choke. Contact your local Red Cross about infant and child cardiopulmonary resuscitation (CPR) classes.

Chapter 11

About Six Months

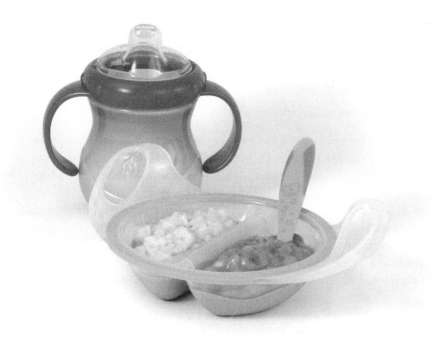

A man finds out what is meant by spitting image
when he tries to feed cereal to his infant.
—Imogene Fey

Is Your Baby Ready?

Beatriz had a feeling that her son, Marco, was ready for solid foods. He could turn his head from side to side, could sit with support, and seemed interested in what she was eating. He didn't seem satisfied with his usual amount of nursing either. Danielle was wondering if daughter, Sofia, was ready for solids, too. Sofia was drinking thirty-six ounces of formula a day and still seemed hungry.

If you think your baby, like Marco and Sofia, might be ready for solids, check the signs of readiness on page 177. If your baby shows all the signs, pick up a spoon, bib, and camera and begin!

Iron and First Foods

Iron is never more important in your baby's life than right now. To fuel his or her phenomenal growth and nervous system development, there's just no substitute for iron, the mineral that's carries oxygen in each of your baby's red blood cells.

Your baby is born with enough stored iron to last about six months—give or take a month or two. The amount of iron in a baby's bank may be reduced under certain conditions:

- Maternal iron deficiency anemia[1]
- Hypertension resulting in decreased fetal growth
- Diabetes
- Prematurity or low birth weight

Once your baby is born, other factors affect iron absorption: the source of the iron and what's eaten with iron. Babies absorb up to twenty-three times more iron from breast milk than from formula, which is why iron deficiency is pretty rare among term infants who are breastfed and healthy.

Feeding complementary iron-rich foods around six months coincides with a baby's natural iron bank depletion. However, which iron-rich food you start with—as well as which foods you serve with it—affect how much iron your baby absorbs. Whole grains are easily digested, but they also contain phytates, which reduce iron absorption. Vitamin C (in fruits and vegetables) counteracts the action of phytates. Meats are rich in both iron and zinc, and the type of iron in meat is well-absorbed. Serving meat with a grain also increases iron absorption from the grain.

So...which food should you give to your baby first? There's still more to learn about infant iron absorption, but I offer you the following advice based on what we do know.

- **If your baby is breastfed,** offer meat first, then whole-grain cereals and/or iron-fortified cereals, then fruits or vegetables.
- **If your baby was premature or is high-risk,** offer meat or iron-fortified cereals first, then veggies or fruit, then whole-grain cereals.
- **If your baby was full-term and is formula-fed,** offer iron-fortified cereal or meat first, then whole-grain cereals, then veggies or fruit.

First Food: Rice Cereal

Why: Many foods could be your baby's first food. In North America, however, it's usually rice cereal. Puréed meat and iron-fortified cereal are recommended because of their iron content. (For more info on babies' iron needs, see page 157.) Rice is typically a baby's first cereal because rice is the grain that's least allergenic. It also contains no gluten, which some experts believe may increase the risk of gluten intolerance and diabetes. (For more info, see the sidebar on page 218.) Fruits and vegetables are also gluten-free and generally non-allergenic, so some parents choose these foods first.

What kind: Cereal made just for infants is best, because it's fortified with iron and other nutrients your baby needs. I recommend starting with the dry instant type so you can mix it to the perfect consistency for your baby's ever-changing needs. Dry cereal may also be easier for your baby to accept, since you'll be mixing it with breast milk or formula (a familiar taste). Later, you might find jarred cereal mixed with fruit more convenient.

When: The exact time of day isn't important. Your baby should be hungry, but not famished. Some parents like to try that monumental first feeding mid-morning, when their baby isn't starving and is still well-rested. You should both be in a good mood. Breastfeed or formula-feed a little first, then try cereal, then finish up with more nursing or formula. Once you find a good time to feed your baby solids, you can work toward a pattern that eventually melds with your family's mealtimes.

How often: At first feed your baby cereal once a day, then work up to a few times a day.

How much: At first give your baby one teaspoon of dry cereal. Build up to one tablespoon or more twice a day. After a month or two of eating cereal, your baby will probably eat about a half-cup per day of dry cereal mixed with breast milk or formula.

If Your Baby's First Food Is Meat

You may decide to start with meat as a first food, especially if you're nursing. Follow the advice here, except offer puréed, thinned beef or lamb (the meats richest in zinc and iron). Your baby won't eat as much meat because it's richer in calories. He or she will probably start with a teaspoon or two and build up to eating 1 to 2 ounces (30 to 60 grams) per day. After a few weeks, when your baby has adjusted to the taste and texture of meat, add rice, then barley and rye cereals. Remember that it's easy to make your own delicious baby food meats. See Chapter 13 for more info.

That First Feeding, Step by Step

1. Mix about one teaspoon of dry cereal with about four or five tablespoons of breast milk or formula. The mixed cereal should be semi-liquid. Don't feed your baby cereal in a bottle or an infant feeder with a nipple. These methods can cause your baby to overeat, and they don't help your baby develop the eating skills he or she needs.

Starting Solids: Is There a Perfect Time?

Pediatricians agree that babies should never start eating solid foods before four months and that it's best to start closer to six months. What happens when cereal with gluten is introduced earlier or later?

Large prospective studies at the University of Colorado Health Sciences Center suggest that introducing gluten, a protein found in wheat, barley, and rye, before four months and after seven months increases the risk of gluten intolerance and islet autoantibodies (a possible marker for type 1 diabetes) in susceptible children.[2,3] The most drastic risk increase occurred in babies given gluten before four months.

While this study cannot draw firm conclusions about increasing the risk of gluten intolerance or type 1 diabetes in children who are not already at risk, it does shed light on the topic. Before four months, when the intestinal wall isn't completely developed, gluten protein can slip through and cause an immune response. When babies are given gluten foods after seven months, it's possible that they are given much larger servings of gluten foods, which may also cause an immune response.

A similar study done by the same researchers in Colorado has preliminary data that may debunk the idea of avoiding wheat to prevent wheat allergies, too. They found that delaying introduction to wheat until after six months *increased* the risk of wheat allergy instead of decreasing it.[4] The study population was a group of children with genetic predisposition for diabetes.

What's the bottom line? Babies are at higher risk of gluten intolerance if first- or second-degree relatives have the disease. This includes parents, siblings, grandparents, aunts, uncles, and half-siblings. Whether your baby is at risk or not, follow the normal timeline for introduction of solids but do introduce the gluten-containing cereals barley, rye, or oats before seven months. Also, it's wise to breastfeed (at least partially) during and after the time your baby is first exposed to gluten-containing foods, as this seems to significantly decrease gluten intolerance[5].

2. Face your baby toward you. Your baby is probably ready to sit in a highchair at six or seven months. You could also try holding your baby on your lap or on your partner's or placing your baby in a bouncy seat or car seat.

3. Fill just the tip of your baby's spoon with cereal. Move the spoon toward your baby's mouth. If your baby opens up, put the cereal in. If not, don't force it. Try one more time and then stop for the day if your baby still refuses.

4. Don't be insulted if your baby won't accept the spoon, makes a face, spits out the cereal, or screams at you! Get used to it—it's just the beginning of turning down food you offer.

It may take ten to fifteen tries for your baby to like a new food, so be patient and keep trying. Resist the temptation to flavor your baby's cereal with salt, sugar, or honey. Your baby's palate is pure, and he or she won't mind plain, bland food—I promise. I'll tell you in Chapter 13 when you can begin to add spices. If you keep trying to feed your baby solids and your baby continues protesting, wait a week or two and try again. Your baby is trying to tell you that he or she isn't ready.

Allergy Check

Remember that you should wait about three to five days between introducing new foods to check for signs of allergy. If your baby is at high risk for allergies, consider waiting up to seven days. According to the American Academy of Pediatrics (AAP), you should look for the following symptoms.[6] (For more information on preventing allergies, see page 136.)

- **Skin symptoms**: hives, rash, or itching
- **Digestive symptoms**: bloating, stomachache, cramping, nausea, vomiting, or diarrhea
- **Respiratory symptoms**: runny nose, wheezing, or coughing

If you think your baby is reacting to cereal (or any food), the AAP recommends avoiding that food for one to three months.[7] And of course, you should discuss the reaction with your baby's doctor.

Research suggests that most babies outgrow their food allergies by the time they're twelve months old. Typically outgrown allergies include milk, egg, soy, and wheat. Children usually don't outgrow allergies to peanuts, tree nuts, fish, and shrimp. If your child reacts to the latter foods, don't reintroduce them—reactions often get more serious with each exposure. Your child's doctor may recommend skin testing to see if your child is still allergic to a specific food.

> ## What's a Tree Nut?
>
> - Almond
> - Beechnut
> - Brazil nut
> - Butternut
> - Cashew
> - Chestnut
> - Chinquapin
> - Coconut
> - Filbert
> - Gingko nut
> - Hazelnut
> - Hickory nut
> - Litchi nut
> - Macadamia nut or bush nut
> - Pecan
> - Pine nut or piñon nut
> - Pili nut
> - Pistachio
> - Sheanut
> - Walnut (heartnut, butternut)

Second Food: Other Cereals

Next, you can expand your baby's menu by adding oat and barley cereals. You can serve these at the same texture as your baby's rice cereal. Remember to wait at least four days between introducing new cereals to check for allergy signs. You may even want to wait a week to let your baby get used to each new flavor and texture.

Let your baby guide the thickness and amount of cereal you feed. (Once your baby's eating thicker cereal, it may be more convenient to use prepared cereal in a jar. However, keep in mind that dry cereal is higher in iron.) Remember that cereal should provide only a small percentage of your baby's calories—breast milk or formula is still a very important source of nutrition for your baby.

Common Questions

Q: What if I do something wrong?

A: Books like this one give you lots of charts and guidelines to follow, but there really isn't a wrong way to do this! Generations ago, there were no charts and guidelines and books (and they weren't necessary) because grandmothers were usually close by to pass along tried-and-true methods. Today we like to follow science-based recommendations (which is a good thing) and many families are scattered, so parenting books have evolved to fill those needs. Try to chill out and remember:

- Guidelines aren't laws. You won't get hauled off if you don't follow them to the letter.

- If you follow a few basic rules (like introducing solids around six months, avoiding allergenic foods, and handling food safely), it's really hard to mess up!

- Your intuition and your baby's needs and cues are good guides.

- You can do this!

Q: There are so many foods to introduce. How can I get through all of them?

A: It's true: There are so many new foods for your baby to try, it can feel overwhelming. To make matters worse, parents just love to compare what their babies are eating and doing. ("My baby started oatmeal. What's your baby eating?") It's tempting to one-up your baby's peers, but don't. This process isn't a race; follow your own pace. If you feel pressured to keep up with the Joneses, just reply vaguely. ("He's eating all kinds of foods." Or, "We're taking it slow because I don't want her to have allergies.")

Sample Menus

A Day in the Diet...

Here's a sample daily menu for a six-month-old eating rice and oat cereal. Remember: This is just a suggestion!

Rise and Shine

Breast milk or formula

Breakfast

Breast milk or formula
One or two tablespoons of rice cereal

Going Gluten-Free

Gluten is a protein found in many grains, such as wheat (includes bran, germ, durum flour, graham flour, and kamut), oats, rye, and barley. Many foods don't seem to contain gluten, but may be contaminated with it through processing. Gluten-free grains include rice, wild rice, rice flour, buckwheat (which isn't really wheat), kasha or kashi, quinoa, millet, taro flour, tapioca, and corn.

Why avoid gluten? Some people who have gluten intolerance (celiac disease) prefer to keep their baby away from it also—at least for the first year. This is wise, since celiac disease definitely has a genetic component. However, introducing a bit of gluten before seven months may also be a good idea. (See more info on page 218.)

One in every 133 Americans has celiac disease—which is characterized in children by diarrhea, failure to thrive, anemia, projectile vomiting, and sometimes behavioral and learning problems. It's more common in women, Caucasians, and those of European ancestry. (For more information, see http://www.nlm.nih.gov/medlineplus/celiacdisease.html.)

If you're trying to keep your baby away from gluten, avoid oat, rye, and barley cereals until between six and seven months, or until your baby's doctor recommends introducing them. Ask your baby's doctor about the appropriate time to introduce wheat. Once your baby appreciates the flavor of these new cereals, you can begin mixing them. Vary the three cereals throughout the day and week.

Mid-morning

Breast milk or formula

Lunch

Breast milk or formula

Afternoon

Breast milk or formula

Dinner

Breast milk or formula
One or two tablespoons of oat cereal

Bedtime

Breast milk or formula

A Month in the Diet...

Here's a sample calendar for introducing cereals. Whether you start with cereal or meat, it'll be your baby's first experience with solid food! Give your baby a week to get used to the taste and texture before going to the next type of cereal (or meat).

Week One

Introduce rice cereal, and serve it daily. If your baby doesn't take to it at first, wait a few days or a week and try again. Don't push it if your baby's not ready.

Week Two

Add oat and barley cereal at whatever time of day suits you and your baby. (If you're avoiding gluten, skip barley for now.) For example:

- *Day one*: oat cereal for breakfast, rice cereal for dinner
- *Day two*: oat cereal for breakfast, rice cereal for dinner
- *Day three*: oat cereal for breakfast, rice cereal for dinner
- *Day four*: oat cereal for breakfast, barley cereal for dinner
- *Day five*: oat cereal for breakfast, rice cereal for dinner
- *Day six*: oat cereal for breakfast, barley cereal for dinner
- *Day seven*: oat cereal for breakfast, rice cereal for dinner

Week Three

Be creative and feed your baby any combination of cereals you like, at breakfast and dinner. Your baby doesn't need high-protein cereals yet.

Week Four

If you're both feeling good about cereal, you can start on veggies next.

Introducing a Cup

Why introduce a cup? The main reason is to prepare your baby for the life-changing event farther down the road when he or she says good-bye to an old friend: the breast (or bottle). Around six months, when your baby is sitting well and is coordinated enough to hold a cup, is a good time to introduce one. (Your baby may be ready earlier or later—don't sweat the precise timing.)

Many references suggest introducing a cup with juice. Personally, I don't think babies really need juice; fruit is a much better source of the same nutrients. Introducing juice as a norm may get babies into a habit that may lead to obesity. (See Chapter 18 for more info on this issue.) If your baby doesn't care for fruit, juice can fill in for some of the nutrients found in fruit. However, vegetable juices, veggie-fruit juices, or vegetables provide even more of those nutrients. (If you do give your baby juice, always put it in a cup, not a bottle.)

So what *should* you put in the cup? I recommend breast milk, formula, or water. If your baby currently drinks breast milk or formula from a bottle, your eventual goal is to get your baby to drink from a cup instead, so breast milk or formula may be the best choice. If you've exclusively breastfed for six months or so, you may have never introduced a bottle; your baby can go straight to a cup (of whatever liquid you choose). Water is another good choice because it gets your child in the habit of drinking water instead of caloric liquids when he or she is thirsty.

Most babies start with sippy cups to minimize spills. Janet Alba, an occupational therapist working in early childhood intervention, says sippy cups with more of a straw than a spout to drink from are better for developing the muscles needed for speech: "The muscles responsible for speech development require strength and coordination that comes from practice in using a straw or a regular cup for drinking."

While we're on the subject of speech... Speech therapists often see toddlers who aren't talking. In the majority of these cases, the children are still drinking from bottles well into their second (or even third) year. To help your baby develop good speech, if your baby drinks from a bottle, start getting psyched up for its disappearance sometime around twelve months. Does it have to be twelve months on the dot? No—but work toward that goal. (My kids finally got rid of their bottles around fourteen months.)

Chapter 12

Six to Eight Months

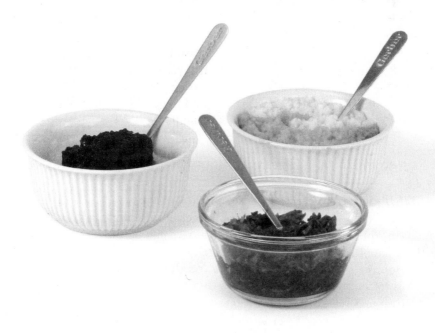

One of the great ironies...is that feeding children,
a task whose misery cannot be overstated,
leads to more diaper changing.

—Gary D. Christenson

In the next few months, your baby will have an incredible diet expansion: home-made whole-grain cereals, vegetables, fruits, and egg yolks. As you begin this nutritional adventure, keep in mind that soon enough, your baby's diet will resemble yours. (That means now's the time to take a closer look at yours—more on that in Chapter 14.) But for now, sit back and enjoy the ride while your baby tries many new foods. I've laid it out step-by-step in this chapter and included some helpful tips and recipes at the end.

Third Food: Homemade Whole-Grain Cereals

As discussed in Chapter 11, the first foods you should introduce to your baby are commercial instant cereals because they're processed, easy to digest, easy to make, and fortified with iron and zinc. Once your baby has no problem eating these cereals, you can introduce homemade whole-grain cereals. However, keep in mind that homemade whole-grain cereals don't contain as much iron as commercial cereals, which are iron-fortified. But you can greatly increase the amount of iron your baby absorbs by serving a vitamin C–rich food at the same time (see page 216). Also, some babies will need more iron than whole grains provide (see page 216). These babies should eat iron-fortified cereal and meats prior to expanding to whole grains.

Whole-grain cereals are actually easy to make, too. You just pour a small amount of dry grain into your blender, blend for a few minutes to turn it into a fine consistency, and then cook with water. The beauty of chopping the grains in the blender is that it speeds up cooking time—by more than half! Lastly, you add breast milk or formula to make it creamier. If you're already preparing whole grains for your family, you can simply use the blender or hand blender to purée them with breast milk or formula. For more details about homemade cereals, see the recipes beginning on page 238.

Why: Whole grains have more minerals, fiber, and antioxidants than processed grains.

What kind: It doesn't matter which you start first—brown rice, whole oats, barley, millet, or quinoa. Visit the bulk section of your local health food store. If you have a blender, just about any whole grain can be blended into small pieces to make a smooth cereal. Barley and oats both contain gluten, although oats have less.

When: At the time you usually give your baby cereal.

How often: Once a day or more.

How much: Begin with a few teaspoons until your baby gets used to the texture—increase per his or her appetite. If any of the grains are new to your baby, wait three to five days before introducing the next food. If you're worried about your baby having adequate iron in his or her diet, alternate whole-grain with iron-fortified cereal or hold off on whole-grain cereals until your baby is eating iron-rich meats.

Storing Grains

Uncooked whole grains can go rancid quickly when at room temperature and exposed to air, so they're best stored in air-tight containers (zipper bags work) in the refrigerator. They're also the favorite cuisine of bugs, so if you have a problem with that in your climate, you might want to store them in the freezer. When you thaw them, add a bit more liquid. As with other homemade baby food, cooked whole grains should be stored no longer than three days. It may be more convenient to make a few batches of different cereals and freeze them in one- to two-ounce portions.

Fourth Food: Vegetables

To see a suggested timeline of when to introduce vegetables to your baby's diet, check out the "A Month in the Diet..." section on page 231.

Why: Vegetables provide vitamins (especially iron, vitamin C, and beta carotene), minerals, antioxidants, and fiber.

What kind: The first vegetables should be cooked and puréed. Begin with sweet and mild flavored varieties: sweet potato, winter squash, carrots, avocado, green beans, peas, zucchini, and asparagus. Then add spinach, cauliflower, broccoli, sweet red or yellow peppers, eggplant, and others. In a few months you can add corn, but wait until one year if your baby is at risk for allergy. (Before introducing homemade vegetables, be sure to read the information about nitrates in the next section.) By your baby's eighth month, don't hesitate to add any other veggies except tomato, which you should hold off until ten months to a year, especially if your baby is allergy prone or has GERD (see page 131).

When: Lunch is a good time to introduce your baby to a new veggie. It's also fine to give them a try at snack time.

How often: Once a day for about a week, then twice a day.

How much: A few teaspoons to a few tablespoons at a time. Gradually increase to one-quarter to one-half cup per day. It never hurts to eat more veggies!

Nitrate Warning

If you make homemade baby food from vegetables, be aware of nitrates and their effects. Nitrates are compounds found in the soil and in well water, and they're naturally present in vegetables. Some nitrates are byproducts of fertilizers. Nitrates can be converted into toxic nitrites with the help of bacteria normally found in the digestive tract of infants under six months old and especially under three months old. This can cause methemoglobinemia (blue baby syndrome), a very rare but sometimes fatal condition. Most cases of infant methemoglobinemia are caused by drinking high-nitrate well water.

Nitrate levels are higher in spinach, carrots, squash, beets, and green beans than in other vegetables. The levels may not be so high when you first make baby foods with these vegetables, but when you store the food, the nitrates can skyrocket. Concentrated forms of the vegetables—such as carrot or beet juice—will be even higher in nitrates, so avoid those. In addition, raw vegetables left at room temperature also convert nitrates to nitrites.

You can reduce the risk of a nitrate problem if you wait to introduce vegetables until your baby is six months or older, especially if he or she was born prematurely. By that age, babies' digestive tracts are better developed, and the bacterial environment is less conducive to conversion of nitrates into nitrites. Because babies under three months old are especially vulnerable to nitrate exposure, the American Academy of Pediatrics (AAP) recommends that you not serve homemade baby food made of spinach, carrots, squash, beets, or green beans to an infant before three months of age.[1] Of course, you shouldn't be giving your baby *any* solids before four months—and preferably closer to six.

When you do introduce spinach, carrots, squash, beets, and green beans, you can further reduce the risk of your baby's having too many nitrates in his or her diet by following these tips:

- Consider using commercial baby food for these vegetables. While nitrates naturally occur in these vegetables, baby food companies monitor nitrate levels.

- If you make homemade baby food with these vegetables, make it from frozen or canned vegetables rather than fresh ones, especially for spinach and beets, which tend to be the highest in nitrates.[2] Frozen and canned vegetables have been processed, so the conversion from nitrate to nitrite doesn't occur as it does with raw veggies during storage time.

- If you make baby food with these vegetables, dish out a serving and *freeze the rest immediately*.

- If you want to use fresh vegetables for baby food, buy organic varieties—they appear to have significantly fewer nitrates.[3]

- If you use private well water, have its nitrate level tested before using it to prepare food for your baby or mixing with formula. The nitrate-nitrogen content of the water should be less than ten parts per million (ppm.)[4] Keep in mind that nitrate levels in well water change with the seasons and are generally higher in early spring and summer after planting season, when fertilizers are applied.[5]

- If you breastfeed, know that breast milk doesn't contain a significant amount of nitrates, even if you happen to drink well water high in nitrates.

- If your baby takes any medication to decrease stomach acid (such as for GERD), ask your doctor about when it will be safe to give your baby high-nitrate vegetables.

New Taste Sensations

If you expect your baby's first bite of green beans to go down with a smile and an open mouth for more, think again! Imagine what you'd do if offered something you'd never eaten in your life. To top it off, imagine what you'd do if that food were a really disgusting color and smelled much different than anything you'd ever eaten. With these first impressions, you'd likely make a funny face. Your baby will probably react the same way, twisting his or her face in yet-to-be-seen expressions. Remember, though—you must keep your poker face through it all. When you dish out puréed broccoli or spinach, you must smile and say "Yummy!" even if you feel like making the same face as your baby!

Also remember that when your baby makes funny expressions at a new food, don't assume it means he or she doesn't like it. Again, think of how you typically try new dishes: With your second taste of a presumably disgusting food, you discover it actually tastes okay. Your third bite tastes pretty good, and by the seventh bite, you're wondering if seconds are available! Even if your baby may not coo for more when he or she eats a new food for the first time, keep trying. Your baby will need some time to get used to the texture, color, smell, and taste.

Gassy Veggies

Let's face it—some of us are gassier than others. And some foods create more gas than others. High-sulfur vegetables like cauliflower, broccoli, Brussels sprouts, raw onions, and cabbage have a reputation, as do beans. Because of this, some parents put off introducing these foods until later.

When you do introduce these gassy foods to your baby, you can reduce their potency by mixing them with another vegetable or a cereal you've already introduced, like potato or rice. If these foods cause gas but your baby doesn't seem to mind it, count your blessings. The gassiest foods are also some of the healthiest! But if your baby still has uncomfortable amounts of gas because of the food, put it off for another month.

Fifth Food: Fruit

After your baby has had a few weeks with a variety of vegetables, it's time to bring fruits into the picture. To see a suggested timeline of when to introduce fruits to your baby's diet, check out the "A Month in the Diet..." section on page 231.

Why: Like vegetables, fruits contain vitamin C, beta carotene, potassium, minerals, antioxidants, and fiber.

What kind: Mild, noncitrus fruits without seeds or peel are good to start, such as cooked and puréed peach, pear, apricot, and apple. Ripe banana and mango can be puréed without cooking. Next you can add cooked and puréed blueberries and strawberries (strained), plus raw puréed melon and cooked dates and raisins. By the time your baby is about eight months old, you can give him or her just about any fruit, except citrus and pineapple because of their acidity. You'll want to wait another month or two for those (longer if your baby has risk of allergies or GERD). By seven months, you can also skip cooking fruit before you purée or mash it, as long as the fruit is very soft and ripe.

When: Give fruit a try at breakfast and snack time, then at lunch or dinner. Once accepted, they go great with cereal. And the vitamin C in fruit helps with iron absorption.

How often: At first offer them once a day, then try twice a day.

How much: A few teaspoons to a few tablespoons at a time. Gradually increase to one-quarter to one-half cup per day.

Favoring Fruits over Vegetables

What if your baby likes fruit more than vegetables—is he or she still getting enough vitamins? It's not unusual for babies to favor fruits. Then again, some babies would rather eat broccoli than bananas. Don't worry, all fruits and vegetables have important vitamins. Some have very similar nutrient contents, so look below to find out which fruits and veggies can be swapped, depending on your baby's preferences.

Rich in Vitamin C

Guava	Bell pepper
Kiwi fruit	All berries
Mango	All melons
Papaya	Cabbage
Broccoli	Kale
Cauliflower	Potato

Rich in Vitamin A (Beta Carotene)

All bell peppers	Collard and turnip greens
Spinach	Cantaloupe
Sweet potato	Broccoli
Pumpkin	Winter squash
Carrots	

Rich in Folic Acid

Beans	Oranges
Asparagus	Green peas
Strawberries	

Sixth Foods: Egg Yolks

At about seven months, it's time to introduce your baby's first protein food: egg yolks. (For some babies, however, egg yolks will be the second protein food if they are already eating meats. See page 217.) Avoid egg white until one year or later, since it's more allergenic. After eight months, you can introduce other protein foods—see Chapter 13 for details.

Why: Egg yolks are perfect for babies, and here's why:

- Egg yolks are an excellent source of protein; fat; vitamins A, B_6, B_{12}, D, and E; folic acid; thiamin; niacin; riboflavin; phosphorus; zinc; and iron. They're also an excellent source of choline—half an egg yolk provides all the choline your baby needs. Choline is a B vitamin recently found to help with the development of the memory center of your baby's brain.

- They have a protein quality that is second only to breast milk.

- They require little chewing and are easily digested.

- They have a delicate taste most babies enjoy.

- They are versatile and economical.

What kind: It's a good idea to choose eggs fortified with DHA. (See the section below for more details.)

When: Anytime. Breakfast is, of course, the typical meal to have eggs, but they're also great as a snack or for lunch or dinner.

How often: As often as every day.

How much: One egg yolk at a time.

What Kind of Eggs Should You Use?

There are several types of "designer" eggs available:

Brown Eggs

Contrary to popular opinion, the shell of the egg has to do with the chicken's breed rather than its diet. Chickens with red feathers and earlobes lay brown eggs. However, hens that lay brown eggs are usually bigger and eat more—hence, the larger price tag of the eggs.

> **Myth or Fact?**
>
> Myth or fact: Golden or orange egg yolks are more nutritious than light yellow yolks. Myth! The color has nothing to do with the nutritional value of the egg and everything to do with the kind of feed given to hens. While artificial colors are not allowed in chicken feed, additives such as marigold petals can give yolks a more golden color.

DHA- and Omega-3 Fortified Eggs

Several brands of eggs have additional vitamin E and DHA, an omega-3 fatty acid (see page 79 for more info). For the eggs to have these additional nutrients, farmers feed the chickens a special diet. Eggland's Best eggs, for example, are produced from chickens fed an all-vegetarian feed that contains healthy grains, canola oil, and an all-natural supplement of rice bran, alfalfa, kelp, and vitamin E. They contain one hundred milligrams of omega-3 fats, including fifty milligrams of DHA per egg as well as ten times more vitamin E and nearly three times more iodine than a typical egg (Eggland's Best also has an organic line.) Gold Circle Farms eggs also contain much more DHA than a typical egg—150 milligrams each. Gold Circle Farm hens are also fed an all-natural vegetarian diet enriched with cold-water microalgae to increase the DHA content. Personally, I like the idea of making a nutritious food much healthier with the addition of DHA, which is important to brain and eye development for infants and heart health for adults. My family eats about eighteen DHA-fortified eggs per week!

Organic Eggs

Organic eggs come from hens given feed with ingredients that were grown without pesticides, fungicides, herbicides, or commercial fertilizers. In addition, the hens are not given antibiotics or growth hormones. However, they don't have any extra nutrients than do nonorganic eggs. Due to higher production costs and lower volume per farm, organic eggs are more expensive than eggs from hens fed conventional feed.

Free-Range Eggs

True free-range eggs are those produced by hens raised outdoors or with daily access to the outdoors. That said, it might be important to note this statement from the American Egg Board: "Due to seasonal conditions, however, few hens are actually raised outdoors. Some egg farms are indoor floor operations and these are sometimes erroneously referred to as free-range operations. Due to higher production costs and lower volume per farm, free-range eggs are generally more expensive. The nutrient content of eggs is not affected by whether hens are raised free-range or in floor or cage operations."[6]

What about Cholesterol?

Egg yolks have an undeserved reputation for being "high in cholesterol" and causing heart problems in adults. If you're concerned about your baby's egg yolk intake, remember that for most people, cholesterol in foods such as egg yolks has little or no effect on "bad" cholesterol levels or plaque buildup in arteries. Also, remember that infants need fat and cholesterol for proper growth and development.

What about Salmonella?

Like any perishable animal protein, eggs can contain food-borne bacteria, especially salmonella. (See page 202.) Babies are more likely than adults to get sick from food-borne bacteria due to their immature immune systems, so you must take care in handling eggs:

- Wash your hands well *before and after* handling raw eggs.
- Don't leave eggs at room temperature.
- Use only clean, uncracked eggs.
- Use eggs no more than four to five weeks after the packing date printed on the package.
- Cook eggs until they reach a temperature of 160°F (71°C).
- Never serve raw or undercooked eggs to your baby.
- Store raw eggs in the refrigerator at 40°F (4°C).
- Once cooked, either chill or keep them warm for serving—but don't let the temperature go between 140° F (60°C) and 40°F (4°C). This is considered the "danger zone" for bacterial growth.
- If you spill raw egg on food preparation areas, first wipe with a paper towel. Follow with an antibacterial wipe or wipe with a diluted bleach solution made from one-half teaspoon (three milliliters) bleach plus two cups (five hundred milliliters) cool water.
- Always use separate utensils for raw eggs than for foods that won't be cooked, such as fresh fruits and vegetables.

A Month in the Diet...

Adding homemade whole-grain cereals, vegetables, and fruits to your baby's diet isn't as hard as it may seem. Here's a suggested timeline for when to introduce these new foods over the course of a month *in addition to the normal mealtimes with breast milk or formula*. You'll see that the whole-grain cereals are added in here and there. (To see how to combine a liquid diet with solids for this age group, see the "A Day in the Diet..." section on page 233.) Note: This timeline recommends waiting three or four days between introducing new foods. If your baby is at high risk for allergies, consider waiting longer. And always remember to watch carefully for reactions to any new food you introduce. For recipes, see pages 238–249.

Week One

Your baby is now a pro with commercial instant cereal, so it's time to add home-made whole-grain cereals to his or her diet. It's also time to add vegetables. Begin with one veggie a day for about a week, then graduate to two a day.

- *Day one*: quinoa cereal for breakfast, winter squash for lunch, rice cereal for dinner
- *Day two*: whole oat cereal for breakfast, winter squash for lunch, quinoa cereal for dinner
- *Day three*: brown rice cereal for breakfast, winter squash for lunch, quinoa cereal for dinner
- *Day four*: quinoa cereal for breakfast, winter squash for lunch, barley cereal for dinner
- *Day five*: brown rice cereal for breakfast, carrots for lunch, whole oat cereal for dinner
- *Day six*: barley cereal for breakfast, carrots for lunch, rice cereal for dinner
- *Day seven*: whole oat cereal for breakfast, carrots for lunch, winter squash and brown rice cereal for dinner

Week Two

If things are going well, keep adding new vegetables. Near the end of the week, add a green vegetable.

- *Day one*: whole-grain mixed cereal for breakfast, winter squash for lunch, strained carrots and rice cereal for dinner
- *Day two*: whole-grain mixed cereal for breakfast, sweet potato for lunch, strained carrots and oat cereal for dinner
- *Day three*: barley cereal for breakfast, sweet potato for lunch, strained carrots and brown rice cereal for dinner
- *Day four*: whole oat cereal for breakfast, winter squash for lunch, sweet potato and whole barley cereal for dinner
- *Day five*: rice cereal for breakfast, peas for lunch, carrots and whole oat cereal for dinner

- *Day six*: barley cereal for breakfast, peas for lunch, sweet potato and whole-grain mixed cereal for dinner
- *Day seven*: rice cereal for breakfast, carrots for lunch, peas and barley cereal for dinner

Week Three

By this time, you can keep adding new green vegetables. You can also give your baby one or two veggies at a meal. Finally, near the end of the week, you'll be ready to introduce fruit.

- *Day one*: whole oat cereal for breakfast, peas and carrots for lunch, green beans and rice cereal for dinner
- *Day two*: barley cereal for breakfast, green beans and carrots for lunch, sweet potato and whole oat cereal for dinner
- *Day three*: brown rice cereal for breakfast, winter squash and peas for lunch, green beans and quinoa cereal for dinner
- *Day four*: whole oat cereal for breakfast, green beans and sweet potato for lunch, carrots and peas for dinner
- *Day five*: quinoa cereal and pears for breakfast, peas and sweet potatoes for lunch, barley and green beans for dinner
- *Day six*: whole oat cereal and pears for breakfast, green beans and peas for lunch, carrots and brown rice cereal for dinner
- *Day seven*: quinoa cereal and pears for breakfast, peas for lunch, carrots and barley cereal for dinner

Week Four

Now you get the idea! Continue adding new fruits and veggies while offering old favorites (and even not-so favorites). The only fruits you should wait a while to add are pineapple and citrus, and the only vegetable you should wait on is tomato.

- *Day one*: barley cereal with pears for breakfast, winter squash and peas for lunch, oat cereal and green beans for dinner
- *Day two*: whole oat cereal for breakfast, peas and broccoli with brown rice for lunch, carrots for dinner
- *Day three*: quinoa cereal with pears for breakfast, broccoli with carrots for lunch, green beans and brown rice for dinner
- *Day four*: whole-grain mixed cereal for breakfast, broccoli with peas for lunch, carrots with oat cereal for dinner
- *Day five*: quinoa cereal for breakfast, broccoli and pears for lunch, winter squash and oatmeal for dinner
- *Day six*: oat cereal and peaches for breakfast, winter squash and peas for lunch, green beans and quinoa cereal for dinner
- *Day seven*: whole oat cereal with peaches for breakfast, barley cereal and green beans for lunch, carrots and winter squash for dinner

A Day in the Diet...

Of a Seven-Month-Old Eating Cereals, Vegetables, and Fruits

Now that you know when to introduce cereals, vegetables, and fruits, here's a snapshot of how it works within a normal day of breastfeeding or formula-feeding. For recipes, see pages 238–249.

Rise and shine

Breast milk or formula

Breakfast

Breast milk or formula
Oat cereal mixed with applesauce

Mid-morning snack

Breast milk or formula

Lunch

Breast milk or formula
Puréed green beans
Puréed peaches

Mid-afternoon snack

Breast milk or formula
Puréed pears

Dinner

Breast milk or formula
Pea and brown rice purée

Bedtime

Breast milk or formula

Of an Eight-Month-Old Eating Cereal, Vegetables, Fruit, and Egg Yolks

Here's a snapshot of a daily menu once egg yolks are added and your baby has also progressed to a little thicker texture. For recipes, see pages 238–249.

Rise and shine

Breast milk or formula

Breakfast

Cereal with Egg Breakfast
Mashed banana

Mid-morning snack

Breast milk or formula

Lunch

Breast milk or formula
Puréed butternut squash
Puréed plums

Mid-afternoon snack

Breast milk or formula
Mashed avocado

Dinner

Puréed asparagus or green beans
Puréed brown rice cereal

Bedtime

Breast milk or formula

Picking Produce

Fresh, frozen, or canned—when it comes to picking produce to make your baby's food, what's the most nutritious choice?

Fresh

Produce picked from your own garden wins hands down in the "fresh" department. It can go from your garden to your baby's mouth with only cooking time in between. But how about fresh produce from the store? In some cases, especially for food out of season in your area, produce may spend as many as seven to fourteen days in transit before making it to the store. Add this to the time it spends in the store before you buy it and then in your crisper before you use it. What started out as *fresh* may not qualify for the term once you cook it! And with this timeline, many of the nutrients you expect from fresh produce are actually gone by the time you prepare it for your baby. (For information about using fresh vegetables that are high in nitrates, see page 225.) If you still prefer to make baby food from fresh produce, follow these tips for getting the most out of it:

Is Organic Best for Baby Food?

Some commercial fruits and veggies have rather high pesticide levels for babies. With organic produce, chemical and synthetic pesticide contamination is reduced to almost zero. Organic produce is also more likely to have higher nutrient content and lower nitrate levels. Check out page 21 for suggestions about which types of produce should be purchased as organic.

- Buy produce in season for your area so it spends less time in transit.

- Buy from a farmer's market, but still ask where the produce comes from to determine its transit time. I've found in Texas, much of the farmer's market produce still comes from California!

- Buy organic to help ensure freshness.

- Go to a "pick-your-own" farm—it's fun, and you can pick the perfect ripeness. Just make sure you're ready to process the produce once you take it home, otherwise you add to the "crisper time."

- Buy produce for baby food no more than one day before you cook it. If you don't have time to prepare it, blanch it briefly in boiling water and freeze it.

Frozen

Many busy parents know that buying frozen produce means you don't have to worry as much about handling or how long you keep it before cooking it for your baby. But while most people assume fresh produce is the healthiest choice to make baby food, the truth is, frozen produce can be just as nutritious—if not more so. In 1998, the government allowed food companies to label frozen produce as "healthy." To use this definition, frozen produce had to have at least the same nutrient content as fresh produce.

However, some data showed that frozen produce had a higher nutrient content than fresh. Dr. Barbara Klein at the University of Illinois found that frozen green beans had twice as much vitamin C as their fresh counterparts. In her study, the fresh green beans spent three days in a display case at a grocery store and three days in a home refrigerator.[7] In a real-life situation, imagine the vitamin C loss if green beans spend even longer in transit to the store and even longer in storage, buried in your crisper at home.

Canned

Commercially canned foods are especially useful when you're in a time crunch or when certain produce is out of season. But what about the nutrient content?

Canned foods have an undeserved reputation for being much less nutritious than fresh. "Canned food is easy-to-use, versatile, and readily accessible," explains Connie Evers, registered dietitian, child-nutrition expert, author of *How to Teach Nutrition to Kids*, and mother of three. "Misconceptions still abound, but the fact is that canned foods do not contain chemical preservatives to retain the nutritional value of the food. Because of their shelf life and naturally-occurring preservatives, canned goods will retain their nutrients and flavor for more than two years in the pantry allowing the efficient cook to stock up for mealtime."

Two university studies have shed light on why canned food can be just as good and in some cases better than fresh. The 1997 University of Illinois study "Nutrient Conservation in Canned, Frozen, and Fresh Foods" uncovered these findings about the nutrients in canned produce:

- **Fiber**: The canning process can make the fiber more soluble and more useful to the body.

- **Vitamin A and carotenoids**: Little of this vitamin is lost. In fact, the heating process of canning can make carotenoids even more beneficial than when the produce is raw.

- **Folate**: This water-soluble vitamin holds up well during the canning process.

- **Vitamin C**: Only small amounts of vitamin C are lost, and most of it can be found in the liquid in the can. Cooking with the liquid will rescue the otherwise lost vitamins.

Getting the Most Out of Canned Produce

To get the most out of canned produce, follow these tips:
- Be sure to buy varieties without added sugar or salt, when possible.
- Keep in mind that "vacuum packed" means more food and less liquid in which to lose vitamins.
- Consider canned if you want to make homemade baby food from beets, carrots, green beans, or spinach, but are worried about nitrate content. The cooking process stops the conversion of nitrates to nitrites that occurs with fresh produce during storage time. (See page 225.)

Cooking Tips

Adding Liquid to Make a Smooth Purée

Beginning on page 239, you'll find recipes for making homemade baby food from whole-grain cereals, vegetables, fruits, and egg yolks. These recipes are very easy: Steam or cook in a small amount of water, purée, add liquid for a smooth consistency, and serve. What could be simpler?

As for adding liquid to smooth the purée, some parents wonder which liquid is best. For the first month, it's best to use either breast milk or formula. Those familiar tastes may help your baby accept new foods more easily.

Another option is to use the cooking liquid. Sometimes it's more convenient, and it's a good way to preserve the vitamins lost during the cooking process rather than throwing them down the sink. As your baby gets older and becomes a pro at eating new foods, go ahead and use the cooking liquids as needed. You may even want to reserve or freeze these liquids and add them to soups and sauces to boost the vitamin content for the rest of your family's dishes.

Microwave Cooking

Although heating your baby's bottle of breast milk or formula in the microwave is not recommended, microwaving your baby's solid food is an ideal and quick cooking method for busy parents. More nutrients are lost in microwaving compared to steaming, but if you use only a small amount of water, you can keep nutrient loss to a minimum. Here are a few tips:

- Always use a glass or microwave-safe ceramic or plastic dish.
- If your dish doesn't have a cover, use plastic wrap, but make sure the wrap doesn't touch the food.
- It's easy to get burned by the steam from microwaved foods, so peel back the plastic wrap or lift the cover just a bit to vent the steam.
- Even microwave-safe dishes can get hot—make sure to have hot pads handy.
- To ensure even cooking, cook the food halfway, then stop and stir it.
- Food continues cooking after the microwave stops, so let it stand about five minutes before puréeing.
- Most foods need only one to two tablespoons (15–30 milliliters) of added liquid.
- Never put closed jars, closed containers, or whole eggs in the microwave—they can explode.
- To keep your baby's food safe, clean spatters in the microwave and always put food in a dish or on a plate for cooking.

How to Separate the Egg Yolk from the White

The white of an egg is more allergenic than the yolk, which is why you should hold off giving it to your baby until one year. Therefore, if you cook egg yolks for your baby, you'll need to separate them from the whites. It's best to use one of these methods:

- Use an egg separator.

- Use a funnel. After cracking the egg, gently pour it into a funnel and let the egg white fall through. You may need to hold up the yolk with a spoon while the white falls through.

- Crack the egg and let some of the white fall into a bowl while keeping the yolk in the other half of the shell. Hold your clean hand flat with your fingers slightly open. Transfer the egg yolk to your hand and allow the rest of the egg white to flow through your fingers into the bowl.

- The traditional method is to crack the shell, separate the halves, and let the white fall into a bowl as you transfer the yolk back and forth between the halves. But keep in mind that this method increases the risk of the yolk coming into contact with bacteria that could be on the shell. If you use this method, rinse the egg well before breaking.

Storage Reminder

Here are the basic rules for storing homemade baby food:

- For homemade cereals, veggies, and fruits, refrigerate what you will use within two days. Freeze any remainders. Exception: When making baby food from high-nitrate vegetables, immediately freeze anything over a serving.

- For eggs, refrigerate what you will use within twenty-four hours. Freeze any remainders, but note that some egg recipes won't freeze well.

Recipes

About the Nutrient Content

I've analyzed the nutrient content of all the recipes in this book with a program called FoodWorks by The Nutrition Company. Each recipe lists the nutrients with 10 percent or more of the Dietary Reference Intakes (DRI) for the appropriate age group. Don't worry that some foods don't have a lot of vitamins listed—most foods have a small amount of many vitamins and minerals, even if they don't reach 10 percent of the daily recommended dose.

Whole Barley Cereal

Yield: 1 cup (250 milliliters)

¼ cup (60 milliliters) whole pearled barley
1¼ cups (310 milliliters) water

1. Blend barley 1–2 minutes or until it resembles a fine flour.
2. Pour water into pan and stir in barley. Bring to a boil, then reduce to a simmer. Cover and cook about 10 minutes, stirring frequently.
3. Remove from heat and let cool, stirring a few more times.
4. Add breast milk or formula as needed to achieve a smooth consistency.

Nutrient content of 2 tablespoons (30 milliliters)

22 calories, 0.5 gram protein, Manganese 15%, Selenium 10%

The Right Blender

Other blenders may take 2 minutes to grind brown rice into a fine flour, but my Braun blender did it in about 30 seconds!

Brown Rice Cereal

Yield: 1 cup (250 milliliters)

¼ cup (60 milliliters) medium- or small-grain brown rice
1 cup (250 milliliters) plus 2 tablespoons (30 milliliters) water

1. Blend brown rice 30 seconds to 2 minutes or until it resembles a fine flour.
2. Pour water in pan. Stir in rice. Bring to a boil, then reduce to a simmer. Cover and cook about 10 minutes, stirring frequently.
3. Remove from heat and let cool, stirring a few more times.
4. Add breast milk or formula as needed to achieve a smooth consistency.

Nutrient content of 2 tablespoons (30 milliliters)

21 calories, 0.5 gram protein, Manganese 40%, Vitamin B$_6$ 10%, Magnesium 10%

Whole Oat Cereal

Yield: 1 cup (250 milliliters)

¼ cup (60 milliliters) whole-grain oats or old-fashioned rolled oats
1¼ cups (310 milliliters) water

1. Blend oats 1–2 minutes or until they resemble a fine flour.
2. Pour water into pan and stir in oats. Bring to a boil, then reduce to a simmer. Cover and cook about 10 minutes, stirring frequently.
3. Remove from heat and let cool, stirring a few more times.
4. Add breast milk or formula as needed to achieve a smooth consistency.

Nutrient content of 2 tablespoons (30 milliliters)

22 calories, 0.5 gram protein, Manganese 25%, Magnesium 10%, Vitamin B$_6$ 10%

Quinoa Cereal

Quinoa is an ancient Incan "grain" (really a seed) with a distinct flavor and texture. It's very nutritious, higher in iron and protein than most grains, and it's wheat- and gluten-free.

Yield: ¾ cup (180 milliliters)

¼ cup (60 milliliters) quinoa
⅔ cup (160 milliliters) water
½ cup (125 milliliters) breast milk, formula, or water

1. Bring quinoa and water to a boil in a saucepan.
2. Reduce heat to low and simmer 10–15 minutes until water is absorbed.
3. Remove from heat and cool slightly.
4. Purée with breast milk, formula, or water. The purée won't be completely smooth, but more like the consistency of cream of wheat. Add additional liquid to achieve a smoother consistency.

Nutrient content of 2 tablespoons (30 milliliters)

17 calories, 0.5 grams protein, Manganese 20%, Magnesium 10%

Millet Cereal

Millet is a highly nutritious, easy-to-digest grain not likely to cause an allergy. It's also high in iron.

Yield: 1 cup (250 milliliters)

3 tablespoons (45 milliliters) millet
1 cup (250 milliliters) water

1. Blend millet 1–2 minutes or until it resembles a fine flour.
2. Pour water into pan and stir in millet. Bring to a boil, then reduce to a simmer. Cover and cook about 10 minutes, stirring frequently.
3. Remove from heat and let cool, stirring a few more times.
4. Add breast milk or formula as needed to achieve a smooth consistency.

Nutrient content of 2 tablespoons (30 milliliters)

22 calories, 1 gram protein, Manganese 40%, Magnesium 10%, Vitamin B$_6$ 10%

Mixed Cereals

Once your baby has successfully eaten the previous cereals (pages 238–239) without sign of allergy symptoms, you can make cereals by mixing the grains.

Yield: 1 cup (250 milliliters)

¼ cup (60 milliliters) of mixed grains, such as brown rice + oats, oats + barley, millet + brown rice, millet + quinoa, and so on
1¼ cups (310 milliliters) water

1. Blend grains 1–2 minutes or until they resemble a fine flour.
2. Pour water into pan and stir in grains. Bring to a boil, then reduce to a simmer. Cover and cook about 10 minutes, stirring frequently.
3. Remove from heat and let cool, stirring a few more times.
4. Add breast milk or formula as needed to achieve a smooth consistency.

Nutrient content of 2 tablespoons (30 milliliters)

Varies depending on grain. See nutrient contents for previous cereal recipes.

Cooking Alternative

If you're cooking whole potatoes for the family, skip chopping your baby's potato into pieces. Instead, cook all the potatoes whole in the microwave. To determine the cooking time, add 6 minutes for the first medium potato plus 2 minutes for each additional potato. Be sure to prick the skins several times to let the steam out. When done, purée your baby's potato as indicated above.

Root Vegetable Purée: White Potatoes and Sweet Potatoes

Yield: Varies, depending on size of potato

Medium white potato or sweet potato, peeled and chopped
1–2 tablespoons (15–30 milliliters) water (optional for microwave cooking)

1. Steam potato above boiling water for 5–8 minutes or until tender. Alternately, place potato in a microwave-safe container with water; cover and microwave on high for about 5–8 minutes or until tender. The smaller you chopped your potato, the quicker it will cook.
2. Purée using a potato ricer or potato masher. Add breast milk or formula to achieve a smooth consistency. Let cool before serving.
3. Freeze what your baby will not eat in 2 days. Root vegetables such as potatoes tend to thicken during freezing, so you may need to add extra liquid to get a smooth consistency after thawing.

Nutrient content of 2 tablespoons (30 milliliters) white potato

13 calories, Manganese 10%, Thiamine 150%, Folate 10%

Nutrient content of 2 tablespoons (30 milliliters) sweet potato

19 calories, 1 gram protein, Vitamin A 100%, Vitamin E 20%, Vitamin B_6 15%

Winter Squash and Pumpkin Purée

There are many types of winter squash: acorn, butternut, spaghetti, delicata, golden nugget, red kuri, sweet dumpling, and kabocha. Give a new one a try! Winter squash as well as pumpkin is packed with nutrients.

Yield: Varies, depending on size of vegetable

Winter squash or pumpkin, peeled, seeded, and chopped
3 tablespoons (45 milliliters) water per pound of vegetable (optional)

1. Cook the squash or pumpkin in one of the following ways:

   • Steam it above boiling water for at least 15 minutes, depending on the freshness of the vegetable and the size of the pieces.

   • Bake for 1½–2 hours at 350°F (176°C).

   • Place pieces face-down in microwave-safe dish. Add 3 tablespoons (45 milliliters) water for each pound. Cover and microwave on high 10–15 minutes. Let stand for another 5 minutes and check for doneness. If not done, cook an additional 3–5 minutes.

2. Purée with breast milk, formula, or water as needed. Let cool before serving.

Nutrient content of 2 tablespoons (30 milliliters) acorn squash

8 calories, Vitamin B$_6$ 10%

Nutrient content of 2 tablespoons (30 milliliters) butternut squash

10 calories, Vitamin A 30%

Nutrient content of 2 tablespoons (30 milliliters) pumpkin

7 calories, Vitamin A 15%, Potassium 10%

Getting through the Peel

Sometimes it's tough to get through the peel of a squash or pumpkin. If you're brave with a sharp knife, use it to peel and chop the squash or to slice a chunk of pumpkin and peel it. Otherwise, cut off a chunk of the veggie, boil or steam it until soft, scoop out the seeds, and then scoop out the flesh. Use a fork to get all the strings out. Still another option is to poke a few holes in the veggie, pop it in the microwave for 5–10 minutes or until it's soft enough to cut open and take out the seeds.

Soft Vegetable Purée: Zucchini, Yellow Squash, Asparagus, Green Beans

These soft veggies are mild flavored and may appeal to your baby.

Yield: About 2 cups (500 milliliters)

1 pound (500 grams) zucchini, yellow squash, asparagus, and green beans*
1–2 tablespoons (15–30 milliliters) water per pound of vegetable

1. Trim ends of squash and green beans. For asparagus, remove the fibrous ends. Cut vegetables into small pieces.
2. Steam over boiling water 6–8 minutes. Or microwave on high 7 minutes with 1–2 tablespoons (15–30 milliliters) water per pound. Either way, green beans take a bit longer.
3. Purée with breast milk, formula, or water as needed. Let cool before serving.

*It's best to wait until your baby is six months old to introduce homemade green beans because they can be high in nitrates (see page 225). Even then, you may want to use frozen or canned green beans rather than fresh. Dish out a serving for your baby and immediately freeze the rest.

Nutrient content of 2 tablespoons (30 milliliters) zucchini or yellow squash

4 calories, Potassium 10%

Nutrient content of 2 tablespoons (30 milliliters) asparagus

7 calories, Folate 50%, Thiamine 10%, Vitamin B_6 10%

Nutrient content of 2 tablespoons (30 milliliters) green beans

8 calories, Manganese 15%

Avocado Purée

Okay, some of us know avocado is really a fruit, but most of us call it a vegetable! Avocado provides a great source of vitamins and monounsaturated fat.

Yield: 6 tablespoons (90 milliliters)

Medium very ripe avocado, washed

1. Cut a small slice into pieces and mash with a fork. Avocado is easily oxidized when exposed to air and doesn't freeze well, so make only as much as your baby will eat at a meal.
2. Add a small amount of breast milk or formula to achieve a smooth consistency.

Nutrient content of 2 tablespoons (30 milliliters)

50 calories, Vitamin B_6 25%, Potassium 25%, Folate 20%, Magnesium 15%, Manganese and vitamin E 10%

Spinach Purée

Wait until your baby is six months or older to introduce homemade spinach because it's a high-nitrate vegetable (see page 225). When you do introduce it, use frozen spinach. Unlike fresh spinach, it's blanched, which stops the nitrate level from increasing.

Yield: 2.5 cups (625 milliliters)

16-ounce (500-gram) package frozen spinach
½–1 cup (125–250 milliliters) liquid

1. Cook spinach according to package directions.
2. Purée, adding breast milk, formula, or water to achieve a smooth consistency. (Don't use the cooking water because it may contain nitrates.)
3. Serve immediately and immediately freeze the rest.

Nutrient content of 2 tablespoons (30 milliliters)

Folate 80%, Potassium 30%, Vitamin A 15%, Vitamin C and iron 10%

Carrot Purée

Carrots are full of beta-carotene and are generally well liked by babies. However, wait until your baby is six months or older to introduce homemade carrots because they are high in nitrates (see page 225). When you do introduce carrots, use frozen instead of fresh.

Yield: 3 cups (750 milliliters)

16-ounce (500-gram) package frozen carrots
1 cup liquid

1. Cook carrots according to package directions.
2. Purée, adding breast milk, formula or water to achieve a smooth consistency.
3. Cool a serving in the refrigerator before use. Immediately freeze the rest. Root vegetables tend to thicken during freezing, so you may need to add extra liquid to get a smooth consistency after thawing.

Nutrient content of 2 tablespoons (30 milliliters)

17 calories, 1 gram fiber, Vitamin A 30%, Manganese 50%, Potassium 10%

Beet Purée

If color is an indication of vitamin content, beets have to be pretty healthy! When handling beets, prepare yourself for staining. Your baby will need a bib that covers well—or perhaps you'll want to feed your baby shirtless with a bib! That bright scarlet hue can also make it into your baby's diaper—either in stool or urine. However, wait until your baby is six months or older to introduce homemade beets because they are high in nitrates (see page 225). When you do introduce beets, use canned or frozen instead of fresh. Plus, because beets take a long time to cook and can lose more nutrients when cooked in water, using canned beets is the easy route!

Yield: About 1 cup (250 milliliters)

15-ounce (150-gram) can of beets

1. Drain beets and rinse several times to remove excess sodium.
2. Purée, adding perhaps a bit of apple juice or water.

Nutrient content of 2 tablespoons (30 milliliters)

13 calories, 1 gram fiber, Folate 30%, Magnesium and potassium 20%

Other Ways to Cook Beets

If you've got time on your hands, try one of these methods. Remember to immediately freeze anything more than a serving since beets are a high-nitrate vegetable.

- Boiling: Beets will keep more of their nutrient content if boiled whole rather than in pieces. However, this can take 45 minutes to 2 hours, depending on the size and age of the beets.
- Baking: This is a great way to lock in the nutrients. Wrap beets in foil and bake for 1½–2 hours at 350–400°F (175–200°C).
- Microwaving: Perhaps the fastest method. For each pound of whole beets, add ¼ cup of water to a microwave-safe dish. Cover and cook 15–20 minutes. Let stand 5 minutes and check doneness.

Soft Fruit Purée: Peaches, Nectarines, Pears, Apricots

At seven months, your baby should be able to eat these fruits without cooking, as long as they're very ripe. Before your baby is seven months or when the fruit isn't ripe, here's how to cook it briefly.

Yield: 1 cup (250 milliliters), depending on size of fruit

2 very ripe peaches, pears, or nectarines, or 4–5 apricots

1. Wash fruit, peel, and cut into pieces.
2. Cook fruit 1 minute in small amount of boiling water or microwave 1½ minutes with 1 teaspoon of water.
3. Purée or mash with a fork and add a small amount of breast milk or formula.

Nutrient content of 2 tablespoons (30 milliliters) peaches

18 calories, Vitamin K 50%, Potassium 10%, Niacin 10%

Nutrient content of 2 tablespoons (30 milliliters) nectarines

17 calories, Potassium 10%

Nutrient content of 2 tablespoons (30 milliliters) pears

24 calories, Potassium 10%

Nutrient content of 2 tablespoons (30 milliliters) apricots

17 calories, Vitamin A 10%, Potassium 12%

Crisp and Chewy Fruits: Apples, Dried Apricots, Dried Plums

When buying dried fruit to make baby food, look for varieties without sulfur additives.

Yield: About 2 cups (500 milliliters)

4 apples or 1 cup dried apricots, dried plums, or other dried fruit
1–2 tablespoons (15–30 milliliters) water

1. Peel fruit if necessary, then chop. Make sure apricots and plums have no small pieces of pits.
2. Place in a saucepan with water and cook 10 minutes or until tender. Or place in microwave-safe dish, cover, and microwave 10 minutes on high. Let stand 5 minutes and check tenderness.
3. Purée, adding a quarter to half cup of breast milk or formula.

Nutrient content of 2 tablespoons (30 milliliters) dried apricots

32 calories, Potassium 20%

Nutrient content of 2 tablespoons (30 milliliters) dried plums

39 calories, 1 gram fiber, Potassium 20%, Vitamin B_6 20%

Nutrient content of 2 tablespoons (30 milliliters) apples

Manganese 20%, Vitamin B_6 20%

Fresh Fruit Purée

Very ripe apricot, cantaloupe, mango, banana, and papaya can be puréed without cooking first. But because fresh fruits don't freeze well, make enough for your baby, then eat the remaining portion yourself!

Yield: Varies with size of fruit–3 cups of sliced or chopped fruit yields about 2 cups purée

Very ripe apricot, cantaloupe, mango, banana, or papaya

1. For mango and papaya, wash outside skin, cut, and scoop out flesh. For banana, peel and cut. For cantaloupe, wash outside skin with a produce brush, cut in half, scoop out seeds, and then scoop out fruit.
2. Purée or mash with a fork, adding a small amount of breast milk or formula as needed.

Nutrient content of 2 tablespoons (30 milliliters) apricot

19 calories, Vitamin A 10%, Vitamin C 10%, Vitamin B_6 10%

Nutrient content of 2 tablespoons (30 milliliters) cantaloupe

16 calories, Vitamin C 15%, Vitamin A 15%, Vitamin K 20%, Vitamin B_6 20%, Folate 10%

Nutrient content of 2 tablespoons (30 milliliters) mango

18 calories, Vitamin C 15%, Vitamin B_6 10%, Vitamin A 10%

Nutrient content of 2 tablespoons (30 milliliters) banana

Vitamin B_6 100%, Potassium 30%, Magnesium 20%, Manganese 10%

Nutrient content of 2 tablespoons (30 milliliters) papaya

Vitamin C 35%, Folate 10%, Potassium 10%

Creative Combinations

Once your baby has eaten whole-grain cereals, veggies, and fruits by him- or herself (without signs of allergies), try these combinations of simple purées. Simply mix about half and half of each food. You can either cook them together or separately. Combine them as you are inspired—the combinations are almost limitless! Fruit is a great natural sweetener for cereal, and the vitamin C helps iron absorption.

Combinations are great if your baby has a preference of one kind of food over another. Use the taste your baby loves to "sneak" in something he or she may not like as much.

Veggie and Grain

Acorn squash with whole barley cereal
Asparagus and whole oat cereal
Avocado with rice
Broccoli and millet
Butternut squash and brown rice cereal
Cauliflower, carrots, and oatmeal cereal
Green beans and mixed cereal
Peas and quinoa cereal
Spinach with brown rice cereal

Veggie Combinations

Acorn squash and carrots
Asparagus and zucchini
Asparagus and green beans
Asparagus with carrots
Beets and potato
Broccoli and carrots

Broccoli, cauliflower, and carrots
Broccoli and potato
Carrot and cauliflower
Carrots and zucchini squash
Cauliflower and yellow squash
Green beans and zucchini
Green beans and broccoli
Green beans and potato
Peas and cauliflower
Peas and carrots
Peas and zucchini
Sweet potato and cauliflower
Potato with carrots
Spinach and potato
Potato, carrot, and turnip
Peas, cauliflower, and zucchini
Broccoli, green beans, and yellow squash

Veggie and Fruit

Acorn squash with apple
Acorn squash with apricots
Apple and beets
Apricot and sweet potato
Butternut squash and apricots
Carrot and apple
Carrots with pear
Green beans with avocado
Sweet potato and pear

Fruit Combinations

Apple and dried plums
Apples and plums
Apples and apricots
Apples and cranberries
Apples and blueberries

Apricot with dried plums
Banana and plums
Banana with blueberries
Mango and pear
Mango and banana
Peaches and apricot
Peaches and apple
Peaches and plum
Pears and bananas
Plums and pears
Plums and bananas

Fruit and Grain

Apple with oatmeal
Apple and dates with quinoa
Avocado with brown rice cereal
Banana and barley cereal
Banana and millet cereal
Cranberry with oatmeal
Dates with mixed cereal
Mango and rice cereal
Pears and whole oat cereal
Peaches and barley cereal
Pears, dates, and brown rice cereal
Plums and millet

Hard-Cooked Egg Yolks

There are many ways to cook egg yolks for your baby. You can either hard-cook the whole egg and then take out the yolk (as explained here), or you can scramble the separated yolk with some liquid. You can also cook the yolk with cereal (as explained on page 249).

Yield: Depends on number of eggs hard-cooked

Uncracked raw eggs

1. Place cold eggs in a single layer in a saucepan. Cover top of eggs with at least 1 inch (2.5 centimeters) cold water.
2. Cover saucepan and bring to a boil quickly over high heat.
3. Immediately remove pan from heat to stop boiling.
4. Let eggs stand in water 20–25 minutes.
5. Drain and immediately run cold water over eggs until cooled.
6. Remove eggs from shell and separate yolks from whites.
7. Purée.

Nutrient content for 1 egg yolk

60 calories, 3 grams protein, Choline 150%, Vitamin B$_{12}$ 90%, Phosphorous 30%, Riboflavin 25%, Folate and zinc 20%, Vitamin E 10%, Iron 5%

Scrambled Egg Yolk

Yield: 2 servings

2 egg yolks
2 teaspoons (10 milliliters) liquid (cooking liquid from vegetables, fruit juice, breast milk, formula, or water)
½ teaspoon (2.5 milliliters) unsalted butter or olive oil

1. Beat egg yolks with liquid in a bowl.
2. Use a nonstick pan or heat butter or oil in pan over medium heat.
3. Add eggs to pan and stir constantly until no liquid egg is visible.
4. Purée with small amount of breast milk or formula.

Nutrient Content for 1 serving

63 calories, 3 grams protein, Choline 150%, Vitamin B$_{12}$ 90%, Phosphorous 30%, Riboflavin, 25%, Folate and zinc 20%, Vitamin E 10%, Iron 5%

Cereal with Egg Breakfast

Yield: 2 servings

½ cup (125 milliliters) cooked cereal
2 egg yolks

1. Heat cereal in saucepan, adding breast milk or formula as needed to achieve a smooth consistency.
2. Add egg yolk to saucepan and stir constantly until mixture reaches 160°F (71°C) or until no liquid egg is visible.

Nutrient Content of 1 serving

99 calories, 5 grams protein, 1 gram fiber, Choline 150%, Manganese 80%, Magnesium 25%, Iron 10%

Fruity-Oat Breakfast

This cereal turns into a balanced meal with the addition of egg and the extra nutrients of dried fruit. It can be made with any cereal.

Yield: 1¼ cups (310 milliliters)

4 small dried apricots, chopped
4 dried plums, chopped
2 dates (pitted with fibrous inner layer removed), chopped
5 tablespoons (74 milliliters) water
⅓ cup uncooked Scottish-cut oats (or any cereal your baby likes)
1 cup (250 milliliters) water
2 beaten egg yolks

1. Put fruit and 5 tablespoons water in medium saucepan. Bring to a boil and then simmer 3 minutes.
2. Add oats, 1 cup water, and egg yolks. Bring back to a boil, then reduce to a simmer.
3. Cover and cook 10 minutes.
4. Remove from heat and let cool. Add breast milk, formula, or water and purée to achieve a smooth consistency.
5. Cool and serve.

Nutrient content of 4 tablespoons (60 milliliters)

88 calories, 3 grams protein, 2 grams fiber, Magnesium 90%, Choline 60%, Manganese and phosphorous 30%, Vitamin B_{12} and thiamine 30%, Zinc and vitamin B_6 20%, Iron 10%

Cereal with Mango or Melon

Adding a vitamin C–rich fruit like mango or melon will increase the amount of iron your baby absorbs from cereal. It's great served cool on a warm summer day.

Yield: 4 tablespoons (60 milliliters)

3 tablespoons (45 milliliters) puréed mango or melon
1 tablespoon (15 milliliters) breast milk, formula, or water
2 tablespoons (30 milliliters) prepared dry iron-fortified infant cereal

1. Mix puréed fruit with breast milk, formula, or water.
2. Stir fruit into cereal.
3. Serve cool or lukewarm.

Nutrient content of 4 tablespoons (prepared with mango)

30 calories, Niacin 35%, Riboflavin 25%, Iron 20%, Vitamin C 10%, Vitamin A 10%

Chapter 13

Eight to Ten Months

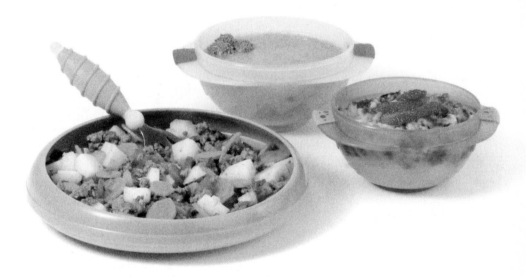

Whatever is on the floor will wind up in your baby's mouth.
Whatever is in your baby's mouth will wind up on the floor.

—Bruce Lansky, parenting book publisher

By this time your little guy or gal should be able to sit well in a highchair. This makes feeding easier (and messier). Your baby can pick things up with her whole hand (plantar grasp) and is fascinated with small objects like crumbs. Your baby also should be showing interest in finger foods and may be trying to grab food off of your plate! It's okay to feed your baby from your plate, but try not to let her eat *after* you or from your utensils. You could pass on unwanted germs this way, and your baby's immune system is still immature.

During the next few months, your baby's diet will continue to expand with the addition of protein foods and wheat, foods that enable you to offer many mixed foods as well as finger foods. You may also add small amounts of dairy, unless your baby is allergic to cow's milk protein or is at high risk for a food allergy.

Seventh Food: Protein Foods

If your baby is allergy-prone, hold off on tofu, soybeans, and processed soy foods until at least twelve months. Hold off on seafood until three years.

Why: Protein foods are, of course, good sources of protein for your baby's growing body. They're also typically good sources of iron, zinc, vitamin B_6, and vitamin B_{12}. Beans provide an extra nutritional punch: fiber, folic acid, niacin, vitamin B_6, manganese, and copper.

What kind: Good protein foods for babies are puréed meats (beef, lamb, pork, fish, chicken, and turkey), legumes (lentils, split peas, and other beans), tofu, and soy foods. If your baby doesn't like the taste of protein foods alone, try mixing them with something your baby likes. When your baby can handle the texture, you can finely chop protein foods instead of puréeing them. Adding them to mashed vegetables or potatoes may help them go down easier.

When: At lunch or dinner

How often: Once or twice a day

How much: Start with a teaspoon or two (5 to 10 milliliters). Work up to one or two tablespoons per day (15 to 30 milliliters), then increase to four tablespoons (60 milliliters) per day.

Protein Power

Protein is especially important during times of growth. It's used to build body tissues you can see, like skin, hair, muscle, and fingernails, as well as those you can't see, like new blood and nerve cells, antibodies, hormones, and many other chemicals that help the body grow.

Most North Americans eat more protein than they need, so you might be tempted to pile the protein on your child. You may be surprised at how little protein he or she needs:

- Infants birth to six months: nine grams of protein
- Infants seven to twelve months: eleven grams of protein
- Children one to three years and twenty-nine pounds: thirteen grams of protein
- Children four to six years and forty-four pounds: nineteen grams of protein

Babies get most—if not all—of their protein from breast milk or formula. Most toddlers can get enough protein just from drinking milk. The benefit of adding meat is not so much its protein content as its iron and zinc content. Research suggests that a six- to eight-month-old breastfed infant needs to get only 23 to 28 percent of his or her required protein from complementary food, but needs to get 99 percent of iron, 72 percent of zinc, 78 percent of vitamin B_{12}, and 43 percent of vitamin C required from complementary food.[1]

Feeding more protein than your baby needs will not improve your baby's health or speed up growth. In fact, over many years a high-protein diet may contribute to osteoporosis and kidney disease. That's because too much protein in the diet alters calcium metabolism, causing some calcium from the bones to be excreted in urine.

Protein-Rich Foods for Eight- to Ten-Month-Olds

- Animal products, such as fish, lean beef, lean pork, poultry, and lamb
- Breast milk and formula
- Cheese and yogurt
- Soymilk, tofu, and other soy products
- Legumes
- Buckwheat and kasha
- Seed butters
- High-protein grains like quinoa, millet, and spelt

The following protein foods are also high in iron and zinc:

- Lean red meats
- Legumes (especially garbanzo beans)
- Tofu

Tales from the Trenches: Meat Spitters

My friend's daughter Ana Maria spits out meat and gets upset when her parents coax her to eat it. Ana Maria is not unusual. In fact, meats are the least popular foods among babies. If your baby is a meat spitter, don't worry: It doesn't mean he or she will never eat meat.

Two cases in point: My older son, Nicolas, didn't care for homemade or jarred puréed meats, but took to them just fine when he could eat them chopped. My younger son, Robert, chose to be vegetarian until about eighteen months. His protein food of choice was refried beans from a can—not what you'd expect from a dietitian's son. But hey—low-fat vegetarian refried beans are good for you! To this day Robert still prefers canned pork and beans over homemade, and his regular order when we go out for Mexican food is a bean burrito.

While your baby's refusing meat, just offer other foods that provide similar nutrients.

Eighth Food: Wheat

If your baby is at high risk for allergies or gluten intolerance, the traditional advice is to delay introducing wheat, as well as processed foods that contain wheat, until your baby is twelve months or older. However, ask your baby's doctor about some new research that suggests earlier introduction might be better. (See page 218 for more info.)

Why: Introducing wheat expands your baby's diet to include more family foods. Wheat also provides fiber and B vitamins.

What kind: Introduce small amounts of single-grain infant wheat cereal first. After four days, if your baby shows no allergy symptoms, you can add other wheat foods, such as pasta, teething biscuits, crackers, bread, and mixed-grain cereals.

When: You might want to try wheat cereal in the morning. Once you see there's no problem, you can add other wheat foods throughout the day.

How much: Start with one tablespoon of cereal mixed to the texture your baby likes and increase to a few tablespoons a day. Serve whole-grain wheat products daily. Whole grains contain more fiber and antioxidants than processed grains.

How often: Serve wheat once or twice a day at first. Eventually your baby's diet will contain many servings of wheat.

Whole Grains

Your baby is probably ready now to try different textures of the foods he or she has had only in puréed or mashed form. For example, your baby can eat regular white or brown rice in addition to rice cereal, and whole barley instead of barley cereal.

This is a great time to begin adding whole grains to your baby's diet. Since your baby is forming lifelong eating habits now, serving whole grains regularly will get your baby started out right. However, eating only whole grains can add so much fiber that it can be too filling for a baby, so you'll still want to give your baby some refined grains like infant cereal and regular pasta.

Good baby-friendly whole-grain foods are:

- Whole-grain cereals (See recipes in Chapter 12.)
- Whole-wheat pasta (including couscous)
- Unhulled barley
- Brown rice
- Ground cornmeal—found in corn tortillas and polenta
- Bulgur wheat
- Quinoa
- Millet
- Whole oats
- Buckwheat (not really a grain, but generally regarded as one)
- Triticale (a cross between rye and wheat)
- Whole-grain crackers
- Corn on the cob
- Puffed wheat
- Puffed kashi

What's So Great about Whole Grains?

Lots. Not so long ago, we thought whole grain's main asset was its fiber. Now research has shown that whole grain has many healthy components.

A grain has three main parts: the bran or outer covering, which is fiber-rich; the starchy endosperm; and the nutrient-rich germ. Whole grains contain fiber and nutrients such as B vitamins, vitamin E, magnesium, iron, and many disease-fighting phytochemicals and antioxidants. Because the many nutrients in whole grains work together to provide health benefits, a whole grain is more than the sum of its parts.

And just what are the benefits? There are plenty:[2]

- Whole grains reduce risk of certain cancers and heart disease, as well as stroke and type 2 diabetes.

- People who eat whole grains have lower body mass index (BMI), lower total cholesterol, and lower waist-to-hip ratio.

- Fiber from whole grains protects against constipation, hemorrhoids, diverticulitis, and appendicitis.

How to Spot a Whole Grain

You can't judge a whole grain by its color. For example, some breads are brown, but from added molasses instead of whole grain.

The best way to find a whole grain is to look at a food's ingredient list. If you don't see the phrase *whole grain*, look for *whole, rolled,* or *steel-cut.* If you see the word *enriched,* it's a clue that the food is not whole-grain; refined grains must have nutrients added back that were lost in processing. The term *fortified* means that additional nutrients have been added to a food that weren't there in the first place. Be aware that bran cereals are composed of just the bran part of a grain and are not considered whole-grain.

You've got a fussy baby in the cart and don't have the luxury to peruse every label? Look for a whole-grain health claim on the front of the package. A health claim may say something like "can help lower cholesterol and reduce the risk of heart disease and some cancers." To put this health claim on its package, a product must:

- Contain all portions of the grain kernel
- Contain at least 51 percent whole grain by weight
- Meet specific fat, saturated fat, and cholesterol restrictions

Although some packages claim the food inside is an "excellent" or "good" source of whole grain, be aware that these claims are not formal Food and Drug Administration (FDA) terms.

Ninth Food: Dairy

If your baby isn't allergy-prone, you can introduce small amounts of dairy starting at nine months. If your baby has a cow's milk protein allergy or is at high risk of allergy, delay all dairy foods until one year or later.

Why: Introducing dairy expands your baby's diet to include more family foods. Dairy also provides protein, calcium, riboflavin, vitamin B_{12}, and other B vitamins. Dairy is a good substitute for kids who don't like meat. Yogurt with live, active cultures provides probiotics (good bacteria), which keep the intestines healthy. Probiotics also help prevent and treat yeast infections (thrush) and antibiotic-induced diarrhea.

What kind: Introduce yogurt, pasteurized cheese, and cottage cheese only. Don't introduce regular cow's milk until one year.

When: Serve dairy at meals or for snacks. Yogurt is a great treat when mixed with fruit or used in a fruit smoothie.

How much: Offer a half-ounce (fifteen grams) of cheese and a quarter-cup (sixty milliliters) of yogurt at first. As your baby gets closer to twelve months, you can increase serving sizes.

How often: Once or twice a day

Tenth Foods: Mixed Foods and Finger Foods

Introduce mixed foods and finger foods at nine months.

Why: Mixed foods and finger foods expand your baby's diet to include more family foods.

What kind: Mixed foods include soft foods like macaroni and cheese, other pasta dishes, stews, and casseroles. Make sure your baby has already tried all the foods in a mixed dish and has no reaction to them. Finger foods can be just about anything cut into baby-safe pieces.

When: You can serve mixed foods and finger foods for both meals and snacks.

How much: Amounts will vary depending on the food.

How often: As often as every meal and snack, depending on your baby's readiness.

Hand to Mouth

Your baby's getting much more talented at picking up and holding things. He or she is also getting more coordinated and curious. Putting objects in his or her mouth is suddenly really easy and fun—not to mention soothing for sore gums—so your baby does it all the time.

It's more important than ever to keep anything that could be a choking hazard away from your baby. (See pages 212–213 for more information about choking prevention.) This includes food. Finger foods can be a healthy addition to your baby's diet—but take care to offer only appropriate textures and sizes.

Good Finger Foods

- Cheerios, Oatios, or other low-sugar cereal Os
- Gerber Veggie Puffs and Fruit Puffs
- Bite-size toast pieces

- Crackers
- Cubed steamed vegetables
- Grated apple
- Well-cooked pasta, cut up
- Scrambled egg yolk
- Small pieces of soft banana, mango, peaches, pear, or avocado
- Very soft or lightly steamed berries
- Cooked peas
- Tofu pieces
- Small pieces of ripe melon
- Slightly mashed peas or beans
- Teething biscuits
- Small pieces of rice cake
- Cooked brown rice or barley
- Bite-size pieces of whole-grain waffle or pancake

Taste and Texture

Adding Spices

If you want your baby to eat what you eat, he or she needs to get used to the spices you typically use. It's now okay to add small amount of spices to your baby's food. Try to keep avoiding salt, hot peppers, and other spicy condiments, but feel free to use small amounts of cooked garlic, shallot, onion, and dry herbs and spices like basil, oregano, thyme, cumin, nutmeg, cinnamon, and even a pinch of pepper. As with all foods, add just one spice at a time to make sure your baby doesn't have an allergic reaction. (If your baby has GERD, stay away from pepper, oregano, and hot spices.)

Changing Textures

It's important to increase and vary the texture of your baby's food now to help him or her get used to the wide range of textures in your family's diet. There's no need to rush, though; as long as you're making progress, the speed isn't important. Follow your baby's lead in working toward more mashed and chunky foods.

> **Tales from the Trenches: My Pet Fear**
>
> Choking. It was my biggest fear when my kids were small.
>
> I saw a news story about a toddler who choked while riding in a stroller and eating whole grapes. Not only was the food hazardous but also the mom couldn't see the child because he was facing away from her. It was a case of everything going wrong: While the mom kept looking for help, the paramedics couldn't locate her. Sadly, that choking incident was fatal.
>
> Well, every parent has a right to go overboard on something. My obsession was choking prevention. I went so far as to peel and chop grapes for Robert when he was ten months old, and I always took care not to give either of my boys any risky foods. My friends thought me quite paranoid because I never let my kids walk around while eating.
>
> But that was okay with me—I felt much better about being freakishly safe than sorry.

A Day in the Diet...

Of a Nine-Month-Old

Here's a sample daily menu for a nine-month-old eating cereals, fruits, vegetables, dairy, and protein foods. At this point, a baby should be starting to have better defined meals plus snacks.

Breakfast

Breast milk or formula
French Toast Strips with Blue-
    berry Sauce (page 282)

Mid-morning snack

Yogurt with chopped pear

Lunch

Breast milk or formula
Baby Beef Stew (page 270)

Mid-afternoon snack

Diluted juice
Cheerios

Dinner

Breast milk or formula
Chicken with Root Vegetables (page 268)

Bedtime snack

Breast milk or formula

Of a Ten-Month-Old

Here's a sample daily menu for a ten-month-old who's starting to eat some mixed foods and finger foods.

Breakfast

Mixed brown rice and
    barley cereal
Blueberries
Breast milk or formula

Mid-morning snack

Strawberry Crème Dip
    (page 302) on crackers
Diluted juice

Lunch

Breast milk or formula
Pork Loin with Butternut Squash
    and Cauliflower (page 268)
Asparagus

Mid-afternoon snack

Breast milk or formula
Teething crackers

Dinner

Macaroni and cheese with beef
Chopped broccoli
Carrot cubes
Fruit Pop (page 326)

Bedtime snack

Breast milk or formula

Of a Vegan Ten-Month-Old

Here's a sample daily menu for a ten-month-old who eats no meat, fish, eggs, or dairy.

Breakfast

Breast milk or formula
Whole-grain waffle strips
Honeydew melon

Mid-morning snack

Soy yogurt with chopped peaches

Lunch

Breast milk or formula
Black Bean Soup (page 303)
   with rice

Mid-afternoon snack

Breast milk or formula
Crackers
Hummus Spread (page 280)

Dinner

Cubed tofu
Chopped broccoli and sweet potato
Toast strips

Bedtime snack

Breast milk or formula

Issues for This Age Group

Setting a Good Example

You've probably noticed that your baby likes to mimic you—whether you're making a funny face or opening your mouth in hopes of getting your baby to do the same. Your baby is also noticing what you eat and naturally wants to share it with you.

It's time to start setting a good example! From here on out, the best way for your kid to learn healthy eating is to watch you model it. (For more information on this topic, see Chapter 18.) There's another good reason to eat well, too: Good eating leads to good health and longevity. You want to care for your child to the best of your ability and stick around long enough to be a grandparent.

If you just *must* have your regular dose of junk food, do it while your baby is sleeping! Junk food will enter your baby's world all too soon on its own; why expose your baby to it any earlier?

Adding Water to the Diet

Your baby is now eating many solid foods and may need more liquids, particularly in hot weather. Breast milk or formula should still be your baby's main beverage, but it's okay to add some water now for quenching thirst. If you establish a good habit of drinking water now, you may head off a bad habit of drinking juice or soda to quench thirst when your child is older.

Make sure your water supply is safe. (See page 86 to learn how.) Some parents choose to give their babies filtered water to avoid any chance of bacterial or chemical contamination.

Plaque Alert

Your baby is now eating solid food more often, and as you add finger foods to your baby's repertoire, your baby's teeth can begin accumulating more plaque. Be sure to clean your baby's teeth twice a day with a toothbrush made for infants.

Cooking for Your Eight- to Ten-Month-Old

Cooking Meat, Poultry, and Fish

Looks Aren't Everything

No baby food looks particularly appetizing, but puréed meats look the worst! The recipes in this book are no exception. But be assured that I've tested and tasted them all, and I think they actually taste good!

Here are some tips for cooking meat, poultry, and fish to make them taste good:

- Sear it at a higher temperature first. Don't brown it; just cook the outside so it changes color.
- Don't boil it.
- Don't overcook it.
- Cook it with a vegetable.
- Add herbs or spices. Once it's clear your baby isn't allergic to a new meat, poultry, or fish, you can begin flavoring it. Here's how:

  - First add a bit of garlic for a few days. Just half a clove, well cooked, provides great flavor and many phytonutrients. Sauté the garlic in a tiny amount of oil before adding it to a recipe. Let your baby get used to the flavor and watch for an allergic reaction.
  - Then add a bit of chopped onion to the garlic. (Or add dehydrated onion to a dish with liquid.)
  - Then add any herbs you normally use, sparingly and one at a time (for example, sage, cumin, oregano, or curry powder).

> **Breast versus Thigh**
>
> In the fat department, chicken breast wins; it's far lower in fat than the thigh. The thigh wins in the nutrient department, though; it has twice the iron and two and a half times the zinc. So go ahead and use the thigh—just make sure to trim it of all fat before you cook it.

Using a Food Thermometer

Using a thermometer seems like a pain, but it really isn't—especially if you've got a decent one. The tiny effort it takes can prevent both undercooking, which often leads to food-borne illness, and overcooking, which dries out food and robs it of flavor and nutrients. (See page 199 for safe cooking temperatures for meat, poultry, eggs, and seafood.)

I was using an old thermometer when I started testing recipes for this book. (How old? Let's just say I got it when I was a dietetics student.) It was slow. I quickly lost patience with the waiting and trying to read the little numbers on the dial. I went to the store to check out new thermometers and walked out with a ten-dollar investment: a Polder digital thermometer that works like a charm—in seconds.

Go ahead and invest in a digital quick-read thermometer—you'll be much more likely to use it!

Seafood Cooking Tips

Seafood is the ultimate fast food; a small portion cooks in just a few minutes in the microwave. Here are a few tips for cooking safe, tasty seafood:

- Feed your baby fish that are low in mercury. See page 209 for a list of fish with high, moderate, and low mercury content.
- If you catch your own fish, follow local fish advisories. (See page 210.)
- Start with mild-flavored seafood (sole, tilapia, trout, cod, flounder, salmon, shrimp, and crab).
- Try mixing seafood with potatoes, grain, or a veggie.
- Choose fish filets, not steaks or whole fish.
- If you do cook whole fish, remove all skin and fat before cooking. (I usually ask the person at the fish counter to do this.)
- Poaching fish in a bit of leftover cooking liquid from vegetables or milk keeps it moist and speeds up cooking time.
- Remember that fish is fragile and is easily overcooked. See page 199 for safe cooking temperatures and tips on checking doneness.
- In general, cook fish (fresh or thawed) about five minutes per half-inch of thickness by poaching, baking, or grilling. Cook fish three to five minutes per pound in the microwave. Be aware that stuffed fish and fish patties take longer.
- Cook frozen fish about ten minutes per half-inch of thickness. Be sure to check the internal temperature.
- You can reserve cooking liquid from mild-flavored fish to make a sauce. Otherwise, discard cooking liquid. Always discard cooking liquid from fish cooked whole or with the skin.

Cooking Beans

Dried Beans

- Most people cook dried beans with something salty like bacon, ham, or salt pork. But extra salt is still off-limits for your baby, so use onion, garlic, spices, and herbs to enhance flavor. If your baby is okay with onion and/or garlic, chances are all the related foods (green onion, shallot, leeks, and chives) will be fine, too. I like cooking with green onions because they're quick to chop and cook and less likely to make me cry. In a pinch, you can use dehydrated onion, shallot, or chives. Or use any of a number of salt-free herb blends, like Mrs. Dash.

- Don't add sweet vegetables or acidic foods like tomato until the beans are tender. Sugar and acid both prevent beans from softening.
- High altitude can double cooking time for beans.
- Pressure-cooking beans takes a fraction of the time it takes to cook beans in a regular pot.
- Always make sure there is enough liquid in the pot to cover the beans.
- The following beans cause less gas than others: Anasazi beans, adzuki beans, black-eyed peas, lentils, pigeon peas, and split peas.
- Cooked beans can keep in the refrigerator for three days.
- Cooked beans freeze well in zipper bags; just cool them first. If you plan to freeze beans, slightly undercook them and then finish cooking with additional liquid after thawing them.
- Introduce beans to your baby in small amounts—a few tablespoons at a time—to help your baby adjust to their high fiber content. Or mix beans generously with another vegetable.

Canned Beans

Raise your hand if you cook beans from scratch once a week. I don't see many hands! Let's face it: Most of us don't have the time or motivation to cook beans from scratch. If you look in my pantry, you'll find a variety of canned beans: fat-free refried beans, black beans, chickpeas (garbanzo beans), white beans, and baked beans. The only beans I regularly cook from scratch are quick-cooking lentils or split peas.

Can you feed canned beans to your baby? Yes! Just follow a few simple guidelines:

- Buy salt-free or low-sodium beans. That way you can use the liquid in the can to boost nutrient content.
- If you use regular (salted) beans, discard the liquid in the can and rinse the beans well to remove excess sodium.
- Use herbs and spices to give canned beans more flavor.

Introducing Dairy

In this chapter, your baby hits a big milestone: he or she can begin eating small amounts of dairy. Previous chapters may have you quite concerned with allergies—you may wonder why dairy is now mentioned as an addition to the diet before one year.

If your baby is at higher risk of allergy or has had any allergic reactions, you'll want to continue to be vigilant about not giving your baby any cow's milk protein until you have your doctor's okay.

On the other hand, if your baby has no risk of allergies and has shown no symptoms of allergy from any of the foods introduced so far, or anything else, it's okay to give small amounts of dairy in the coming months. That's because your baby's more mature gastrointestinal tract acts as a barrier to proteins that might have gotten through and caused an allergic reaction a few months ago.

Here's a primer on how and what dairy foods you should introduce first:

- **Yogurt**: As I've said before, yogurt is one of the healthiest foods around. It's a good idea to present yogurt to your baby as the first dairy food. The live active cultures in yogurt break down the lactose (milk sugar), making it more digestible, even for babies who've had previous problems with lactose intolerance. The milk proteins are also modified by the culturing process, making them easier to digest as well. By now you know all about the wonderful probiotics in yogurt that are very healthy for your baby (especially if your baby is taking antibiotics). Yogurt can also be used in cooking in place of milk (though it loses its thickness).

- **Cheese**: Milk is heated to high temperatures and is also cultured to produce cheese. This makes the protein easier to digest and also lowers the lactose. Unless your child has been diagnosed with a milk allergy, cheese should pose no problem. However, it tends to be high in sodium and saturated fat, making it something you give to your baby in small amounts: one-fourth– to one-half–ounce servings of hard cheese, or one-fourth of a cup of cottage cheese.

- **Milk**: Milk is not recommended as a beverage until one year, when it would be consumed in large amounts, because it doesn't contain the nutrient mix your baby needs. Consuming large amounts of milk can irritate the lining of the digestive tract, causing small iron losses. However, at this age, small amounts of milk can be introduced in foods after you've introduced yogurt and found no problems. Your baby will be eating finger foods and table foods, too; some of these will also contain small amounts of milk protein.

You can use any type of milk in these recipes (even skim milk), because your baby is still getting the necessary fat from breast milk or formula and other foods. You can also use cream; it's higher in fat but lower in protein. If you're avoiding or delaying dairy, you can substitute breast milk, soymilk, soy formula, or cooking liquid from meat or vegetables. (Cooking will, however, destroy or reduce some of the good things in breast milk.)

Storage Reminder

Here are the basic rules for storing homemade baby food:

- For homemade cereals, veggies, and fruits, refrigerate what you will use within two days. Freeze any remainders. Exception: When making baby food from high-nitrate vegetables, immediately freeze anything over a serving.

- For eggs, refrigerate what you will use within twenty-four hours. Freeze any remainders, but note that some egg recipes won't freeze well.

Basic Meat Recipe

Yield: ¼ cup (60 milliliters)

2 ounces (60 grams) chicken breast, chicken thigh, pork loin, or lamb with all fat removed, cut into small pieces
3 tablespoons (45 milliliters) water or other cooking liquid
½ minced garlic clove (optional)
1 tablespoon (15 milliliters) minced green onion (optional)
½ teaspoon (2.5 milliliters) vegetable oil

1. Sauté chicken over medium-high heat for 1 to 2 minutes, stirring constantly, until all sides are seared. (Optional: Add garlic or onion sautéed in ½ teaspoon oil first.)
2. Add 3 tablespoons (45 milliliters) water. Lower heat to medium and cover. Cook for 2 minutes or until meat reaches the proper internal temperature. (See page 199.)
3. Chop meat very finely or purée with 1–2 tablespoons (15 to 30 milliliters) of additional water, breast milk, or formula.

Nutrient content of 2 tablespoons (30 milliliters) chicken breast

42 calories, 8 grams protein, Niacin 60%, Vitamin B$_6$ 30%, Zinc 10%, Vitamin B$_{12}$ 10%

Nutrient content of 2 tablespoons (30 milliliters) chicken thigh

59 calories, 7 grams protein, Niacin 50%, Vitamin B$_6$ 30%, Vitamin B$_{12}$ 20%, Zinc 25%

Nutrient content of 2 tablespoons (30 milliliters) beef round

60 calories, 9 grams protein, Vitamin B$_{12}$ 140%, Zinc 50%, Selenium 40%, Phosphorous, niacin, and vitamin B$_6$ 30%, Iron 10%

Nutrient content of 2 tablespoons (30 milliliters) lamb loin

53 calories, 8 grams protein, Vitamin B$_{12}$ 180%, Zinc 50%, Niacin and vitamin B$_6$ 40%, Selenium 15%

Nutrient content of 2 tablespoons (30 milliliters) pork loin

60 calories, 8 grams protein, Selenium 60%, Thiamine 50%, Niacin and vitamin B$_6$ 30%, Vitamin B$_{12}$ 25%, Zinc 20%

Basic Fish Recipe

Yield: ½ cup (125 milliliters)

4 ounces (120 grams) boneless, skinless fish
½ cup (125 milliliters) water, broth, milk, or other cooking liquid
1 sprig parsley or cilantro
1 green onion

1. In a small pan, bring cooking liquid and herbs to a boil.
2. Add fish and lower heat to a simmer.
3. Cook 3 to 4 minutes or until fish flakes easily.
4. Discard herbs. Reserve liquid to make a sauce if desired.
5. Chop fish very finely or purée with 1 to 2 tablespoons (15 to 30 milliliters) of cooking liquid.

Nutrient content of 2 tablespoons (30 milliliters) flounder purée

40 calories, 6 grams protein, Vitamin B$_{12}$ 90%, Niacin, vitamin B$_6$, potassium, and phosphorous 20%, Vitamin E 15%

Nutrient content of 2 tablespoons (30 milliliters) salmon purée

60 calories, 6 grams protein, 640 milligrams omega-3 fatty acids, Vitamin B$_{12}$ 130%, Selenium and niacin 60%, Thiamine and phosphorous 30%, Potassium 20%, Folate 10%

Basic Bean Purée

How to Cook Beans from Scratch

Step One: Sort and Rinse

Occasionally during harvesting, a small pebble gets into the mix, so it's important to quickly sort through the beans to look for rocks. Rinsing gets any post-harvest dirt off, too. I usually do this by pouring the beans in a colander, then sorting and rinsing at the same time.

Step Two: Soak

After soaking, your beans will triple in size; plan accordingly. Slow Soak: If you plan ahead, you can soak the beans 8 hours or overnight in the refrigerator. In a large pot, cover one pound of dry beans with about 10 cups (2.5 liters) of cold water. Measuring isn't important. Just put your beans in a large pot and cover amply with water. Quick Soak: For those spontaneous cooks, place one pound of beans in a large pot with about 10 cups (2.5 liters) of hot water. Bring to a boil and let boil 2 to 3 minutes. Turn off heat and let stand for at least one hour.

Beans, Beans, Beans

Common and Other Names	Attributes	Cooking Ideas	Cooking Time
Adzuki beans	Strong, nutty, sweet flavor	Popular in Asia; ingredient in sweet red bean paste	40 to 60 minutes
Baby lima beans	Smooth creamy texture	Soups and casseroles	1 hour
Black beans (turtle beans)	Rich and creamy	South/Central American cuisine	1 to 1.5 hours
Black-eyed peas (cowpeas)	Savory flavor	Southern recipes, eaten in the South on New Year's for good luck	30 minutes to 1 hour
Dark red kidney beans	Firm texture	Chili, soups, salads, red beans and rice	1.5 to 2 hours
Garbanzo beans (chickpeas)	Nutty flavor, firm texture	Main ingredient in Middle Eastern dishes: hummus and falafel	1 to 1.5 hours
Navy beans	Small and white	Used in baked beans	1 hour
Pinto beans	Turn brown when cooked	Staple in Latin cooking; burritos, tacos	1.5 to 2 hours
Lentils	Don't need soaking. Can be firm or soft, depending on variety	Used in many cuisines, especially Indian and Middle Eastern	25 to 45 minutes
Split peas	Don't need soaking. Are smooth and creamy when puréed.	Main ingredient in split pea soup	45 to 60 minutes

Letting it stand up to another hour may make the beans easier to digest.

Step Three: Cook

Drain soaking water from beans and rinse. Cover with fresh water and add spices (see next step). Cook 30 minutes to 2 hours, depending on the bean. Read bean package for specific information. Check occasionally to make sure there is water left in the pot. Taste test to ensure softness.

Step Four: Spice

The sky's the limit when it comes to flavoring your beans. For the batch your baby eats, put in only the spices your baby tolerates and keep out the hot spices and salt. Here are just a few of the herbs and spices that go well with beans. Bay leaves are a nice addition to all beans—remove before serving.

- Garlic
- Onion
- Thyme and oregano
- Italian seasoning
- Basil
- Marjoram
- Fresh cilantro
- Curry powder
- Cumin

Don't add any acidic foods like tomatoes or vinegar until beans are tender.

Bean Math

One 15-ounce can of beans = 1.5 cups (750 milliliters) cooked beans
One pound dry beans = 2 cups (500 milliliters) dry beans
One pound dry beans = 6 cups (1.5 liters) cooked beans
One cup dry beans = 3 cups (750 milliliters) cooked beans, drained

Cooking Note: The longer you keep dry beans and peas in your pantry, the longer they take to cook!

Lentil and Split Pea Cooking

These peas are still in the legume family but are smaller and rounder than dry beans. Neither needs to be soaked before cooking, but they should be sorted to pick out any rocks and then rinsed.

- There are several varieties of lentils; some are best for certain purposes.
- Brown lentils are the garden variety you find at the grocery store. They hold their shape unless overcooked and then become mushy.
- Green and French green lentils keep a firm texture after cooking— making them perfect for salads.
- Orange lentils are hulled and split so they cook even faster than other lentils. They are often used in Middle Eastern and Indian dishes.
- Red lentils cook quickly but don't hold their shape. The hulled red lentil is known as the *massoor dal* and is most common in Indian dishes.

To Cook Lentils

1. Pour 1.5 cups (375 milliliters) of water or broth for every 1 cup of dry lentils into a saucepan.

2. Add desired seasonings. (Salt added during cooking toughens them, so add after you take out your child's portion.)

3. Bring liquid with lentils to a boil. Boil for 2 to 3 minutes and then reduce to a simmer.

4. Cook until tender: about 45 minutes for green lentils and brown lentils and 25 minutes for red and orange lentils. Check for tenderness 15 minutes before the end of suggested cooking time, which can vary depending on moisture content.

Split Peas

Split peas are actually field peas split in half; they're raised for drying and are often made into split pea soup.

To Cook Split Peas

1. Pour 2 cups (500 milliliters) of low-sodium broth or water into pot for each cup of split peas.
2. Bring water and peas to a boil and boil 3 minutes. Continue simmering until peas are tender—45 to 60 minutes.
3. For split pea soup, add chopped onion, carrots, and celery as desired and cook until vegetables are tender.

Bean Purée

Once beans or peas are well-cooked, they can be puréed with a small amount of cooking liquid, breast milk, or formula. They can also be added to other vegetables your baby likes—carrots, potato, and so on. For babies who like more texture, beans can be mashed with a fork or potato masher. And eventually, well-cooked beans make great finger foods.

Nutrient content of 4 tablespoons (60 milliliters) white beans

48 calories, 3 grams protein, 4 grams fiber, Folate 30%, Magnesium and manganese 15%, Thiamine 10%

Nutrient content of 4 tablespoons (60 milliliters) lentils

47 calories, 4 grams protein, 3 grams fiber, Folate 90%, Zinc, vitamin B$_6$, riboflavin, magnesium, and potassium 20%, Iron 10%

Nutrient content of 4 tablespoons (60 milliliters) Adzuki beans

55 calories, 3 grams protein, 3 grams fiber, Folate 65%, Potassium and magnesium 30%, Zinc 25%, Iron 10%

Nutrient content of 4 tablespoons (60 milliliters) split peas

49 calories, 3 grams protein, 2 grams fiber, Folate and thiamine 30%, Potassium and magnesium 20%

Basic Creamy Veggie Soup

Yield: about 8 cups (2 liters)

2 pounds (1 kilogram) any raw vegetable, chopped into 1-inch pieces (smaller for faster cooking). Some vegetables that work well are asparagus, broccoli and carrots, spinach and carrots, and spinach, broccoli, and carrots

1 pound (500 grams) new potatoes, peeled and cut into 1-inch pieces

2 to 3 cups (500 to 750 milliliters) liquid such as cooking liquid, soymilk, rice milk, breast milk, or formula (If your baby is one year or older, you can use whole milk.)

1 to 2 ounces (30–60 grams) soft pasteurized cheese, such as cream cheese or Laughing Cow (optional)

1. Time the cooking of the vegetables and potatoes according to the vegetables you use. (For example, spinach cooks quicker than the potatoes, so you'd need to start cooking the potatoes first, then add the spinach.) Cook in a minimal amount of liquid until vegetables and potatoes are tender.
2. Purée in batches in a blender, adding liquid as needed. If you like, add cheese while puréeing.
3. Pour soup back in pan and stir to mix all batches. Reheat if needed.

Nutrient content

Varies with vegetables used

Pork Loin with Butternut Squash and Cauliflower

Yield: about ¾ cup (180 milliliters)

2 ounces (60 grams) cooked pork loin, fat removed
¼ cup (60 milliliters) butternut squash, cooked
¼ cup (60 milliliters) cauliflower, cooked

1. Purée pork and vegetables with 1 to 2 tablespoons (15 to 30 milliliters) of leftover cooking liquid.

Nutrient content of ¼ cup or 4 tablespoons (60 milliliters)

49 calories, 6 grams protein, Selenium and thiamine 40%, Potassiuim and niacin 20%, Zinc 15%

Chicken with Broccoli

Yield: ½ cup (125 milliliters)

2 ounces (60 grams) chicken, cooked
1 heaping cup (250 milliliters) broccoli florets, cooked

1. Purée with 1 to 2 tablespoons (15 to 30 milliliters) of leftover cooking liquid.

Nutrient content of ¼ cup (60 milliliters)

58 calories, 10 grams protein, Vitamin C 80%, Niacin 70%, Vitamin B$_6$ and niacin 60%, Magnesium, potassium, and phosphorous 30%, Calcium 10%

Chicken and Peas

Yield: 1 heaping cup (250 milliliters)

½ cup (125 milliliters) water
½ cup (125 milliliters) frozen peas
3 ounces (90 grams) chicken, cut into pieces

1. Bring water to boil in small saucepan.
2. Cook peas until almost tender, about 5 minutes.
3. Lower heat and add chicken. Stir constantly and cook about 2 minutes, or until chicken has reached 165°F (74° C).
4. Purée chicken and peas using cooking liquid and additional liquid as needed.

Nutrient content of ¼ cup (60 milliliters)

48 calories, 7 grams protein, 1 gram fiber, Niacin 50%, Vitamin B$_6$ 30%, Thiamine and phosphorous 20%, Folate, magnesium, and manganese 15%

Chicken with Root Vegetables

Yield: 1 cup chopped (250 milliliters) or heaping ½ cup puréed (125 milliliters)

⅓ cup (80 milliliters) chopped carrots
⅓ cup (80 milliliters) chopped parsnips
2 ounces (60 grams) chicken

1. Cook carrots and parsnips in small amount of water or steam them.
2. Lower heat and add chicken and cook about 2 minutes, or until chicken has reached 165°F (74°C).
3. Purée chicken and vegetables using cooking liquid and additional liquid as needed.

Nutrient content of ¼ heaping cup (60 milliliters)

Vitamin B$_6$ 60%, Niacin 50%, Zinc, folate, and potassium 30%, Vitamin B$_{12}$ 20%

Turkey with Prunes

Yield: about 4 cups (1 liter)

1 onion, sliced
1 teaspoon (15 milliliters) canola or
  olive oil
5 boneless, skinless chicken thighs
  (about 1 pound or 500 grams)
2 cloves garlic, minced
24 prunes
2 cups apple juice or water

1. In non-stick skillet, heat oil. Add
   onions and garlic; sauté over
   medium-high heat about 5 minutes
   until translucent.
2. Move onions to edge of pan and
   add chicken. Lightly brown 2 to 3
   minutes on each side.
3. Add apple juice or water. Cover
   skillet and simmer 15 minutes, or
   until chicken has reached an internal temperature of 165°F (74°C).
4. Remove chicken from pan. Pour
   pan juices and prunes into dish
   and refrigerate until oil separates.
   Skim off fat.
5. Cut chicken into small pieces. Place
   half the chicken and pan juices in
   blender with as much onion and
   prune as desired. Add additional
   juice or water as needed. Repeat.
6. For this recipe, purée part of it for
   your baby; serve the rest to your
   family. It's very tasty!

Nutrient content of 4 tablespoons (60 milliliters)

100 calories, 8 grams protein, 1 gram fiber, Copper
45%, Niacin 40%, Vitamin B_6 35%, Zinc, selenium, and
potassium 25%

Lamb and White Beans

Yield: ⅔ cup (160 milliliters) puréed

½ teaspoon (2.5 milliliters) oil
1 small clove garlic, minced
2 ounces (60 grams) lamb chop or ten-
  derloin, cut into pieces
½ cup (125 milliliters) cooked or canned
  great northern or navy beans

1. Heat oil in small saucepan.
   Add garlic and sauté for about
   1 minute or until transparent.
2. Add lamb and cook to a minimum
   internal temperature of 160°F
   (71° C), about 2 minutes.
3. Add beans to lamb and stir
   until heated.
4. Chop or purée to desired consistency using liquid from beans.

Nutrient content of 4 tablespoons (60 milliliters)

90 calories, 2 grams fiber, Vitamin B_{12} 120%, Zinc 50%,
Folate, potassium, and magnesium 30%, Iron 15%

Baby Beef Stew

Yield: 2 cups (500 milliliters) stew or 1 heaping cup (250 milliliters) purée

1 medium potato, peeled and chopped
  (about ½ heaping cup)
½ cup (125 milliliters) sliced carrots
  (about 12 baby carrots)
1 stalk celery, chopped
2 tablespoons (30 milliliters) water
½ teaspoon (2.5 milliliters) olive or
  canola oil
1 clove garlic
½ green onion
3 red bell pepper strips, chopped
  (about ⅛ cup)
3½ ounces (100 grams) extra-lean
  natural ground beef

1. Place potato, carrots, celery,
   and water in a microwave-safe
   dish. Cover and microwave 3
   minutes on high or until tender.
   Let stand covered.
2. Over medium heat, sauté garlic,
   green onion, and bell pepper with
   oil. Add beef and cook 2 to 3 minutes or until it reaches an internal
   temperature of 160°F (71° C).
3. Combine vegetables and beef
   mixture. Chop to the appropriate
   texture for your baby or purée.

Nutrient content of ¼ cup (60 milliliters)

50 calories, 7 grams protein, Vitamin B$_{12}$ 150%,
Zinc 55%, Niacin 40%, Selenium 30%, Potassium,
phosphorous, and vitamin C 20%

Finely chopping veggies cuts cooking time,
but it also makes it easy to over-cook them—
leading to lost nutrients. Use minimal water
when veggies are finely chopped and
expect shorter cooking time.

Cheesy Sauce

Yield: a little over ½ cup (125 milliliters)

½ cup (125 milliliters) chopped butternut squash
½ cup (125 milliliters) broth, formula,
  or low-fat milk
1 ounce (30 grams) or ¼ cup grated
  Cheddar cheese
Garlic powder
Onion powder

1. Put squash in microwave-safe dish.
   Add 1 tablespoon of water. Cover
   and cook on high for 1½ minutes.
   Let stand several minutes.
2. Purée squash using hand blender.
   Gradually add ½ cup liquid while
   puréeing.
3. Transfer mixture to small
   saucepan. Stir in cheese until
   melted. Add a shake of garlic and
   onion powder and stir.

Nutrient content of 2 tablespoons (30 milliliters)

53 calories, 3 grams protein, 1 gram fiber, Calcium
and vitamin B$_{12}$ 30%, Potassium and riboflavin 20%,
Folate and zinc 15%

Wheat-Free White Sauce

Yield: 1 heaping cup (250 milliliters) or 8 2-tablespoon (30-milliliter) servings

1 tablespoon (15 milliliters) butter
2½ tablespoons (35 milliliters) sweet rice flour
1 cup (250 milliliters) liquid (milk, reserved cooking liquid, soymilk, formula, or combination)
3 tablespoons (45 milliliters) additional liquid
Herbs and/or spices to taste

1. Over low heat in small saucepan warm 1 cup of liquid and butter.
2. In separate bowl, make a paste with rice flour and 3 tablespoons milk or other liquid.
3. Scoop paste into saucepan, stirring into liquid. Cook over low heat, stirring constantly with a whisk.
4. Cook about 4 minutes to desired thickness.

Nutrient content of 2 tablespoons (30 milliliters)

37 calories, 1 gram protein, Calcium 15%, Vitamin B$_{12}$ 15%

Chicken-Avocado Spread

Yield: ½ cup (125 milliliters) or 4 2-tablespoon (30-milliliter) servings

4 tablespoons (60 milliliters) cooked and puréed chicken
4 tablespoons (60 milliliters) well-mashed avocado
Dash of garlic powder

1. Mix well and serve. Spoon-feed to a younger baby or spread onto toast pieces or crackers for an older baby.

Nutrient content of 2 tablespoons (30 milliliters)

46 calories, 4 grams protein, 1 gram fiber, Niacin 40%, Vitamin B$_6$ 30%, Potassium 15%, Zinc and magnesium 10%

Avocado-Chicken-Cheese Spread

Yield: ½ cup (125 milliliters) or 4 2-tablespoon (30-milliliter) servings

¼ cup (60 milliliters) chopped cooked chicken (or other cooked meat)
¼ cup (60 milliliters) cottage cheese
1 medium avocado, pitted and sliced
Dash of minced dehydrated onion
Dash of garlic powder
Dash of dill

1. Mix well and serve. Spoon-feed to a younger baby or spread onto toast pieces or crackers for an older baby.

Nutrient content of 2 tablespoons (30 milliliters)

95 calories, 5 grams protein, 2 grams fiber, Niacin 40%, Magnesium 20%, Vitamin B$_6$ 50%, Zinc 10%

Fruit Custard

Yield: about 1¼ cups (300 milliliters)

1 tablespoon (15 milliliters) sweet rice flour (found in Asian section of grocery store)
¾ cup milk (180 milliliters)
2 egg yolks
½ cup (125 milliliters) puréed fruit
¼ teaspoon (1 milliliter) vanilla

1. Mix rice flour and ¼ cup (60 milliliters) milk in saucepan. Stir in additional ½ cup milk (125 milliliters) and both egg yolks. Cook over medium heat, stirring constantly.
2. Mixture will begin to thicken after about 3 minutes. Cook 30 seconds more or until it reaches a temperature of 160°F (71°C).
3. Stir in fruit and vanilla.

Nutrient content of ¼ (60 milliliters) custard made with peaches

68 calories, 3 grams protein, Vitamin B_{12} 60%, Riboflavin 30%, Calcium 20%, Zinc 15%

Sweet Potato Custard

Yield: about 1 cup (250 milliliters)

⅓ cup (80 milliliters) puréed sweet potatoes
½ cup (125 milliliters) formula or milk
1 egg yolk
¼ teaspoon (1 milliliter) vanilla

1. Mix first three ingredients in small saucepan. Cook over medium heat, stirring constantly, until thickened (about 3 minutes).
2. Cook an additional 30 seconds—until 160°F (71°C) is reached. Remove from heat and stir in vanilla.
3. Let cool and serve.

Nutrient content of ¼ cup (60 milliliters)

62 calories, 2 grams protein, Vitamin A 50%, Vitamin B_{12} 40%, Riboflavin and vitamin B_6 30%, Calcium and manganese 20%

Smooth Split-Pea Soup

Yield: 6 cups (1.2 liters)

1 pound (500 grams) dry split peas
2 bay leaves
1 medium onion, chopped
½ teaspoon thyme
Water

1. Wash peas thoroughly in a strainer and pick through them to make sure there are no small stones.
2. Place peas and other ingredients in large pan and add enough water so that there's an inch of water over the top of the peas.
3. Bring peas to a boil and reduce to a simmer. Cover.
4. Cook 50 to 60 minutes or until peas are tender.
5. Purée the mixture in a blender, adding enough water, milk, or other liquid to make it smooth.

Nutrient content of ½ cup (125 milliliters)

44 calories, 3 grams protein, 1.5 grams fiber, Folate 30%, Magnesium and potassium 20%

Chapter 14

Ten to Twelve Months

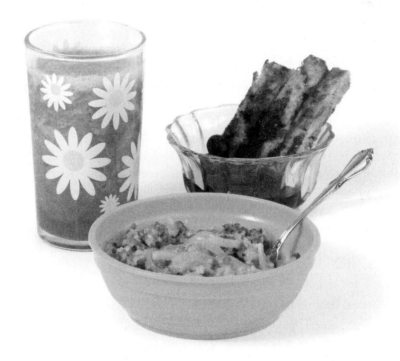

*I was doing the family grocery shopping accompanied by two children,
an event I hope to see included in the Olympics in the near future.*

—Anna Quindlen, Pulitzer-prize winning columnist

Changes in Attitude, Changes in Appetite

It's amazing how much your baby's eating habits have changed in just a few months! At ten months, your baby will be eating just about everything you eat. Your baby will be eating many finger foods and will probably show interest in self-feeding with a spoon. You may also notice that your baby's appetite is waning. This is normal; growth slows down as the first birthday approaches. Here are some other typical eating developments at this age:

- Your baby is able to eat mashed foods and chunkier foods.
- Your baby has more teeth and can bite and chew soft pieces of vegetables and fruits.
- Your baby is perfecting the pincer gasp and getting very good at picking up small finger foods.
- Your baby is eating three meals a day with a few small snacks.
- Your baby is starting to master drinking from a cup.
- It takes longer to feed your baby when he or she insists on self-feeding. It's also messier.

Your Baby's Declaration of Independence

On the homestretch to one year, your baby's personality and independence blossom. Your baby may now point to or ask for some foods by name, or say no to an unwanted food. Your baby may decide bibs are for the birds. You may have a hard time getting your baby to sit long enough to eat. (Try to keep a firm rule of sitting while eating. It's a great way to prevent choking, and you don't want to get into the habit of chasing your baby around the house with a plate and spoon.) Your baby is probably also beginning to show his or her true tastes in food. My son Nicolas loved every flavor of baby food, but once he started eating the same vegetables from the table, the number of veggies he liked took a nosedive.

Transitioning to the Family Diet

Remember to Add Spices

If you haven't already, I suggest you start adding small amounts of herbs and spices to your baby's food—but not salt. A touch of cinnamon or a shake of garlic powder or oregano will make your baby's food taste better—and may help your baby warm up to your favorite foods. However, just add one different spice at a time and wait a few days between introducing new spices, in the rare case that your baby has a reaction. (If your baby has GERD, hold off on pepper and other hot spices, which could increase reflux symptoms.)

If you're feeding your baby table food, continue to set aside some food for your baby before you season the family's portion. The salty foods most adults eat are still not a good idea for babies.

Is Your Family's Diet Healthy?

As your baby begins eating what you eat, it's a good time to assess the example you're setting. So what *is* a healthy diet? Check out the following advice, which is based on the latest U.S. Department of Agriculture (USDA) dietary guidelines. The guidelines apply to everyone over two years (with smaller servings for children).[1]

Choose Wisely from Every Food Group

The best way to give your body the balanced nutrition it needs is by eating a variety of nutrient packed foods every day. Here's how:

- **Focus on fruits**. Eat a variety of fruits—whether fresh, frozen, canned, or dried—rather than drinking fruit juice.
- **Vary your veggies**. Eat more dark green veggies, such as broccoli, kale, and other dark leafy greens; more orange veggies, such as carrots, sweet potatoes, pumpkin, and winter squash; and more beans and peas, such as pinto beans, kidney beans, black beans, garbanzo beans (chickpeas), split peas, and lentils.
- **Make half your grains whole**. Eat at least three ounces (90 grams) of whole-grain cereals, breads, crackers, rice, pasta, or other grain foods every day. For packaged food, make sure grains are referred to as "whole" in the list of ingredients.
- **Go lean with protein**. Choose lean meats and poultry. Bake it, broil it, or grill it. And vary your protein sources by eating more fish, beans, peas, nuts, and seeds.
- **Don't forget calcium-rich foods**. Drink three cups of low-fat or fat-free milk every day. (For kids two to eight years, it's two cups of milk.) Or eat the same amount of low-fat yogurt or an ounce and a half of low-fat cheese. If you don't like or can't have milk, choose lactose-free dairy products and/or calcium-fortified foods and beverages.

Balance Food and Physical Activity

Regular physical activity is important for your overall health and fitness. It also helps you control your body weight by burning up the calories you take in each day.

- **Exercise daily**. Be physically active for at least thirty minutes most days of the week.
- **Challenge yourself**. Increasing your exercise intensity or time can provide even greater health benefits, and may be needed to control body weight. (You may need about sixty minutes a day to prevent weight gain.)
- **Get your kids involved**. Children and teenagers should be physically active for sixty minutes every day (or almost every day).

Get the Most Nutrition from Your Calories

There is a right number of calories for you to eat each day. This number depends on your age, activity level, and whether you're trying to gain, maintain, or lose weight. (Two thousand calories per day is used as a general reference for food labels. You can calculate your unique calorie needs at http://www.bcm.edu/cnrc/caloriesneed.htm.)

You could get all those calories by eating a few high-calorie foods, but chances are they won't give you the full range of nutrients your body needs to be healthy. Instead, follow these tips:

- **Reality-check your servings and calories**. Compare the recommended serving size for foods you eat to the amount you're actually eating. If you double the servings, you also double the calories and nutrients.

- **Make your calories count**. Compare calorie content with nutrient content to determine whether a food is worth eating. Every day, choose the most nutrient-rich foods you can from each food group—those that are packed with vitamins, minerals, fiber, and other nutrients but are lower in calories. Pick foods like fruits, vegetables, whole grains, and fat-free or low-fat dairy products often.

- **Don't sugarcoat it**. Since sugars provide lots of calories with few or no nutrients, look for foods and beverages low in added sugars. Read the ingredient list for a food and make sure added sugars aren't among the first few ingredients. Some names to look for are *sucrose, glucose, high-fructose corn syrup, corn syrup, maple syrup,* and *fructose.*

- **Know your fats**. Look for foods low in saturated fats, trans fats, and cholesterol to reduce your risk of heart disease. (5 percent daily value or less is low; 20 percent daily value or more is high.) The goal for trans fat should be as close to zero as possible. Most of the fats you eat should be polyunsaturated and monounsaturated fats. Keep your total fat intake between 20 and 35 percent of the calories you eat.

- **Reduce sodium; increase potassium**. Research shows that eating less than 2,300 milligrams of sodium per day may reduce your risk of high blood pressure. Be aware that most of the sodium people eat comes from processed foods, not from a saltshaker. Also look for foods high in potassium, which counteracts some of sodium's effects on blood pressure.

Play It Safe with Food

Know how to prepare, handle, and store food safely to prevent food-borne illness. Heed the following tips and see Chapter 10 for more details.

- **Clean** hands, food-contact surfaces, fruits, and vegetables. To avoid spreading bacteria to other foods, don't wash or rinse meat, poultry, or fish.

- **Separate** raw, cooked, and ready-to-eat foods while shopping, preparing, and storing them.

Healthy Eating Cheat Sheet

The USDA dietary guidelines are excellent rules to eat by—but it can be hard to remember them all, especially when you're busy and sleep-deprived. Here's a six-step cheat sheet to help you.

1. Eat fruits and veggies at every meal.
2. Eat a variety of protein: Go meatless at least once a week, eat fish twice a week, eat red meat once or twice a week, and fill in the rest with poultry and pork.
3. Eat avocado, nuts, seeds, and wheat germ often.
4. Choose healthy snacks: yogurt, fruits, veggies, whole-grain crackers, and cheese.
5. Use canola or olive oil for cooking.
6. Eat whole grains three times a day and whole foods as often as possible.

- **Cook** meat, poultry, and fish to safe internal temperatures to kill bacteria.
- **Chill** perishable foods promptly and thaw foods properly.

Ten Tips for Feeding Older Babies and Toddlers

There's a lot to learn in this book about your role as a parent feeding your child. I've summarized your most important tasks in these ten little tips. Copy this list and keep it on your fridge!

1. Don't force or bribe your child to eat.
2. Set a good example by eating at least seven fruits and vegetables a day yourself.
3. Make mealtimes pleasant.
4. Encourage your child to help with meal planning, preparation, and cleanup.
5. Back off when eating becomes a power struggle.
6. Accept food jags as phases that will eventually pass.
7. Accept that your child is an individual and will dislike certain foods (and there may be many). Your kid is not doing this to annoy you— I promise!
8. Don't give up when introducing foods to your child. Research shows it can take ten to fifteen exposures to a new food for a child to accept it.
9. Use this division of responsibility: As a parent, you decide when to eat and what to serve. Your child is responsible for deciding how much (if any) to eat. Remember that your child is naturally able to eat what his or her body needs.
10. It's okay to give your child a multivitamin-mineral supplement, especially if he or she is a picky eater.

A Day in the Diet...

Of an Eleven-Month-Old

Here's a sample daily menu for an eleven-month-old who's eating everything.

Breakfast

Oatmeal with cooked plums
Half piece whole-wheat toast
Breast milk or formula

Mid-morning snack

Kiwi fruit chunks with string cheese

Lunch

Cheesy Stars (page 280) with
    chopped salmon
Steamed broccoli trees
Breast milk or formula

Mid-afternoon snack

Half whole-grain waffle with Avocado
    Chicken-Cheese spread (page 271)
Breast milk or formula

Dinner

Mushroom-Cheeseburger Bulgur (page 279)
Green peas
Pears

Bedtime snack

Breast milk or formula

Of a Nursing Twelve-Month-Old

Rise and Shine

Breast milk

Breakfast

Mixed cereal with mashed
  mango

Mid-morning snack

Yogurt with apricots

Lunch

Lentil soup with carrots
One-half sandwich with roast beef
Raspberries
Whole milk

Mid-afternoon snack

Guacamole on crackers
Diluted juice

Naptime snack

Breast milk

Dinner

New England Fish Chowder (page 281)
Cornbread
Maui Smoothie (page 303)

Bedtime snack

Breast milk

Of a Weaned Twelve-Month-Old

Here's a sample daily menu for a weaned twelve-month-old who's drinking whole
milk and eating eggs and citrus.

Breakfast

Half-cup ready-to-eat iron-fortified
  cereal with sliced strawberries
Whole milk

Mid-morning snack

Mandarin orange sections
Small slice Cheddar cheese

Lunch

Chicken Couscous (page 279)
Chopped romaine lettuce with
  tomatoes and ranch dressing
Whole milk

Mid-afternoon snack

Rice cake with Crunchy Cream Cheese
  Spread (page 303)
Diluted juice

Dinner

Chopped spaghetti with Smooth and
  Healthy Meat Sauce (page 315)
Cooked chopped spinach
Creamy Carrot Soup (page 267)
Whole milk

Bedtime snack

Whole milk
One graham cracker

Storage Reminder

Here are the basic rules for storing homemade baby food:

- For homemade cereals, veggies, and fruits, refrigerate what you will use within
  two days. Freeze any remainders. Exception: When making baby food from
  high-nitrate vegetables, immediately freeze anything over a serving.

- For eggs, refrigerate what you will use within twenty-four hours. Freeze any
  remainders, but note that some egg recipes won't freeze well.

Mushroom-Cheeseburger Bulgur

Yield: 2 cups (500 milliliters)

½ cup (125 milliliters) natural extra-lean
   ground beef
3 large mushrooms, finely chopped
½ teaspoon oil
1 cup (250 milliliters) water
½ cup (125 milliliters) bulgur (cracked
   wheat), cooked brown rice, quinoa,
   or white rice
½ cup (125 milliliters) grated cheese
   (about 2 ounces or 60 grams)

1. In small saucepan, cook ground
   beef over medium heat, stirring
   well to give it a fine texture. Cook
   until it reaches an internal temperature of 160°F or 71° C. Drain
   grease. Remove beef to dish and
   wash pan or wipe grease from it
   with a paper towel.
2. Add oil to pan. Sauté mushrooms
   on medium-high heat for 1 minute,
   stirring constantly.
3. Add bulgur (or other grain) and
   water. Bring to a boil. Reduce to a
   simmer and cook covered for 15
   minutes, stirring occasionally.
4. Mix in beef and cheese until
   cheese melts.

Nutrient content of ¼ cup (60 milliliters)

73 calories, 6 grams protein, 1 gram fiber, Vitamin B_{12}
70%, Zinc 40%, Niacin and vitamin B_6 30%, Manganese
25%, Calcium 20%

Chicken Couscous

Yield: 3 cups (750 milliliters)

⅓ cup (80 milliliters) chopped carrots
⅓ cup (80 milliliters) chopped turnips
   or parsnips
⅓ cup (80 milliliters) chopped zucchini
1 teaspoon olive oil
¼ cup (60 milliliters) chopped red
   bell pepper
2 cloves garlic
1 chopped green onion
1 pinch pepper
3 ounces (90 grams) chicken, cut
   into pieces
1 cup (250 milliliters) water
½ cup (125 milliliters) whole-wheat
   couscous

1. Steam carrots, parsnips, and
   zucchini. Or cook covered in
   microwave-safe container for 2
   to 3 minutes until tender.
2. In medium saucepan, heat oil
   and add garlic, green onion, and
   pepper. Sauté 1 minute.
3. Add chicken to saucepan and cook
   for 2 minutes or to an internal
   temperature of 165°F or 74°C,
   stirring frequently.
4. Add steamed vegetables, water,
   and couscous.
5. Bring to a boil and then turn
   heat to low. Cover and cook until
   the water is absorbed—about 2
   minutes. Remove from heat and
   let stand 5 minutes.

Nutrient content of ⅓ cup (80 milliliters)

53 calories, 4 grams protein, 1 gram fiber, Niacin and
vitamin B_6 20%, Vitamin C 15%

Cheesy Stars

Yield: 1 cup (250 milliliters)

¼ cup (60 milliliters) star-shaped pasta
2 cups (500 milliliters) water
½ cup (125 milliliters) prepared Cheesy
  Sauce (page 270)

1. In small saucepan, bring water to a
   boil. Add stars, return to a simmer.
2. Cook 10 to 12 minutes or until tender.
3. Drain. Add ½ cup (125 milliliters)
   cheesy sauce and mix.

Nutrient content of ¼ cup (60 milliliters)

108 calories, 5 grams protein, 1 gram fiber, Folate and
selenium 50%, Calcium, potassium, niacin, vitamin
B$_{12}$, and riboflavin 30%

Creamy Spinach

Yield: 1½ cups (375 milliliters)

1 10-ounce (280 grams) package
  frozen spinach
4 ounces (120 grams) low-fat
  cream cheese
¼ teaspoon (1 milliliter) garlic powder
Dash of pepper

1. Cook spinach over low heat until
   warmed through. Drain liquid.
2. Add cream cheese and garlic
   powder and stir until combined.
3. Serve as is or purée.

Nutrient content of ¼ cup (60 milliliters)

55 calories, 3 grams protein, Folate 90%, Magnesium
60%, Vitamin A and vitamin B$_6$ 40%, Calcium 30%

Shrimpy Spread or Dip

Yield: 5 1-tablespoon (15-milliliter) servings

¼ cup (60 milliliters) whole-milk
  cottage cheese
¼ cup (60 milliliters) baby shrimp
  (½ cup shrimp for a thicker dip)
Dash of dried or fresh dill

1. Purée the cheese, shrimp, and
   dill together.

Nutrient content of 1 tablespoon (15 milliliters)

27 calories, 4 grams protein, Vitamin B$_{12}$ 30%

Hummus Spread

Yield: about 2 cups (500 milliliters)

1 15-ounce can (425 grams) chickpeas
  (garbanzo beans)
¼ cup (60 milliliters) water
3 tablespoons (45 milliliters) tahini
  (sesame seed butter)
¼ teaspoon (1 milliliter) garlic powder

1. Drain chickpeas and rinse.
2. Pour beans in blender or food
   processor with ¼ cup water
   and tahini.
3. Blend until smooth.

Nutrient content of 2 tablespoons (30 milliliters)

44 calories, 2 grams protein, Folate and thiamine 20%,
Magnesium and zinc 10%

New England Fish Chowder

(modified from *Quick and Healthy: Low-Fat, Carb-Conscious Cooking* by Brenda Ponichtera)

Yield: 6 cups (1.42 liters)

1½ cups (375 milliliters) diced new potatoes
1 cup (250 milliliters) water
½ cup (125 milliliters) chopped
    green pepper
½ cup (125 milliliters) chopped onion
½ teaspoon (2.5 milliliters) dried thyme
2 cups (500 milliliters) whole milk
2 tablespoons (30 milliliters) cornstarch
⅛ teaspoon (.5 milliliters) ground pepper
1 pound (500 grams) fish filets, cut into
    1-inch pieces
½ teaspoon (2.5 milliliters) salt

1. In a medium saucepan, combine the first five ingredients and bring to a boil.
2. Reduce heat to low and simmer, covered, for 15 minutes or until potatoes are tender.
3. Mix cornstarch with milk and remaining seasonings except salt. Stir into soup and bring to a boil, stirring constantly, until slightly thickened.
4. Reduce heat and add fish; simmer until fish is cooked (to internal temperature of 145°F or 63°C).
5. Set aside a portion for your baby and add salt to the rest of the family's portion.
6. If you like, further mash or purée your baby's portion.

Nutrient content of ½ cup (125 milliliters)

130 calories, 10 grams protein, 870 milligrams omega-3 fatty acids, Vitamin B$_{12}$ 240%, Vitamin B$_6$ 100%, Niacin 90%, Selenium 80%, Thiamine 60%, Calcium 20%, Zinc 10%

Winter Squash Soup

Yield: about 6 cups (1.5 liters)

4 cups (1 liter) cooked butternut squash
1 cup (250 milliliters) milk
1 cup (250 milliliters) applesauce
1 tablespoon (1 milliliter) butter
Dash of nutmeg

1. Put all ingredients into blender and blend until smooth. Add more milk for a thinner soup.

Nutrient content of ½ cup (125 milliliters)

50 calories, 2 grams protein, Vitamin A and manganese 30%, Vitamin B$_6$ and vitamin B$_{12}$ 20%, Calcium 15%

Berry n'Ice

Yield: 12 ounces (375 milliliters) or 3 ½-cup (125-milliliter) servings

1 cup (250 milliliters) whole unsweetened
    frozen strawberries
½ cup (125 milliliters) blueberry-cranberry
    juice, cranberry-raspberry juice, or
    other berry juice
¼ cup (60 milliliters) sliced pears
    (½ a medium-size pear)
¼ teaspoon sugar (optional)

1. In blender or small food processor, blend all ingredients on low and then high speed until smooth.
2. Drink now or freeze as fruit pops.

Nutrient content of ½ cup (125 milliliters)

60 calories, 1 gram fiber, Vitamin C 70%

French Toast Strips

Yield: 1 piece, 3 strips

1 egg yolk
2 tablespoons (30 milliliters) water
1 slice whole-grain bread, crust removed
Dash of cinnamon or pumpkin pie spice

1. In shallow bowl, mix egg yolk with water and spice.
2. Place bread in bowl briefly, turning to soak up egg mixture.
3. Place bread in nonstick pan over medium heat.
4. Cook about 2 minutes on each side or until toast is cooked through and brown.
5. Slice into 3 strips.
6. Serve with Blueberry Sauce (see right) or puréed fruit.

Nutrient content of 3 strips

124 calories, 5 grams protein, 2 grams fiber, Choline 150%, Vitamin B$_{12}$ 100%, Magnesium and folate 40%, Zinc 30%, Iron 10%

Blueberry Sauce

Yield: ½ cup (125 milliliters) or 4 2-tablespoon (30-milliliter) servings

1 cup (½ pint or 250 milliliters) fresh blueberries
3 tablespoons (45 milliliters) blueberry-cranberry juice, cranberry-raspberry juice, or other berry juice
½ teaspoon (2.5 milliliters) sugar (optional)
Dash of cinnamon and nutmeg (optional)
Squeeze of lemon or orange juice for zest (optional, for babies older than a year)

1. Place all ingredients in a saucepan over medium-high heat.
2. Simmer, stirring often and popping the blueberries with the spoon, until cooked to the desired thickness (5 or 6 minutes). If you'd like your sauce to be thinner, add an extra tablespoon or two of juice.

Nutrient content of 2 tablespoons (30 milliliters)

27 calories, 1 gram fiber, Vitamin C 15%

Chapter 15

Twelve to Eighteen Months

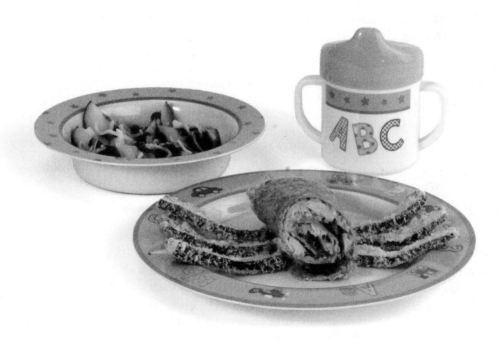

*Cleaning your house while your kids are still growing
is like shoveling the walk before it stops snowing.*
—Phyllis Diller

Your baby's first birthday came quickly, didn't it? At one year, your baby can eat just about anything you do, with a few exceptions for allergy-prone kids. It's also time to get rid of a thing or two. If you're formula-feeding, you can replace formula with whole milk or full-fat, vitamin-enriched soymilk. If you're breastfeeding and either you or your baby is ready to wean, you can replace breast milk with the same options. You can toss the baby bottle, too.

Following I've summarized the main changes in your baby's diet and typical eating habits at this age.

- Baby's diet at one year
    - Grains: all grains okay
    - Vegetables: all vegetables okay
    - Fruits: citrus, pineapple okay
    - Protein foods: egg white, peanut butter, and other nut butters okay
    - Dairy: whole milk okay
    - Extras: Honey and corn syrup okay
- Typical eating habits at this age
    - Mealtime takes longer as your baby self-feeds.
    - Picky eating begins.
    - Your family's eating habits become your child's.
    - Growth is slow and steady.
    - Your baby is now active!
    - Your baby can ask for foods by name.
    - Your baby can throw a tantrum when given an unwanted food (or not given a wanted food).

Kids in the Kitchen

As your baby becomes more mobile, invite him or her to join the fun of food preparation. When my boys were small, we often had them in a jumper hanging from the kitchen doorway. Today there are lots of ways for your older baby or toddler to have fun in the kitchen under your watchful eye—from Jumperoos to Exersaucers to Learning Towers. Listening to you talk about what you're doing is a great way for your baby to bond with you and learn from you.

At the Grocery Store

Your local market is a great place to teach so many concepts: colors, shapes, numbers, names, textures, smells, and sometimes even tastes. The produce department is an especially interesting place. Let your baby hold a big smooth orange or a fuzzy little kiwi fruit. (Keep an eye out to prevent nibbling!) Let your baby sniff a bunch of cilantro. In the dry foods area, hand over a box of pasta to shake or a bag of beans to play with. It's never too early to get your child involved in making good choices.

For example, as soon as he or she can talk or gesture, you can ask if your baby wants peaches or pears.

At Home

The most important thing about having your child "help" in the kitchen is to make it fun. Every task will probably take longer and be messier. But it's worth it when you consider the quality time you're spending together and the nifty skills your child is learning.

From the beginning, it's important to teach your child about safety. Take care not to transfer hot food from the stove or oven when your child is nearby. And remember that good cooks of all ages wash their hands before getting to work!

Keep the cooking jobs fun and brief if you want your child to come back for more. Your child may beg to make cookies from scratch, but may have only enough patience for the slice-and-bake type!

Following are a few ideas to get you and your child started.

Jobs for One-Year-Olds

- Practice measuring water with measuring cups at the kitchen sink.
- Sprinkle cheese on top of vegetables or salad.
- Dump premeasured ingredients into a bowl
- Shape cookie dough into balls or push a cookie cutter into rolled-out dough.
- Watch a timer and tell you when it goes off.
- Dump chopped vegetables into a salad.
- Hand you an egg or other ingredients.
- Shut the microwave door.
- Sprinkle raisins into batter.
- Poke chocolate chips onto cookies or drop blueberries into pancake batter.

Jobs for Two-Year-Olds

- Wash vegetables and fruits.
- Help set the table—put spoons or napkins in place.
- Tear lettuce for salads.
- Break bread into pieces for stuffing.
- Spread peanut butter on a cracker.
- Put the top on the blender and push the button.
- Snap fresh green beans.
- Put crackers or cookies on a serving plate.
- Pour premeasured salad dressing on a salad.

- Help mix a fresh fruit salad.
- Roll up cloth napkins.
- Fold paper napkins.

Jobs for Three-Year-Olds

- Help measure ingredients.
- Help crack eggs.
- Shape cookies.
- Help pour batter into pan.
- Hold a hand mixer.
- Push buttons on the microwave.
- Make a yogurt parfait.
- Knead bread.
- Shape dough.
- Roll cookie dough into balls.

The Picky Eater

So far, you may have felt lucky regarding your baby's eating habits. But don't get too comfortable; about the time when a baby's growth slows down and baby foods take a back seat to table foods, eating habits often change. Here are some new picky eating behaviors you might start seeing:

- Your baby temporarily refuses a specific food.
- Your baby wants only one color of food (usually beige).
- Your baby wants a specific food prepared only one way.
- Your baby refuses a whole group of foods (like veggies or meats).
- Your baby eats only a specific food or food group, like bread or cereal. (This is called a food jag.)
- Your baby doesn't eat much of anything.

How Should You React to Picky Eating?

1. Grant your baby's every food wish.
2. Make a big fuss over your baby's new eating habits.
3. Throw up your hands and decide your baby will never eat healthy again.
4. Treat this as a temporary phase that will pass.
5. Beg, barter, or bribe your baby to eat what you want him or her to eat.
6. Let eating become a power struggle between you.

How you react to your picky eater could make or break your baby's future eating habits. Check out the possible results of each choice:

1. If you always give into your baby's food desires, you become a short order cook. Occasionally giving your baby what he or she wants is fine, but don't make it a habit.

2. If you give your baby's new eating habit a lot of extra attention, your baby will figure out that this new behavior is a good way to get attention and will keep doing it! Instead, treat it as no big deal.

3. If you give up on your baby's ever eating healthy again, your baby probably *won't* ever eat healthy again. Instead, keep plugging away. Keep offering old favorites and healthy new foods in different ways. Don't give up!

4. If you treat this behavior as a phase, your little guy or gal will realize that it's no big deal. Your baby will know that you respect his or her appetite opinions about food.

5. If you beg, barter, or bribe your child, you teach him or her to ignore internal appetite cues. Sorry, Mom or Dad, you may be setting your child up for future disordered eating.

6. If you let eating become a power struggle, you'll regret it. You can't win this one! It makes eating an unhappy experience for everyone.

Parents' Behavior and Kids' Food Preferences

Research is uncovering some very interesting information on this subject. Never underestimate your role in developing your child's preference for or avoidance of foods:[1]

- Children are more likely to eat in a positive atmosphere.

- Restricting access to certain foods increases a child's preference for this food.

- Forcing a child to eat certain foods decreases the child's liking for the foods.

Of course, parents don't shape all their kids' food preferences. Flavor is a big factor—and flavor is determined by taste buds, which are shaped by genes.

Taste receptor genes account for some kids' preferences for sweet or bitter foods. Kids who have a certain taste receptor gene can taste bitter foods more intensely; kids without the gene may not taste bitterness at all. This may explain why a few kids go for broccoli over potatoes.

What happens when kids and parents have different taste buds? Research suggests that this difference could affect parent-child interactions. Mothers who did not have the bitter taste receptor gene tended to think of their kids who did as more emotional.[2]

Bear in mind that you just may not taste things the same way your child does. Try to be sensitive to his or her taste buds.

The Ground Rules

First, realize that it's impossible to always be perfect. There will be times when you'll ask, "What would you like for dinner?" And being the loving parent that you are, you'll proceed to make the requested food (unless it requires an extra trip to the grocery store). And there will be times when you're too tired to do anything but give in: "Yes, you can have cereal for dinner. Have all the cereal you want!" Don't worry if you veer from the rules sometimes. If you follow them most of the time, you and your child will do just fine.

As your child exerts more independence and eats less, you'll surely be tempted to intervene more. Don't. If you become either overly restrictive or overly encouraging, you teach your child not to trust his or her appetite. This can lead to disordered eating, which can lead to overweight or underweight.

Parents' Responsibilities

- Serve regular meals and snacks that include a variety of foods.
- Decide what to serve and where.
- Eat with your child to promote good eating habits as well as family bonding.
- Try to include one food that your child likes at each meal.
- Have no expectations about how much your child should eat.
- Trust that your child will eat what he or she needs, even if it seems like too much or too little.
- Remember that over time, your child will get the nutrients he or she needs, even if it's not all in one day. (It'll be more like a week.)

Children's Responsibilities

- Your child decides what to eat and how much.
- Your child eats what he or she needs to grow.
- Your child eventually learns how to behave at the table.
- If your child doesn't eat well at one meal, he or she will have another opportunity at the next snack or meal.

What You Shouldn't Do at Mealtime

- Don't coax or bribe your child to eat more.
- Don't be overly restrictive on the amount of healthy food your child eats. (It's always okay to limit less healthy foods, but you shouldn't overly restrict those either.)
- Don't keep offering alternatives if your child doesn't like what you've served.
- Don't reward desired mealtime behavior with food. (In fact, you should *never use food as a reward*.)

The Results

- Your darling daughter or son gets the message that it's okay not to eat a certain food, but that you will keep dishing it out. One day he or she wakes up and actually likes it! (There'll be foods your child may never like, especially if they're bitter. Or your child may grow into them as an adult.)

- Your child learns it's also okay to like certain foods and to ask for more.

- Your child may eat much more or much less than usual at certain times, and he or she knows it's okay. Your child may fall into a pattern, or your child's eating may be totally unpredictable.

- Over time, your child gets the calories he or she needs from the regular meals and small, healthy snacks you consistently serve.

Resisting Ads for Unhealthy Eating

If your child watches TV, you may need to screen the commercials as well as the programs. Better yet, turn off the TV altogether.

Why? According to Juliet Schor, sociologist and author of *Born to Buy*, fifteen billion dollars in TV advertising was aimed at children in 2004. This is an astronomical increase over the one hundred million spent just twenty years earlier.[3] Much of the ads aimed at kids are, unfortunately, for junk foods. Kids are watching more TV today, too—and at an earlier age. About 70 percent of childcare centers use TV in a typical day. Kids in the United States watch an average of four hours of TV a day.[4]

The problem with advertising to young children is that before the age of eight, children lack the skills necessary to tell commercial from noncommercial content and to recognize the persuasive techniques of advertising. I realized this was true when my five-year-old said I should buy a certain brand of detergent and went on to describe— verbatim from the commercial—why it was best! Kids have big buying power. They spend two hundred billion dollars annually on foods and drinks—and this doesn't count their influence on their parents at the grocery store!

Marketing to children is a concern around the world. The relentless advertising of unhealthy food to kids, plus the wide availability of these foods, could be partially responsible for the rise in childhood obesity. In fact, there is strong evidence that exposure to food and beverage advertising is associated with body fatness in children from two to eighteen years.[5] Studies in the United Kingdom show that marketing to kids affects their food preferences, purchase behaviors, and what they eat—not just for specific brands, but for categories of food and beverages.[6]

Be aware of marketing in other media, too. Children's magazines, websites, and merchandise are all potential ad vehicles. Even parents sometimes advertise unhealthy foods to their kids. Research shows that parents who use baby bottles decorated with soft drinks logos are four times more likely to put these sweet liquids into their baby's bottle.[7]

What can you do to resist all this marketing?

- Put off TV watching for as long as possible. The American Academy of Pediatrics (AAP) discourages TV watching for children under two and encourages brain-building activities like playing and reading instead.

- When and if your child does begin watching TV:

  - Limit it to one hour per day. The AAP recommends that children have no more than one to two hours of high-quality entertainment media per day.[8] (This includes all screen time: TV, movies, computer games, and video games.) Definitely do not put a TV in your child's bedroom.

  - Check out public broadcasting. It's usually a great source of high-quality programs for young children; it's also commercial-free.

  - Try to save TV programs for adults until after your child's bedtime.

  - Record your child's show(s) without the commercials.

  - Rent, buy, or borrow (from the library) videos or DVDs that you approve of. Skip the commercials at the beginning of a movie.

- Support lawmakers working on legislation giving the Federal Trade Commission (FTC) the authority to regulate marketing to kids.

- For more information, read a report on food marketing to children by the National Academy of Sciences at http://www.nap.edu/books/0309097134/html.

Breastfeeding and Weaning after One Year

It's Up to You

Many women choose to stop nursing around their baby's first birthday. However, breastfeeding past one year is becoming more and more common.

The AAP recommends that moms continue breastfeeding past the first year if it's mutually agreeable to mom and baby. The World Health Organization (WHO) urges women to nurse until their babies are at least two years old.

Research shows that your milk continues to change to meet your baby's needs during the second year and continues to be an excellent source of nutrition. Also, breastfeeding seems to have a dose effect. The longer you nurse, the more health benefits you and your baby get. Extended breastfeeding may be especially beneficial if your baby was born prematurely or has chronic health problems.

How long you'll breastfeed after one year is up to you. But of course, your education, culture, upbringing, and life experiences—as well as your partner's—will affect your decision. Your other family members' opinions can play into this, too. If you disagree with your partner or family members, express your reasons for wanting to keep breastfeeding

Tales from the Trenches: Weaning at One Year

"When Aidan was a year old, he nursed only a few times a day: at wake-up, naptime, and bedtime," said Kitee. "Suddenly he lost interest; he was too busy looking around and didn't want to slow down to nurse. I was sad, but also relieved that weaning wasn't a big issue."

or to wean. Don't be afraid to quote the AAP, WHO, and/or your doctor or lactation consultant. And remember that in the end, the decision lies between you and your baby.

Weaning

Some moms practice child-led weaning; that is, they continue nursing until their child voluntarily gives up feedings due to greater interest in other foods and liquids or greater interest in other activities.

You may decide to start the weaning process before your baby does for your own reasons. Perhaps you're going to be away from home longer or have job challenges. Or perhaps you're just ready to stop.

Whatever the reason for weaning, moms tend to experience the same varied emotions. You may be sad to stop, because you enjoyed the unique bonding of breastfeeding. You may be looking forward to your child's growing independence and your growing freedom. And you may feel guilty if you're ready to stop and your baby isn't. You may feel all those emotions and more; whatever you feel, know that it's normal. Weaning is a big life transition—especially if this is your last baby.

Tales from the Trenches: Extended Nursing

Sofia is a pro at extended nursing. She nursed her first son, Jimmy, for two years, up to the last month of her pregnancy with Sammy, her second son. She nursed Sammy almost three years.

Once each boy was well into solids, she nursed only in the morning, at naptime, and at bedtime. Why did she continue? "Because of the nutritional aspects— milk is alive," Sofia said. "I could also nurse through illnesses to help them get better faster."

Support at home made it easy to keep breastfeeding. Sofia's father was very supportive; he saw it as a positive experience that wasn't popular for his generation. Sofia's husband, sister, and other family and friends were also behind her.

Sofia's advice: "Forget about what everyone else thinks. If you feel comfortable doing it, then continue. As soon as you feel uncomfortable, it's a sign to start weaning."

A Gradual Goodbye: Weaning Tips

- Go gently. Your child and you will need to adjust, both physically and emotionally. You'll need to substitute extra love and attention for your nursing times together.

- Don't rush it. The length of the weaning process depends on how many times a day you're nursing right now and also how much solid food your child is eating. The whole process should take *at least* two weeks.

- If you don't have a deadline and want to wean your child cooperatively, try the "don't offer, don't refuse" method. It's not exactly child-led weaning, but it's not mom-led either. If your child wants to nurse, do so. But don't offer to nurse when your child hasn't requested it. This method usually results in fewer nursing sessions and creates a very slow, gentle weaning process.

- If you do have a deadline or want to wean your child more proactively, drop one feeding at a time.

- You might start with skipping the mid-morning or midday feeding, when you'd both rather be doing something else.

- Offer your child a cup of water before a usual nursing time to quench his or her thirst. Offer small snacks of healthy finger foods to satisfy your child's hunger.

- During a usual nursing time, distract your child with another activity, such as a library or bookstore storytime or a walk to the park.

• Avoid situations that may remind your child of nursing, such as cuddling in your favorite nursing chair.

- Once you've successfully dropped one nursing session, wait about four days to let your body adjust. Pump only enough to relieve discomfort. Then drop another feeding.

- Many women drop the bedtime feeding last. It's a special bonding time that's hard to give up. When you do give up that last feeding, start another bedtime ritual. Perhaps your partner can read a book and offer a nutritious snack, or an older sibling can sing a song after your child is all tucked into bed.

• Be flexible. If your child is very unhappy about giving up a specific feeding, continue it for a while. If he or she gets sick or needs extra comforting for another reason, expect regression. Approach such situations with love and realize that your baby may have a harder time with weaning than you do.

• Don't toss your nursing pads. It's normal to leak breast milk for a week or two after you finish weaning.

Saying "See Ya" to the Bottle

I know we've already talked about this, but now is the time to act! If you're bottle-feeding when your baby turns one, you need to make a serious effort to switch to a cup. If you've already done so, good job! If you're still reading, you've either found that your baby has no intention of switching or you need additional motivation.

Let's address first things first: Though your baby hasn't made the switch yet, that doesn't mean it'll never happen. Your baby's ability to switch from a bottle to a cup depends on the need to suck, eye-hand coordination, and small motor development. Keep all this in mind if you've met—or continue to meet—opposition.

Now here's some extra motivation for you:

• Drinking from a cup can reduce dental problems such as crooked teeth and tooth decay.

• Drinking from a cup can promote healthy jaw muscles, which your baby needs for proper speech development.

• Drinking from a cup means you spend less time cleaning! No more scrubbing out bottles and nipples caked with milk.

The following practical suggestions and info may help you and your baby make this transition.

- Wait for a calm time to start the permanent switch. For example, don't do it on the first day of daycare or when your child is sick.

- Tell your child that drinking from a cup is for big boys and girls. Positively reinforce your child's accomplishments with the cup, however small. Don't shame your child.

- Let your child pick out several new cups at the store.

- Have a picnic (indoors on a blanket in winter) using your child's special new cups.

- Buy two or three different cups and fill them all with water. Let your child try all to see which one he or she likes the best.

- Use other kids as role models: "Look: Emily is drinking from a cup! That's awesome!"

- Along with your child, ceremoniously give away the last bottle to a stuffed animal or to a younger baby.

- Many toddlers like the soft spout of the Nuby cup. Other babies like The First Years Take and Toss cups. Avent and Gerber both offer interchangeable bottle/cup systems; with these, the feel of the cup is the same as the bottle.

- Don't be surprised if your child will drink water or juice from a cup, but not milk. Drinking milk from a bottle can be a hard habit to break.

- Some hang on to the bottle because their kids just don't drink milk from a cup. Try this trick: Give your baby a choice of water from the bottle or milk from the cup.

- Don't panic if your child's milk intake drops when he or she switches to a cup. That's okay. At this age, kids need just sixteen to twenty-four ounces of milk a day. Your baby can get similar nutrients from cheese and yogurt if necessary.

- A cup with a straw is a great alternative to a sippy cup. Fancy straws may appeal to your child.

- It's okay to keep your child's bedtime bottle for a few more months, as long as you brush your child's teeth before he or she goes to sleep.

- When you drop the bedtime bottle, exchange it for another pleasant ritual, like a book and a bedtime snack.

Switching to Whole Cow's Milk

Why?

Why switch your child to whole cow's milk? If your child is weaning from breast milk or formula, whole cow's milk provides a healthy replacement. When your child is one year old, he or she can better handle the extra minerals, protein, and sodium in cow's milk. And at this age an allergy to cow's milk protein is much less likely. Whole milk is recommended because in their second year, babies continue to need a majority of their calories from fat.

In North America, cow's milk is typically well accepted by kids and fills in many nutritional gaps for picky eaters. Nutrients like calcium, riboflavin, vitamin

Tales from the Trenches: Thuy, Emily, and Joshua

My niece, Thuy, had no problem switching either of her kids from formula to whole milk at one year. The first day, she gave four ounces of whole milk and kept an eye out for any intolerance. The next day, she gave a little more, reducing the amount of formula accordingly. Her kids liked the taste of milk, so it was easy. Within a few days, they were drinking no formula—only milk.

D, and protein can be found in other foods, but cow's milk is so widely available and so well accepted by most kids that it provides the easiest way for kids to get those nutrients.

For most children, making the switch to cow's milk is no big deal. After your baby's first birthday, you can introduce whole milk in a cup. If your child doesn't seem to like the taste, mix it with a bit of expressed breast milk or formula to help your child get used to the new flavor.

If you're breastfeeding and following a restricted diet due to suspected allergies, or if your baby currently drinks soy formula or a hypoallergenic formula, don't switch to cow's milk without checking with your baby's doctor. Most babies do outgrow cow's milk protein allergies, but a few don't.

Comparing the Options

Some parents would rather give their babies something other than cow's milk, such as soymilk, goat's milk, or rice milk. While soymilk has some good things going for it, its fortification levels aren't ideal. Goat's milk is similar nutritionally to cow's milk, but it's harder to find and more expensive. Rice milk isn't a good alternative because it lacks many important nutrients.

What about follow-up formula? Several companies make formulas intended for older babies and toddlers (nine to twenty-four months) who are eating solids. The AAP believes most children don't need follow-up formula. However, if your older baby is eating very few solids, has a history of poor growth, or has food allergies, he or she could benefit from follow-up formula. (For example, a one-year-old who can't have cow's milk and is a very picky eater might benefit from a soy follow-up formula.)

See the following chart to compare the calories and nutrients of whole cow's milk with cow's milk alternatives.

Drinking Dinner

You don't think your baby is eating enough, so you give him more milk. Then your baby isn't hungry for solids and keeps eating less than you'd like. It's a vicious cycle. Or perhaps your baby is drinking more than one cup of juice a day; it's sweet and filling and can easily curb your baby's appetite for solids.

It can be tough to strike a balance between liquids and solids. If either of the situations I've just described sounds familiar, try giving your baby water in place of some of the milk or juice and see if his or her appetite improves. Or try timing your baby's liquids so they don't interfere with meals. Also, keep in mind that your baby should be drinking sixteen ounces of some type of milk, but not more than twenty-four ounces.

Whole Cow's Milk and Alternatives: Nutrient Comparison

Nutrients in 16 Ounces (480 Milliliters) and Percent of DRI for One- to Three-Year-Olds

Nutrient	DRI	Silk Soymilk	Goat's Milk	Rice Dream	Whole Milk	Similac Isomil Advance 2 Soy Formula	Baby's Only Organic Soy Toddler Formula
Calories	About 1000	200 (20%)	337 (34%)	240 (24%)	293 (29%)	320 (32%)	320 (32%)
Fat	About 55 g	8 g (15%)	20 g (36%)	3.97 g (7%)	16 g (29%)	17 g (30%)	17 g (30%)
Protein	13 g	14 g (107%)	17 g (130%)	0.83 g (6%)	16 g (114%)	8 g (57%)	9 g (64%)
Vitamin B_{12}	0.9 mcg	6 mcg (660%)	.34 mcg (37%)	0 mcg (0%)	2.15 mcg (238%)	1.44 mcg (160%)	1.44 mcg (160%)
Riboflavin	0.5 mg	1.02 mg (200%)	.67 mg (134%)	0.025 mg (4%)	0.89 mg (178%)	2.88 mg (576%)	3.2 mg (640%)
Choline	200 mg	†	†	†	69 mg (35%)	38 mg (19%)	38 mg (19%)
Iron	7 mg	2.16 mg (30%)	0.24 mg (3%)	0.39 mg (6%)	0.15 mg (2%)	6 mg (86%)	5.76 mg (82%)
Zinc	3 mg	1.2 mg (40%)	1.46 mg (49%)	0.49 mg (16%)	1.95 mg (65%)	2.4 mg (80%)	3.2 mg (106%)
Calcium	500 mg	600 mg (120%)	654 mg (131%)	39 mg (8%)	600 mg (120%)	432 mg (86%)	432 mg (86%)
Vitamin D	200 IU	240 IU (120%)	59 IU (30%)	0 IU (0%)	195 IU (98%)	192 IU (96%)	192 IU (96%)

† Choline content unknown.

Using Leftover Baby Food

Now your baby is eating table food, and you're thrilled! The only problem is that huge supply of baby food you got on sale, or perhaps the case of blueberry buckle your little one hated. What can you do with leftover baby food?

My first choice would be to give it to a homeless shelter or food bank. These agencies are often short of baby food. There are also many ways to use baby food in cooking for your whole family:

- Add jarred vegetables to a blended soup. To boost protein, you could also add puréed chicken, pork, beef, or mixed dinners.

- Add a bit of milk, fat-free sour cream, or fat-free plain yogurt along with herbs, garlic, onion, or your flavoring of choice to a puréed vegetable, and voilà: a cream sauce for meat or fish. It might even be a fun topping for mashed potatoes. Green taters, anyone?

- Use mixed dinners as the base for a casserole or pot pie. Add diced meat, chopped veggies, and rice or noodles.

- Use puréed fruit as a base for sauce to be used on chicken or pork. You can also reduce the fat in quick breads by replacing the oil with puréed fruit. Or add puréed fruit to pancake mix in place of some liquid.

- Add junior vegetables to brothy vegetable soups.

- Add chunky fruits and cobbler desserts to homemade cobbler, or use them to top frozen yogurt.

The Importance of the Family Dinner Table

In the last two decades, I believe we've lost sight of how important it is to eat together as a family—and we don't make it a priority in our busy lives. Dinner is often eating around the TV or in the car on the way to sports and activities. Sometimes we are just too tired to make the effort.

But believe me, it's worth it. Even if it's ham sandwiches and fruit on a paper plate, it's still family time! Sharing a meal is more than just breaking bread together; it's where family bonds are woven. Here are just a few good reasons to eat together:

- At the dinner table, kids see and learn many things, including table manners and how to carry on a conversation.

- Children model the eating habits they watch at the dinner table.

- Children develop language skills at the table. The more talking they hear, the easier it is for them to learn how to talk.

- The dinner table is where you share family values and make family unity.

- Many fond memories are made at the table.

- Family traditions often revolve around eating together—think holiday dinners.

- The table is where the family reconnects, sharing stories of the day and discussing plans.

- The dinner table is the one place where you can guarantee high-quality family time. All you have to do is get everyone there.

- Mealtime conversations during the preschool years help with early literacy skills. Research shows that mealtime conversations improve vocabulary better than listening to stories or reading out loud.[9, 10]

- Good communication during a child's younger years can improve parental communication with kids as they turn into teenagers.

- Research and teen surveys consistently show that the more often children eat dinner with their parents, the less likely they are to smoke, drink, or use illegal drugs.[11]

- Eating together as a family may reduce the incidence of teenage eating disorders. In a recent study called Project EAT at the University of Minnesota, adolescents who reported more frequent family meals, high priority for family meals, a positive atmosphere at family meals, and a more structured family meal environment were less likely to engage in disordered eating.[12]

- Eating together is even good for mental health. For boys, eating as a family more often is associated with less cigarette, alcohol, and marijuana use, as well as less depression. For girls, eating family meals more often is associated with less cigarette, alcohol, and marijuana use, as well as higher grade point averages, less depression, and lower likelihood of suicidal thoughts or attempts.[13]

What can you do to make family dinners happen more often? Here are some tips:

- Make menus and shop from them as often as possible, so cooking is less stressful.
- Keep some frozen, easy-prep foods on hand for when you really don't have time to cook (frozen cooked chicken, frozen veggies, and so on).
- Even if dinner is takeout, you can still eat it together at the table.
- Have everyone pitch in. Dinner comes together much quicker that way, and it adds to togetherness.
- If opposite work schedules or other factors make dinner together almost impossible, plan special dinners when you'll be together. Put them on the calendar.
- It doesn't have to be dinner—it could be breakfast or lunch.
- If you can't make a meal together every day, plan a few every week and make them a priority.
- Don't feel guilty if you can't eat together every day. Just do the best you can with as many family members as you can. A table for two can be just as special as a table for four!

How can you make the most of the time you spend together? Here's more advice:

- Let toddlers leave the table after a set time period; they have short attention spans. As kids get older they should be able to stay at the table longer.
- Make dinner a positive, relaxed event where everyone feels comfortable.
- Don't use this time for scolding or lecturing.
- Let everyone have equal talk time.
- Be good listeners, even when it requires patience!
- Ask your children open-ended questions: What did you do at preschool today? What did you play? Who did you play with? What was your favorite thing you did today?
- Weave stories and family values into the conversation. For example: "I know sometimes kids aren't nice at school and hit or bite. What should you do?"
- Turn off the TV. Record your favorite shows if you must.
- Don't answer the phone. Let the answering machine get it.
- Don't allow electronics or reading material at the table.
- Avoid toys at the table—except for babies, to extend the time they can stay with you.

Storage Reminder

Here are the basic rules for storing homemade baby food:

- For homemade cereals, veggies, and fruits, refrigerate what you will use within two days. Freeze any remainders. Exception: When making baby food from high-nitrate vegetables, immediately freeze anything over a serving.

- For eggs, refrigerate what you will use within twenty-four hours. Freeze any remainders, but note that some egg recipes won't freeze well.

Whole-Grain Risotto with Sweet Potato

Yield: about 2 cups (500 milliliters)

½ cup (125 milliliters) chopped sweet potato, other sweet vegetable, or dried fruit
2 tablespoons (30 milliliters) water
1 medium garlic clove, minced
1 teaspoon (5 milliliters) olive oil
½ cup (125 milliliters) cracked wheat (bulgur) or arborio rice
2 cups (500 milliliters) water
½ cup (125 milliliters) milk
Dash of cinnamon and nutmeg

1. Place sweet potato or other vegetable in microwave-safe dish. Add water and cook 2 minutes. Let stand.
2. In medium saucepan, sauté garlic in oil for 1 minute. (Omit garlic if you're making a fruit risotto.)
3. Add bulgur or rice and continue cooking 2 minutes, stirring constantly.
4. Meanwhile, heat 2 cups (500 milliliters) of water in a measuring cup in microwave to boiling.
5. Stir ½ cup (125 milliliters) of water into bulgur over low heat. Stir often while simmering until water is absorbed. Repeat with rest of water, ½ cup (125 milliliters) at a time. This will take about 20 to 25 minutes. You'll have to put the water back in the microwave when it cools off, or you can put it in a separate pan on the stove to keep it warm.
6. Heat ½ cup (125 milliliters) milk. Pour into bulgur. (If you're making a fruit risotto, add fruit and a dash of cinnamon and nutmeg now.) Stir constantly until all the milk is absorbed.

Nutrient content of ¼ cup (60 milliliters)

43 calories, 2 grams protein, Magnesium and manganese 15%

Baked Oatmeal

Yield: 16 ¼-cup (60-milliliter) servings

3 cups (750 milliliters or 468 grams) whole (not instant) oats
2 tablespoons (30 milliliters) toasted wheat germ
1 cup (250 milliliters) low-fat milk
2 teaspoons (10 milliliters) baking powder
½ teaspoon (2.5 milliliters) cinnamon
½ teaspoon (2.5 milliliters) salt
½ cup (125 milliliters or 110 grams) brown sugar
½ cup (125 milliliters) applesauce or other puréed fruit
2 eggs (lightly beaten)
1 cup (250 milliliters) other fruit (fresh or dried)
1 teaspoon (5 milliliters) vanilla

1. Preheat oven to 350°F (175°C). Mix dry and wet ingredients together.
2. Stir in fruit.
3. Pour into 8-by-8-inch glass pan sprayed with cooking spray. Cook 30 to 40 minutes

Nutrient content of ¼ cup (60 milliliters)

157 calories, 6 grams protein, 4 grams fiber, Manganese 130%, Magnesium 80%, Thiamine 50%, Zinc 50%, Folate 25%, Iron and riboflavin 20%

Italian Potatoes

Yield: 1 serving

1 small new potato
2 tablespoons (30 milliliters) grated
    mozzarella or Italian cheese mix
3 tablespoons (45 milliliters)
    marinara sauce

1. Scrub potato and poke with fork.
2. Cook 2 to 3 minutes, or until soft.
3. Let stand a few minutes. Slice into
    pieces the right size for your child.
4. Top with warm marinara sauce
    and cheese.

Nutrient content per serving

165 calories, 10 grams protein, 2 grams fiber, Vitamin
C 120%, Vitamin B_6 70%, Calcium and magnesium 40%,
Vitamin B_{12} 30%

Spinach Dip

Yield: 5 1-tablespoon servings

¼ cup (60 milliliters) cooked, drained,
    chopped spinach
¼ cup (60 milliliters) cottage cheese
Dash of dehydrated minced onion
Dash of garlic powder
Dash of dill

1. Blend all ingredients. For a
    milder spinach flavor, add more
    cottage cheese.

Nutrient content of 1 tablespoon (15 milliliters)

13 calories, 2 grams protein, Vitamin A 10%

Oven-Fried Zucchini Sticks

Yield: 6 ½-cup (125-milliliter) servings

½ cup (125 milliliters) Italian
    bread crumbs
2 tablespoons (30 milliliters)
    Parmesan cheese
¼ teaspoon (1 milliliter) garlic powder
3 medium zucchini
Milk or beaten egg yolk
1 cup (250 milliliters) prepared
    marinara sauce or ranch dressing

1. Slice zucchini into rounds or long
    sticks. Preheat oven to 450°F or
    232°C. Spray cooking sheet with
    cooking spray.
2. Mix bread crumbs, cheese, and
    garlic powder in large zipper bag.
3. Dip each zucchini slice in milk or
    egg, then drop into bag and shake
    until coated with crumbs.
4. Bake 10 to 15 minutes or until
    brown and tender.
5. Serve with warm marinara sauce
    or ranch dressing.

**Nutrient content of ½ cup (125 milliliters) zucchini
with 1½ tablespoons (20 milliliters) marinara sauce**

43 calories, 2 grams protein, 1 gram fiber, Vitamin C
25%, Magnesium 20%

Creamy Carrot-Cauliflower Soup

Yield: about 4½ cups (about 1 liter) or 9 ½-cup (125-milliliter) servings

1¾ cups (420 milliliters) water
¼ teaspoon salt
1 pound (500 grams) baby carrots or peeled carrots, cut in 2-inch pieces
½ bunch cauliflower (about ¾ pound or 360 grams), cut into pieces
2 medium red potatoes, (a little over 1 pound), peeled and cubed
1 large clove garlic, chopped
1¾ cups (430 milliliters) whole milk, soymilk, or cooking liquid
1 teaspoon tarragon
½ teaspoon (2.5 milliliters) salt
Pinch of pepper

1. In 6-quart (1-liter) pot, bring water to boil. Add carrots and simmer on high for 15 minutes.
2. Add cauliflower and potatoes. Cook 20 minutes or until tender.
3. Remove from heat. Purée vegetables and milk in batches with spices in blender until completely smooth. Pour into large mixing bowl.
4. Mix with spoon to distribute spices evenly.
5. Garnish with grated carrot and fresh tarragon, if desired. You may also swirl a tablespoon of fat-free sour cream or plain yogurt into each bowl.

Nutrient content ½ cup (125 milliliters)

93 calories, 3 grams protein, 3 grams fiber, Vitamin A 200%, Vitamin C 150%, Vitamin B_6 60%, Vitamin K, magnesium, and manganese 30%, Zinc 20%

Sweet Potato Fries

Yield: About 8 ½-cup (125-milliliter) servings

1½ tablespoons (20 milliliters) canola or olive oil
¼ teaspoon pumpkin pie spice
¼ teaspoon ground cinnamon
¼ teaspoon salt
Cinnamon-sugar mixture or vanilla yogurt (optional)
2 large sweet potatoes (about 1½ pounds or 680 grams), peeled and cut into wedges

1. Preheat oven to 425°F or 220°C.
2. Whisk together first 4 ingredients in a large bowl.
3. Add sweet potatoes and toss to coat evenly with oil.
4. Place on cookie sheet and bake about 20 to 25 minutes, or until tender.
5. Sprinkle with cinnamon-sugar mixture or vanilla yogurt for a sweet treat.

Nutrient content of ½ cup (125 milliliters)

110 calories, 1 gram protein, 2.5 grams fiber, Vitamin A 170%, Vitamin C 130%, Vitamin E 70%, Vitamin B_6 40%, Riboflavin and magnesium 20%

Home Fries

Yield: about 5 ½-cup (125-milliliter) servings

1 pound (500 grams) new potatoes or baking potatoes, well scrubbed
1½ tablespoons (20 milliliters) canola or olive oil
1 clove garlic, crushed
½ teaspoon (2.5 milliliters) seasoned salt

1. Preheat oven to 425°F or 220°C.
2. Cut potatoes into long wedges; do not peel.
3. Mix oil with spices. Toss with potatoes in large bowl until potatoes are well coated.
4. Bake for 20 to 25 minutes or until tender and golden brown.

Nutrient content of ½ cup (125 milliliters)

120 calories, 2 grams protein, 1 gram fiber, Vitamin C 80%, Vitamin B$_6$ 60%, Magnesium 30%

Cinnamon Chips

Yield: 12 large chips

2 whole-wheat or corn tortillas
1½ tablespoons (20 milliliters) cinnamon-sugar mixture
Canola oil or melted butter (optional)

1. Preheat oven to 450°F or 232°C.
2. Using knife or kitchen shears, cut each tortilla into strips or triangles.
3. Brush tortillas with water, canola oil, or melted butter. Sprinkle with cinnamon-sugar mixture.
4. Bake on cookie sheet for about 10 minutes until crisp.

Serve with fruit salsa or Strawberry Crème Dip (see right).

Nutrient content of 3 large tortilla chips (½ tortilla)

50 calories, 1 gram fiber

Fruit Salsa

Yield: about 5 cups (1.25 liters) or 10 ½-cup (125-milliliter) servings

1 8-ounce (240gram) can crushed pineapple
1 cup (250 milliliters) chopped seedless grapes
1 cup (250 milliliters) chopped fresh oranges or canned mandarin oranges
1 large or 2 small bananas, chopped
1 apple, peeled and finely chopped

1. Mix all and serve alone or with Cinnamon Chips (see left).

Nutrient content of ½ cup (125 milliliters)

53 calories, 0.5 grams protein, 1 gram fiber, Vitamin C 80%, Manganese 30%

Strawberry Crème Dip

Yield: ½ cup (125 milliliters) or 8 1-tablespoon (15-milliliter) servings

4 large strawberries
3 ounces (90 grams) low-fat cream cheese

1. Use hand blender or a fork to mash strawberries and stir them into cream cheese. Mix well.

Nutrient content of 1 tablespoon (15 milliliters)

27 calories, 1 gram protein, Vitamin C 10%

Black Bean Soup

Yield: about 5 cups (1.25 liters)

1 teaspoon (5 milliliters) olive oil
1 medium onion, chopped
3 cloves garlic, chopped
1 teaspoon (5 milliliters) dried
    whole oregano
½ teaspoon (2.5 milliliters) dried
    whole thyme
½ teaspoon (2.5 milliliters) cumin
3 cups cooked black beans (750 milliliters)
    or 2 15-ounce (450-gram) cans, drained
    and rinsed
2½ to 3 cups (625 to 750 milliliters) nat-
    ural reduced-sodium chicken broth

Garnish

2 tomatoes, finely chopped
2 tablespoons (30 milliliters)
    chopped cilantro
3 tablespoons (45 milliliters)
    fat-free sour cream (optional)
¼ avocado, mashed
½ cup (125 milliliters) corn

1. Heat oil in medium pan and sauté
    onion and garlic until tender—
    about 5 minutes.
2. Stir in spices, cook 2 to 3 minutes.
3. Meanwhile, purée beans in blender
    or food processor, adding broth to
    reach the desired consistency.
4. Return to pan and simmer 10 min-
    utes or until warmed through.
5. To garnish: Mix avocado with sour
    cream and swirl a spoonful into
    soup. Add corn, tomatoes, and a
    pinch of cilantro on top.

Nutrient content of ½ cup (125 milliliters)

103 calories, 6 grams protein, 5 grams fiber, Folate
60%, Magnesium 50%, Zinc, vitamin C, and thiamine
30%, Iron 20%

Crunchy Cream-Cheese Spread

*Yield: ¾ cup (180 milliliters) or 12 1-tablespoon (15-milli-
liter) servings*

½ cup (125 milliliters) reduced-fat
    cream cheese
¼ cup (60 milliliters) finely grated carrot

1. Mix together. Spread on bread
    or crackers.

Nutrient content of 1 tablespoon (15 milliliters)

23 calories, 1 gram protein

Maui Smoothie

Yield: almost 2 cups (500 milliliters)

½ cup (125 milliliters) pineapple packed
    in juice, frozen
½ frozen banana
1 cup (250 milliliters) plain yogurt
1 ½ teaspoon coconut extract (optional)
Honey to taste (for babies older than
    1 year)

1. Blend all ingredients and serve.

Nutrient content of ½ cup (125 milliliters)

80 calories, 4 grams protein, Vitamin C and vitamin
B$_{12}$ 40%, Vitamin B$_6$ and riboflavin 30%, Zinc 20%

Mom's Apple Pie Smoothie

Yield: 2 cups

1 cup (250 milliliters) applesauce, frozen
1 cup (250 milliliters) vanilla yogurt
¼ teaspoons (1 milliliter) apple pie spice
½ teaspoons (2.5 milliliters) vanilla extract

1. Blend all and serve immediately.

Nutrient content of ½ cup (125 milliliters)

78 calories, 3 grams protein, Vitamin B_{12} 36%,
Riboflavin 28%, Calcium 20%

Salmon Wraps

Yield: 2 wraps

½ cup (125 milliliters) cooked
   salmon, flaked
¼ cup (60 milliliters) reduced-fat
   ranch dressing
2 tablespoons (30 milliliters)
   grated carrots
¼ cup (60 milliliters) chopped
   spinach leaves

1. Mix salmon, carrots, and dressing.
2. Divide between tortillas, and top
   with spinach, and roll tightly.
3. If you like, try these other wrap ideas:
   chicken, avocado, and grated savoy
   cabbage; low-fat refried beans, cheese,
   and tomato; hummus spread with
   finely grated red cabbage; or grated
   cheese and pasta sauce.

Nutrient content of ½ salmon wrap

137 calories, 8 grams protein, 1 gram fiber, Vitamin
B_{12} 90%, Selenium 60%, Vitamin B_6 and niacin 50%,
Zinc, iron, and folate 10%

Chapter 16

Eighteen to Twenty-Four Months

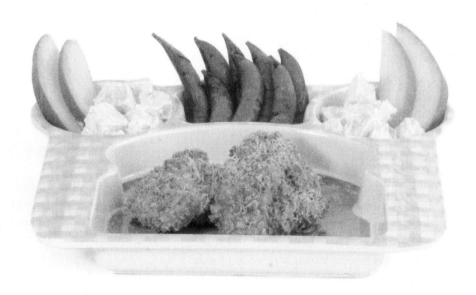

*The age of your children is a key factor in how quickly you are served in a
restaurant. We once had a waiter in Canada who said, "Could I get you your check?"
and we answered, "How about the menu first?"*

—Erma Bombeck

Food Jags and Other Annoying Eating Behaviors

Ethan wants Cheerios for every meal. Addie won't eat meat—or much of anything. Nicolas absolutely can't have his peas touch his carrots. Emma Claire refuses peaches—although it was her favorite food yesterday!

If these scenarios sound familiar—you must have a toddler! Your baby's developing eating personality, new opinions about food, growing awareness of the world, and burgeoning independence can all cause changes in food attitudes.

Is it worth fussing or worrying about? No. I know: That's easy to say, but not so easy to do. But honestly: These eating behaviors are perfectly normal. In fact, I would worry if my child didn't have any. (On second thought...I'd count my blessings.) I've heard stories of toddlers who would rather eat broccoli than cookies, but those kids are rare!

You can count on at least some of the following behaviors from your terrific toddler. And you can handle them, too!

- **Your child is a food purist.** Your kid gets bent out of shape when the broccoli touches the chicken. This is an easy behavior to deal with—simply serve your child's food on a divided plate.

- **Your child wants only one food for days on end.** It's hard not to give in to some extent—but also remember that you're the one in charge. Use this opportunity to teach your child about nutrition; explain that he or she needs other foods to grow. Put a new twist on a favorite food, like adding peas to mac and cheese. If your child insists on chicken, offer turkey.

- **Your child is allergic to green.** Don't sweat this one. Many orange veggies and fruits have the same nutrient profile as green veggies.

- **Your child likes all foods smooth.** Whether it's texture aversion or just personal preference, offer meals that are both smooth and textured. For example, give your child an animal cracker to dip in applesauce. Or serve creamy soup, and let your child float peas, veggie chunks, or saltine cracker pieces on the top and try to eat them with a spoon before they sink. (You can try this same technique with applesauce or blended yogurt.)

- **Your child wants food of only one color.** This is another teachable moment. Encourage your child to eat all the colors of the rainbow so he or she will have the energy to run and catch one. You can also let your child help you plan meals—sometimes your child gets to choose the colors, and sometimes you get to.

- **Your child rejects strongly flavored foods.** Play a game to show your child that a food sometimes tastes much different from its smell. Hold your nose and try the food, then try it while smelling it. Have your child do the same. He or she may find that a food tastes good, even if it smells bad. Let your child hold his or her nose while eating it.

- **Your child can't stand herbs and spices.** It can take a while to get used to the taste of herbs and spices. Remember that for the first eight months to a year, no salt, herbs, or spices crossed your baby's lips. Your child has some catching up to do, so go slowly on food flavorings for your little one. Stay away from pepper and spicy seasonings, and experiment with other herbs and spices to find a middle ground the whole family can enjoy. If your child really prefers food with no flavorings, keep setting aside his or her portion before you add herbs or spices.

Your Child's Food Personality

Observing your child can help you determine if he or she has a particular food personality, which in turn may help you provide healthy foods that'll be eaten. Following are just a few food personalities your child may exhibit.

- **The bird**: Your kid may not each much, but at least he or she is consistent at each meal. You wonder how your child can survive on such a small amount of food. Keep an eye on growth, give a vitamin supplement, and keep encouraging, but don't pressure your child. He or she will eat more when hunger strikes.

- **The one-mealer**: Your kid eats one really good meal a day. There's no need to worry about this unless it happens at every meal. Make sure your child is still hungry when he or she asks for more. And don't be surprised if your child doesn't eat much at other meals.

- **The drinker**: Your little one much prefers drinking to eating. Try to nip this habit in the bud—a toddler can't get enough nutrients from milk or formula alone. If necessary, make sure your child is off the bottle; this can prolong a heavy drinking habit. (See page 293 for tips on ditching the bottle.)

- **The meat and potatoes eater**: You've got a carnivore on your hands; no veggies ever cross your child's lips. If veggies are verboten, offer fruit—it provides many of the same nutrients. Also give your carnivore a chance to help you choose foods at the store and prepare them. This may motivate your child to expand his or her diet a bit.

- **The cereal eater**: Cereal (especially the whole-grain kind) makes a great meal or snack...but cereal for every meal? You'll have to limit how often your child has cereal each day, perhaps to breakfast and a snack or two. Also limit the amount: a half-cup of cereal is a snack, but two cups is a meal! Add a fruit like blueberries or sliced bananas to round it out.

- **The vegan**: This isn't a bad thing—but it may seem like it if the rest of your family are meat lovers. As long as your child drinks two cups of milk a day and eats other sources of iron and zinc like beans, he or she will be fine. (For more info on vegan eating, see page 157.)

- **The fine diner**: Somewhere along the line, your child started ordering specific meals and his or her private chef accommodated him or her. Take my advice and shut the short-order line down now. The longer you cater to your child's whims, the more picky and demanding your child will be. Life doesn't always give us what we want, and the sooner your child learns that the better.

- **The no-mixed-foods eater**: Not only does your child insist that foods not touch each other; they can't be cooked together either. Forget one-dish meals like stews and casseroles! There's a way around this: Use your blender. That's right: Put your chili in the blender and make a smooth soup out of it. Or separate a few ingredients from a casserole before or after cooking it. If this type of food is what you normally cook, however, you'll want your child to get used to it eventually.

De-Stressing Dinnertime

You've had a long day at work, your toddler is tired and wants your attention, and someone's got to put dinner on the table. If you have older children, there's homework to supervise and maybe piano lessons.

Sound familiar? A trip to the nearest drive-through for dinner sounds pretty good about now. But you know it's not healthy or cheap to eat out a lot. And in the long run it often takes longer, too.

You can de-stress the dinner hour without eating out or ordering in every night. All it takes is some planning and getting into a routine.

Planning Ahead

I admire those folks who are so organized that they cook every weekend and freeze a week's worth of meals or plan a month of meals at a time and shop accordingly. I like to plan ahead a week or so, while others can see only two or three days ahead. Whatever your planning personality, here are a few tips:

- Plan menus and meals ahead of time, then make a master list of ingredients and shop from it.
- Double or triple your recipes and freeze the extra food.
- Use a Crock-Pot. Prep the food before bed, then throw it in the pot in the morning, switch it on, and forget about it until you smell your yummy dinner all cooked and ready to eat several hours later.
- Make foods that create leftovers you can use for a different dish. For example, use the chili you made on Monday for tacos or a potato topping on Thursday.
- Keep convenience foods on hand for nights when time is especially tight (cooked chicken breast or shrimp, pasta, canned tuna or chicken, and so on).
- Make meals and snacks regularly scheduled events. Empty tummies mean grouchy toddlers—not a pretty sight. If you know that dinner will be delayed, plan an extra snack.

Preparing Dinner

- Let your child know what to expect. If you're driving home from daycare, announce that your child can help you make dinner or play, but that dinner will be soon. (Toddlers have no concept of time, so it won't help to say that dinner is in a half-hour.)

- Encourage your child to work or play in the kitchen. He or she may enjoy having a job like setting the table or putting food in the dog's bowl. Your child's job could also be to sit at the table and work a puzzle or draw you a picture. If your child is in the kitchen, you can keep an eye on him or her and at the same time, your child gets some (if not all) of your attention. (Do try to keep your little one away from the cooking area to avoid accidents.)
- While you're cooking, give your child choices that help him or her buy into the meal: "Do you want broccoli or carrots?" "Shall we make macaroni or spaghetti?"
- When dinnertime is imminent, give a five-minute warning and set a timer. This will give your child time to transition from playing to cleaning up and sitting at the table.
- Meals with a toddler will continue to be messy. Don't sweat it; just be ready for it. Put a plastic mat under your child's chair and a bib on your toddler.

At the Table

- Make sure your child's chair and utensils are appropriate for his or her size and skills. Sometimes a new plate that your child picks out can provide new motivation for dining.
- Dish up your child's food a few minutes before giving it to him or her, so it's not too hot. Cut the food so your child can self-feed.
- Arrange the food nicely on your child's plate. (When you're planning menus, keep a variety of colors in mind.)
- Serve small portions and let your child ask for more.
- Turn off the TV and avoid other distractions so your family can concentrate on eating and talking together.

When Your Child Is Done Eating

- When your little one signals that mealtime is over, it's over. Trying to extend it... don't go there.
- If your child throws his or her plate, cup, or spoon, discourage this behavior with a reprimand. Encourage your child to use words instead: *all done* or *no more*.
- Don't worry if your child hasn't eaten much at a meal. He or she will have another opportunity to tank up at the next snack.
- Once you clean up your child and his or her eating area, return to the table with a toy so that your toddler can get used to spending more time with the family at the table.
- As your toddler gets older, you can also give him or her after-dinner chores, such as throwing away dirty napkins. Every little bit helps!

Toddler-Size Servings

How big a serving should you expect your toddler to eat? Just because your child is walking and talking doesn't mean he or she's ready for big-kid servings yet. In general, a toddler serving is a tablespoon of each food per year of age at each meal. A toddler portion is also about one-quarter the size of an adult portion.

Here are typical serving sizes of common foods for children one to three years old, along with a guide to how many servings of each food group toddlers should eat in a day. Remember that your child may have more than one serving of a food type at a meal and that the recommended numbers of servings may seem large due to the smaller serving sizes.

A Day in the Diet of a Toddler

Breakfast
½ cup (125 milliliters) cereal
½ cup (125 milliliters) milk
¼ cup (60 milliliters) sliced fruit

Mid-morning snack
½ ounce (15 grams) cheese
3 whole grain crackers
Matchstick-size steamed carrots
¼ cup (60 milliliters) apple juice

Lunch
¾ cup bean and vegetable soup
   (180 milliliters)
1 slice wheat toast
¾ cup (180 milliliters) milk
½ sliced apple

Mid-afternoon snack
½ cup (125 milliliters) yogurt
½ slice fruit bread

Dinner
1½ ounces (45 grams) fish
¼ cup (60 milliliters) broccoli
¼ cup (60 milliliters) sweet potato
½ wheat roll

Bedtime snack
¼ banana
½ cup (125 milliliters) milk
2 graham crackers

Healthy Snacks for Toddlers

For young kids, snacks are a necessity; they fill nutrient gaps in your toddler's diet. Toddlers' tiny tummies make it hard for them to get all they need from just three meals, so for them grazing is the way to go.

Just make sure your toddler's snacks are as healthy as the meals you serve. And while you're dishing out a snack, have a healthy snack of your own! Here are some ideas to get you started:

Toddler-Size Servings

Food Group (Recommended Number of Daily Servings)	Food (Typical Serving Size)
Grains (6 or more)	Bread (½ to 1 slice); small roll or muffin (½ roll or muffin); bun or pita bread (¼ to ½ piece); cereal, rice, or pasta (¼ cup); dry cereal (⅓ cup); crackers (3 crackers)
Vegetables (3 or more)	Cooked (¼ cup); salad (½ cup); juice (¼ cup)
Fruits (3 or more)	Cooked or canned (¼ cup); fresh (½ piece); juice (¼ cup)
Dairy food (4 to 6)	Milk (½ cup); cheese (½ ounce); yogurt (⅓ cup)
Protein foods (2)	Meat, fish, poultry, tofu (1 ounce or 2 1-inch cubes); beans, dried and cooked (¼ cup); egg (½ to 1 egg)

Modified from "Pyramid Power: Portions not Platefuls. Guide to Your Child's Nutrition." American Academy of Pediatrics. 1999.

- **Grain snacks**:
  - Whole-grain crackers
  - Whole-grain cereal
  - Toast
  - Tortilla strips
  - Baked tortilla chips
  - Rice cakes
- **Fruit snacks**:
  - Fresh fruit
  - Canned fruit
  - Stewed dried fruit
- **Veggie snacks**:
  - Steamed veggies like carrots and zucchini
  - Steamed veggies with dip
  - Vegetable juice
  - Mild salsa with crackers
  - Cooked cubed sweet potato
  - Avocado pieces or spread
- **Dairy snacks**:
  - Yogurt
  - Yogurt smoothie
  - Yogurt with fresh fruit
  - Pasteurized cheese
  - Cheese dip

- **Protein snacks**:
  - Refried beans
  - String cheese
  - Cottage cheese or cream cheese
  - Other hard cheese
  - Boiled egg
  - Nut or seed spread (mixed with fruit, only if child isn't allergy-prone)
  - Leftover chicken
  - Thinly sliced roast beef
  - Tofu
- **Processed snacks**:
  - Goldfish crackers
  - Plain cookies like animal crackers or teething crackers
  - Gerber Fruit Puffs or Veggie Puffs

Junk Food Substitutes and Healthier Fast-Food Choices

Junk food and unhealthy fast food are always visible and always available, which makes them hard to avoid. You can quell the urge for unhealthy snacks while you're out and about by making sure your child has a healthy one before you leave the house. Or take a healthy snack with you and take a break to eat it while you're shopping or running errands. Here are some strategies for keeping your child junk food–free!

- **In the car**:
  - Keep snacks like whole-grain crackers, fruits, juice boxes, animal crackers, and cereal with you. It's best not to let your child eat while you're driving, so you can supervise your child and prevent choking.
  - Carry an insulated lunch bag with an ice pack for perishable snacks like sandwiches, string cheese, yogurt, and milk.
  - Keep ready-to-eat entrées with you, too.

- **At the mall**:
  - Soft pretzels without salt
  - Frozen yogurt
  - Baked potato
  - Noodles
  - Cheese pizza or cheese bread with marinara sauce
  - Bean burrito

- **At the drive-through**:
  - Bean burrito or refried beans
  - Grilled chicken sandwich
  - Veggie burger
  - Frozen yogurt or half a small milkshake

Veggie Adventures

By now your toddler has probably had all the normal veggies served in all the normal ways. Now it's time for something completely different!

- **Artichokes**: Trim the prickly ends of the leaves and steam whole artichokes. Let your toddler pluck off the leaves and dip them into salad dressing or lemon butter. Show your child how to strip the edible portion from the leaf by placing between your teeth and pulling the leaf.
- **Veggie slaws**: There's no limit to what you can put in a veggie slaw. If your toddler can't chew slaw yet, steam the veggies briefly first. Try these combinations:
  - Cabbage, mayo, and vinegar
  - Chopped apple, cabbage, and carrot with mayo and a touch of apple juice
  - Carrot, raisin, and pineapple with vanilla yogurt and mayo
  - Grated cabbage and carrot with ranch dressing
  - Broccoli with your favorite vinaigrette

- **Salads**: At the ripe old age of almost-two, your toddler should be able to appreciate salads. Here are some salad-making tips to keep in mind:
  - Remember that the darker the greens, the healthier they are—spinach being best.
  - Finely chop salads to make eating easier. The inner portion of romaine leaf may be too hard for your toddler to chew.
  - Make a meal of your salad with additions like grated cheese, chopped chicken, thinly sliced beef, cooked shrimp, tofu, and/or beans.
  - Use salad dressings that aren't too vinegary. Most kids like ranch. If a vinaigrette is too vinegary, add a bit of water, fruit juice, or oil. Rice vinegar is milder than most.
- **Veggie sticks**: Raw veggies can be a choking hazard, but if you steam them to soften them just a bit, they're fine. Try steaming these veggies for dipping:
  - Julienne carrots or parsnips
  - Broccoli florets
  - Zucchini sticks
  - Bell pepper strips
  - Julienne butternut squash or pumpkin
  - Sweet potato sticks
- **Dips**: And here are some yummy dips for those veggies:
  - Ranch dressing
  - Cheesy Sauce (page 270)
  - Maple syrup (for sweet potato and squash)
  - Applesauce
  - Ketchup
  - Strawberry Crème Dip (page 302)
  - Hummus Dip (page 280)
  - Spinach Dip (page 300)
  - Crunchy Cream-Cheese Spread (page 303)
  - Chicken-Avocado Spread (page 271)
  - Avocado-Chicken-Cheese Spread (page 271)
- **Stir-fry**: Your toddler may enjoy watching you stir up supper with the flair of a Chinese chef! Here are some tips to make stir-fries toddler-friendly:
  - Stir-fried vegetables may not be cooked enough for a toddler. Cook your child's portion a bit longer than the rest of the family's.
  - Chop veggies a little smaller than usual to speed cooking time and make them easier for your little one to eat.
  - Serve stir-fried food with healthy brown rice.

Stir-Fried Sugar Snap Peas

Yield: about 1½ cups (375 milliliters)

1 package (8 ounces or 240 grams)
stringless sugar snap peas (about
1½ cups)
2 teaspoons (10 milliliters) olive oil
½ teaspoon (2.5 milliliters) toasted
sesame oil
2 tablespoons (30 milliliters)
hoisin sauce

1. Heat both oils over medium-high
   heat in a wok or large skillet.
2. Add snap peas and cook over
   medium-high heat, stirring often.
3. For adults, cook 1 to 2 minutes.
   Cook until tender for your baby.
4. Remove from heat and coat with
   hoisin sauce.

Nutrient content of ¼ cup (60 milliliters)

42 calories, 1 gram protein, 1 gram fiber, Vitamin C
40%, Vitamin B₆, vitamin K, thiamine, and folate 20%

Northwest Smoothie

Yield: about 2 cups (500 milliliters)

1 cup (250 milliliters) fresh raspberries,
frozen (or ⅔ cup commercially
frozen raspberries)
2 fresh nectarines, peeled and
chopped, frozen
1 cup (250 milliliters) plain or vanilla
low-fat yogurt

1. Blend all ingredients and serve
   immediately.

Nutrient content of ½ cup (125 milliliters)

80 calories, 4 grams protein, Vitamin C 60%, Vitamin
B₆, Vitamin B₁₂, and riboflavin 30%, Zinc and
magnesium 20%

Chopped Autumn Salad

6 cups (1.5 liters) shredded mixed greens
2 carrots, grated
1 Granny Smith apple, peeled and chopped
1 gala or other crispy red apple, peeled
and chopped
1 lemon wedge
2 ounces (60 grams) or ½ cup shredded
reduced-fat Cheddar cheese

Salad Dressing

1 tablespoon (15 milliliters) apple juice
1 tablespoon (15 milliliters) rice vinegar
or apple cider vinegar
1 teaspoon (5 milliliters) sugar
¼ cup (60 milliliters) olive oil
Shake of salt and pepper

1. Squeeze fresh lemon over apples.
2. Toss with greens, carrots, and cheese
3. Mix salad dressing ingredients and
   toss with salad. Serve immediately.

Nutrient content of ½ cup (125 milliliters)

79 calories, 2 grams protein, 1 gram fiber, Vitamin K
100%, Folate 40%, Calcium 20%, Vitamin E 15%, Zinc 10%

Chicken Salad with Mango

Yield: about 6 cups (1.5 liters)

¼ cup (60 milliliters) mayonnaise
½ cup (125 milliliters) fat-free sour
 cream (or plain yogurt)
½ teaspoon (2.5 milliliters) garlic salt
½ teaspoon (2.5 milliliters) onion powder
¼ teaspoon (1 milliliter) curry powder
1 mango (or peach, nectarine, or apricot), peeled, seeded, and chopped,
 or about ⅔ cup (160 milliliters)
4 cooked boneless, skinless chicken
 breasts, chopped (5 cups [1.25 liter]
 or 2 pounds [1 kilogram] chopped
 leftover or canned chicken) or
 5 cups cubed tofu

1. Mix first 5 ingredients; stir
   in mango.
2. Fold in chicken. If your child
   prefers smooth food, purée.
3. Serve in a tortilla or wholewheat
   pita pocket, or spread on crackers.
4. For older children and for adults
   portions, add raisins, chopped
   walnuts, and chopped celery if
   you like.

Nutrient content of ¼ cup (60 milliliters)

81 calories, 10 grams protein, Niacin 60%, Vitamin B$_6$ 40%, Vitamin C 20%, Magnesium, zinc, and vitamin B$_{12}$ 10%

Smooth and Healthy Meat Sauce

Yield 3½ cups (900 milliliters)

1 teaspoon (5 milliliters) olive oil
½ onion, chopped
3 cloves garlic, chopped
1 cup (125 milliliters) sliced mushrooms
1 red bell pepper, seeded and chopped
½ pound (250 grams) natural, extra-lean
 ground beef
2 cooked carrots
2 cups (500 milliliters) prepared or
 homemade spaghetti sauce

1. Heat oil in medium pan over
   medium heat. Add onion and garlic
   and sauté for several minutes.
2. Add bell pepper and mushrooms
   and increase heat to medium-
   high. Cook, stirring often, for
   several minutes.
3. Add ground beef and cook until it
   reaches an internal temperature of
   160°F or 71°C.
4. In a blender or with a hand
   blender, purée meat mixture with
   heated spaghetti sauce.
5. Serve over pasta, rice, or potatoes
   or use as a dip for veggies.

Nutrient content of ¼ cup (60 milliliters)

Vitamin C 170%, Vitamin A 20%, Vitamin B$_{12}$ 50%, Zinc 40%, Vitamin B$_6$ and niacin 30%, Iron 10%

Chicken or Fish Nuggets

Yield: about 8 2-ounce (60-gram) servings

1 pound (500 grams) chicken tenders
   or chicken breasts, cut into nuggets
1½ cups (375 milliliters) corn flakes
1½ cups (375 milliliters) oat or wheat
   bran flakes
¼ cup (125 milliliters) grated
   parmesan cheese
¼ teaspoon (1 milliliter) garlic powder
½ teaspoon (2.5 milliliters) seasoned salt
Shake of lemon pepper
2 large eggs, beaten or ½ cup (125
   milliliters) milk
⅓ cup (80 milliliters) flour

1. Preheat oven to 425°F (220°C).
2. Pulverize the cereal flakes into crumbs by putting in a plastic bag and crushing with a rolling pin or the back of a pan. Or pulse in a food processor.
3. Mix cereal flake crumbs with rest of dry ingredients.
4. Dip nuggets into flour, then egg, then crumb mixture.
5. Bake on cookie sheet sprayed with cooking spray for 10 to 15 minutes or until nuggets reach an internal temperature of 165°F (74°C).

Nutrient content of 2 ounces (60 grams)

99 calories, 11 grams protein, 1 gram fiber, Niacin 90%, Vitamin B$_6$ 60%, Vitamin B$_{12}$ 50%, Riboflavin 40%, Zinc, iron, and thiamine 30%

Quick and Healthy Tortilla Soup

(modified from *Quick and Healthy: Low-Fat, Carb-Conscious Cooking* by Brenda Ponichtera)

½ pound (250 grams) boneless,
   skinless chicken breasts, cut into
   bite-size pieces
3½ cups (825 milliliters) natural,
   reduced-sodium chicken broth
1 can (15 ounces or 425 grams) black
   beans, drained and rinsed
1 can (14 ounces or 397 grams)
   low-sodium diced tomatoes
1 can (4 ounces or 113 grams) mild
   diced green chilies (optional)
3 corn tortillas (cut into eighths)

1. In a medium saucepan over medium heat, sauté chicken for 3 minutes.
2. Add broth, beans, corn, tomatoes, and chilies. Simmer for 10 minutes.
3. Add tortillas and simmer for an additional 10 minutes.
4. For kids who like their food smooth, purée the soup in the blender.

Nutrient content of ½ cup (125 milliliters)

81 calories, 8 grams protein, 2 grams fiber, Niacin and vitamin C 40%, Magnesium and folate 30%, Zinc and vitamin B$_6$ 20%, Iron 10%

Tropical Fish

Yield: 8 2-ounce (60-gram) servings

1 pound (500 grams) mild white
  fish filets
3 tablespoons (45 milliliters)
  fresh-squeezed lime juice
2 cloves garlic, crushed
1 tablespoon (15 milliliters) olive oil
Pepper and garlic salt to taste

1. Mix garlic with lemon juice; pour
   into a resealable bag. Add fish,
   squeeze out air, close bag, and
   gently shake so marinade coats all
   filets. Refrigerate at least 1 hour.
2. Heat oil in medium skillet over
   high heat. Remove fish from bag
   and discard marinade. Sprinkle
   with pepper and garlic salt. Cook
   on both sides until it flakes easily
   or reaches an internal temperature
   of 145°F (63°C.)

Nutrient content of 2 ounces (60 grams)

80 calories, 13 grams protein, Vitamin B_{12} 100%, Magnesium, vitamin E, and vitamin B_6 250%, Vitamin C and zinc 10%

Lamb Kebab

Yield: 4 large or 8 small kebabs

1 lamb sirloin (1½ pounds or 0.75
  kilograms lamb chops with meat
  trimmed from bone)
1½ pounds (about 0.75 kilograms)
  small new potatoes
1 red bell pepper
2 teaspoons (10 milliliters) olive oil
1 tablespoon (15 milliliters) fresh
  lemon juice
2 tablespoons (30 milliliters) red wine
  or 1 tablespoon (15 milliliters) red
  wine vinegar and 1 tablespoon (15
  milliliters) water
1 teaspoon (5 milliliters) Herbes de
  Provence or Italian seasoning
1–2 cloves garlic, crushed

1. Cut lamb and red pepper into 1-inch
   pieces. Mix last 4 ingredients in
   resealable plastic bag. Add lamb
   and marinate at least 1 hour but
   preferably longer.
2. When ready to cook lamb: Preheat
   grill and wash potatoes. If potatoes
   are bigger than 1½ inches, cut in
   half. Precook in microwave for 5
   to 6 minutes.
3. Remove lamb and pepper from
   marinade and thread on skewers.
   Thread potatoes on skewers.
4. Grill kebabs on medium-high heat
   until both sides are seared, then
   turn heat down to medium-low.
   Lamb is done when it reaches
   an internal temperature of 160°F
   (71°C). Cook potatoes until tender.
5. If your child cannot chew meat well
   yet, finely chop a portion of lamb
   and mix with potatoes.

Nutrient content of ½ large or 1 small kebab

195 calories, 17 grams protein, 1 grams fiber, Vitamin C 228%, Vitamin B_{12} 120%, Vitamin B_6 110%, Zinc 70%, Magnesium, riboflavin, and pantothenic acid 40% Iron 20%

Super Sauce

Yield: 5 cups (1.25 liters)

2 tablespoons (30 milliliters) oil
3 stalks celery, chopped
4 ounces mushrooms (120 grams), sliced
1 small onion, chopped
10 small cloves of garlic, pressed
½ cup (125 milliliters) chopped parsley
2 red peppers, roasted with skin, seeded, and chopped
2 teaspoons (10 milliliters) Italian seasoning
½ teaspoon (2.5 milliliters) dried basil
1 8-ounce (240-gram) can tomato sauce
1 28-ounce (850-grams) can diced tomatoes in juice
½ teaspoon (2.5 milliliters) pepper

1. Heat oil in large saucepan. Add celery, onion, garlic, parsley, mushrooms, and red peppers. Cook until onions are translucent, about 5 minutes.
2. Add rest of ingredients and simmer for 30 minutes.
3. Pour into blender and purée.
4. Serve over ravioli or tortellini.

Nutrient content of ½ cup (125 milliliters)

70 calories, 2 grams protein, 2 grams fiber, Vitamin C 340%, Vitamin B$_6$ 30%, Magnesium 30%, Vitamin E 20%, Vitamin A 10%, Iron and zinc 10%

Nutrient content of ½ cup (125 milliliters) sauce and ¼ cup (60 milliliters) cheese ravioli

177 calories, 7 grams protein, 2 grams fiber, Vitamin C 340%, Iron 30%, Zinc and vitamin E 250%, Calcium 20%, Vitamin A 10%

Strawberry-Orange Pops

Yield: about 1.5 cups (375 milliliters) or 6 ¼-cup (60-milliliter) pops

1 cup (250 milliliters—about 8) whole strawberries
½ cup (125 milliliters) plain or vanilla yogurt
¼ cup (60 milliliters) mandarin oranges

1. Blend all ingredients and pour into molds, or drink some and freeze the rest.

Nutrient content of one pop

21 calories, Vitamin C 80%

Pear Pops

Yield: about 2 cups (500 milliliters) or 8 ¼-cup (60-milliliter) pops

1 cup (250 milliliters) sliced pears (about 2 fresh or canned pears)
1 cup plain yogurt

1. Blend all ingredients and pour into molds, or drink some and freeze the rest.

Nutrient content of one pop

39 calories, 1 gram protein, Calcium 10%

Watermelon Ice

Yield: about 1½ cups or 6 ¼-cup (60-milliliter) pops

2 cups (500 milliliters) cubed seeded watermelon (or cantaloupe, honey-dew, or other melon)
Juice of ¼ lime
1 teaspoon sugar

1. Blend all ingredients and pour into molds, or drink some and freeze the rest.

Nutrient content of ¼ cup (60 milliliters)

16 calories, Vitamin C 35%, Vitamin A 30%

Chapter 17

Two Years and Older

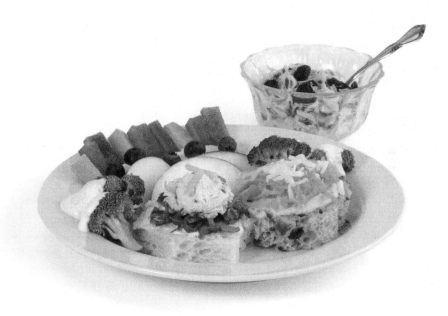

A three-year-old gave this reaction to her Christmas dinner:
"I don't like the turkey, but I like the bread he ate."
—Author unknown

You've made it to the terrific twos—congratulations! No one said it would be easy...but the rewards are well worth it.

Growth and Appearance

Your child's rate of growth will slow between the second and third birthdays, but you'll see a major change in how your child looks. Your child's legs and trunk will lengthen (adding substantial height), and your child will thin out. The fat that made your baby so cute and cuddly will start to disappear; by age five, your child will have half the body fat he or she had at the age of one. You'll notice your child's arms, legs, and face getting slimmer. As your child develops more muscle tone, he or she will look longer, leaner, and stronger all over.

Preschoolers grow about two and a half inches (6.2 centimeters) a year and put on about four pounds (almost two kilograms) a year. Some preschoolers grow slower or faster than others. Some kids slow down their growth in height and don't reach normal height for their age until adolescence, when the next big growth spurt occurs. If you plot your child's growth on a chart and you see a big drop in growth rate, discuss it with your child's doctor. If you think your child is accumulating excess weight or is preoccupied with food, discuss this with your child's doctor, too. Early eating habits can influence the risk of obesity throughout life. (See Chapter 18 for more information on preventing childhood obesity.)

The Preschooler's Diet

Eating Habits and Skills

Because your child's growth is still slow, he or she will probably eat about the same amount of food as during the past year.

Your child's eating skills should be pretty fine-tuned by now. Your kid is probably handling a spoon like a pro and even holding a cup one-handed. At age three, he or she should also eat well with a fork.

Although your child can chew and swallow well, bear in mind that he or she is still learning. Grinding skills for tough meats will come later. Be aware that toddlers are sometimes in a hurry to eat so they can go play, so you'll need to be vigilant to prevent choking. You'll also need to remind your child to slow down and chew, and not talk with food in his or her mouth.

Cutting the Fat

From birth, your child has needed about half his or her calories from fat. Now that your child's brain growth and other growth have slowed down, it's time to reduce the fat in his or her diet. How do you do that?

- **Choose low-fat milk.** One thing that will reduce your child's dietary fat significantly is to buy low-fat or even skim dairy products. You should now make the switch from whole cow's milk to 2-percent milk or from full-fat to low-fat soymilk. This change will reduce your child's fat intake by three grams for every cup of milk. If you switch your child to 1-percent or skim milk, keep in mind that your child will need more fat from vegetable sources (like avocado, canola oil, and olive oil).

- **Choose low-fat dairy products.** If you have been feeding your toddler whole-milk yogurt, you can now switch to low-fat. You can also choose low-fat cheese.

> ### Food Conversation with a Two-Year-Old
>
> Kid: "I don't like it!"
>
> Mom: "Have you tried it?"
>
> Kid: "No."
>
> Mom: "How do you know you don't like it?"
>
> Kid: "I just don't!"

A Day in the Diet of a Two-Year-Old

An Ideal Day

Breakfast

Baked Oatmeal (page 249)
½ cup (125 milliliters) milk
1 teaspoon (15 milliliters) margarine
½ sliced orange

Mid-morning snack

½ ounce to 1 ounce (15 to 30 grams) Monterey jack cheese
4 whole-grain crackers
½ cup (125 milliliters) 2-percent or 1-percent milk

Lunch

½ sandwich with ½ ounce (15 grams) chicken, 1 teaspoon mayonnaise, and 4 spinach leaves
Pear Pop (page 318)
Water

Mid-afternoon snack

Shrimpy Spread (page 280)
Whole-grain crackers
½ cup 2-percent or 1-percent milk

Dinner

1 cup (250 milliliters) Black Bean Soup (page 303) with tortilla chips and cheese
2 large strawberries, cut into pieces
½ cup (125 milliliters) 2-percent or 1-percent milk

Bedtime snack

Berry N'Ice (page 281)

A More Likely Day

Breakfast

2 tablespoons (30 milliliters) egg
1 bite banana
1 cup (250 milliliters) 2-percent or
    1-percent milk

Mid-morning snack

1 cup (250 milliliters) grapes,
    quartered

Lunch

1 ounce (30 grams) meat
¾ cup (180 milliliters) yogurt

Dinner

1 cup (250 milliliters) macaroni and cheese
2 lettuce leaves
½ cup (125 milliliters) juice

Snack

½ cup (125 milliliters) cereal
½ cup (125 milliliters) 2-percent or
    1-percent milk

Myah's Day

Rise and shine

7 ounces milk

Breakfast

1½ pieces of French toast with
    powdered sugar; ¼ apple, cut
    into slices
or ½ to ¾ cup (125 to 180 milli-
    liters) cold cereal with milk

Lunch

½ to ¾ cup (125 to 180 milliliters)
    macaroni and cheese
or 1 to 2 chicken strips
Apple juice

Dinner

½ to ¾ cup (125 to 180 milliliters) spaghetti
    with sauce
⅓ cup (80 milliliters) green beans

Snacks

Carrot slivers and sliced cucumbers
Cheese
½ banana

Aidan's Day

Breakfast

8 ounces (250 milliliters) orange juice
½ banana and 3 strawberries in 1 cup strawberry yogurt
or 1 waffle and ½ banana
or 1 piece of wheat toast with peanut butter and ½ banana

Lunch

12 ounces (375 milliliters) chocolate milk
1 egg, cheese, peas, chopped ham, cup of yogurt
or ½ grilled cheese with ham on wheat bread, cup of apple sauce

Dinner

2 ounces (60 grams) meat loaf with peas and sliced tomatoes.
Mixed berries and whipped cream
or spaghetti with green beans and cheese, cup of applesauce
or ½ chicken breast with mushroom soup, brown rice, green beans, yogurt

Snacks

All-fruit Popsicle
or Chopped-up peeled apples
or A few vanilla wafers

Can't-Miss Tips to Foster Good Eating

It's hard to believe that the eating habits your child is forming now will stick with him or her for life. Of course, it'll change to some extent as your child gets older and peer pressure rears its ugly head or as society norms change. But family and home environment in a child's early years are the greatest predictors of future eating habits.

At this point you may be throwing your hands in the air. What can you do to keep your child on the right track if your child isn't exactly a poster child for good eating? Just keep following these can't-miss tips:

- Continue serving a variety of foods. Even if your child doesn't partake, he or she sees you eating it.

- Always offer fruit for dessert. Most kids will go for it.

- As a family, stay away from fried foods and fast foods as much as possible.

- Eat as many whole foods as possible. Keep processed foods to a minimum.

- Limit caloric drinks to milk or soymilk, dairy drinks, and small amounts of juice.

Taking Care of Teeth

Here's some bad news: Little kids have cavities. One in every ten toddlers has a cavity, 25 percent of three-year-olds do, and 50 percent of five-year-olds do.

The good news is that there's a simple way to prevent your child from becoming a cavity kid: Brush your child's teeth twice a day and limit sweet drinks and candy. Also watch out for starchy foods between meals.

Your toddler *shouldn't* be eating sweets, but realistically he or she may be. They're really hard to avoid in our culture. Keep them as an occasional treat and make sure to brush your child's teeth right afterward. Or at least have your child drink water or rinse with it.

You should now use a small (pea-size) amount of fluoride toothpaste when you brush your child's teeth. Make brushing fun! A battery-operated toothbrush adds a thrill to the mundane task of brushing teeth, as does sparkly or yummy toothpaste. If your child doesn't like toothpaste, just keep trying. Keep in mind that the brushing and rinsing is more important than the toothpaste. Use a timer to help your child brush long enough and a reward system (such as stickers) to help motivate him or her to brush well.

A Word about Candy

I'd have to be really thick to believe that many kids aren't introduced to candy before the age of two. A kid's calendar seems to revolve around sweet stuff; think about all the treats that accompany Valentine's Day, Easter, Halloween, Christmas, and Chanukah. If there's a holiday, I guarantee there's a color-coordinated candy to go with it.

I know it's really hard to avoid candy—but you should put it off as long as possible. Not only is it an empty-calorie food, it can also rot teeth.

Is there any candy that's worse or better than the rest? For the crime of rotting teeth, chewy or slow-dissolving candy is the worst offender. What about general health effects? I recommend staying away from artificial colors as much as possible. Some kids are sensitive to synthetic colors, and some artificial food colorings have been linked to cancer.

Which leaves us with...chocolate. There's actually good news about this candy! Chocolate contains antioxidants that fight against heart disease and cancer. The darker the chocolate (that is, the more cocoa solids it contains), the more antioxidants it has. One study has shown that the antioxidant level of cocoa is higher than that of red wine or green tea.[1] But even if chocolate has some redeeming values (besides its taste), it's still not a nutrient-dense food—so limit your child's intake. I think a chocolate kiss is the perfect size for a sweet treat!

Getting Sneaky with Food

Sometimes we have to get sneaky. Yes, we'd all love to just dish out the broccoli and Brussels sprouts and have our children gobble them up! But few kids over two years old actually do that! So, it's up to us to find creative ways to get fruits and veggies into those tiny tummies. Following are some suggestions.

Veggies

- **Hide it!**
  - Purée a variety of cooked veggies into soups and sauces. Check out these recipes: Cheesy Sauce (page 270), Winter Squash Soup (page 281) Creamy Carrot-Cauliflower Soup (page 301), and Black Bean Soup (page 303).
  - Add finely chopped or puréed veggies to pasta sauce. See Smooth and Healthy Meat Sauce (page 315) and Super Sauce (page 318).
  - Add cooked carrots to mashed potatoes before mashing.
  - Add colorful chopped veggies to rice or other grain before cooking. See Whole-Grain Risotto with Sweet Potato (page 299) and Chicken Couscous (page 279).

- Use shell-shaped noodles for pasta dishes that include chopped vegetables; shells are veggie grabbers! Your kid will gobble up the veggies without even thinking, because they're stuck inside the shells. With other types of pasta, your child may eat the noodles and leave a pile of veggies behind—but with shells, the veggies magically disappear.

- **Dip it!** Let your little one dip veggies into ranch dressing, ketchup, salsa, melted cheese, guacamole, or bean dip. See Oven-Fried Zucchini Sticks (page 300) and Sweet Potato Fries (page 301).

- **Experiment!**
  - Try veggies that aren't typical kid foods. Amazingly, many kids like dipping the leaves from steamed artichokes into salad dressing or lemon butter.
  - Try new foods from other cultures. Hummus Spread (page 280) is one that many kids like.

- **Make it more fun!**
  - Skewer steamed veggies on a straw.
  - Serve veggies in a vegetable bowl. For example, serve pumpkin soup in a hollowed-out baby pumpkin. Tomatoes and red bell peppers also make beautiful bowls.
  - Serve veggie soup in a roll bowl. Hollow out a large whole-grain roll and fill it with creamy soup. Toast the bread you removed and serve it on the side.

- **Fry it!** No, not *that* kind of frying! Oven-fried veggies are healthier (and not so messy). See Oven-Fried Zucchini Sticks (page 300) and Sweet Potato Fries (page 301).

- **Leaf it!**
  - Kids often like salads, even if they don't like cooked veggies. Kids can also help make salads; they're good at tearing greens into pieces.
  - Spinach is packed with vitamins; put it on sandwiches!

- **Grate it!**
  - Shredded cabbage with a sweet dressing is tempting.
  - Carrot salad with raisins or cranberries and pineapple is also fun.

- **Wrap it!**
  - Sometimes different packaging is enticing. Stuff salad or grated veggies in tortillas with the usual sandwich fixings.
  - You can also use egg roll wrappers to make pot stickers. Chopped cabbage and broccoli mix easily with ground meat.

- **Drink it!**
  - Some kids like tomato juice and V8.
  - Your kid might like veggie-fruit juice. A brand called Vruit is available in most natural food stores.

- Make your own veggie-fruit combinations with a juicer. Carrot juice is sweet and can easily be added to fruit juice. Challenge your kid to think up different yummy combinations.

- **Slurp it!**
    - Some kids eat more veggies if they're floating in soup. Even if your child just slurps the broth, he or she is still getting some vitamins from the vegetables cooked in it.
    - Make a cold veggie soup like gazpacho. If your little one likes salsa, he or she will probably like gazpacho.

Fruits

- Put fruits in unexpected places.
    - Make fruit salsas to top meat, chicken, or fish. See Fruit Salsa (page 302).
    - Cook dried fruit in grain pilafs.
    - Put chopped apple, strawberries, mandarin oranges, or dried fruit in chicken salad or a green salad. See Chicken Salad with Mango (page 315).
- Offer exciting tropical fruits like mango and papaya.
- Prepare fruit in a different way.
    - Cook bananas with orange juice and brown sugar.
    - Freeze bananas or grape slices—they taste like sorbet!
    - Bake an apple with cinnamon in the microwave.
- Put fruit in pancakes, quick bread, and waffle batter.
- Use cooked or puréed fruit instead of syrup on pancakes and waffles, or use it to top low-fat ice cream or tapioca pudding.
- Make a smoothie or frozen fruit pop using fruit and yogurt or milk. See the following recipes:
    - Maui Smoothie (page 303)
    - Northwest Smoothie (page 314)
    - Strawberry-Orange Pops (page 318)
    - Pear Pops page 318)
    - Watermelon Ice page 318)
    - Berry n'Ice (page 281)
- Make homemade sorbet.
- Add fresh or dried fruits to hot cereals like oatmeal.
- Use canned and frozen fruit in the winter to add to the limited fresh fruit that's in season.

Packing a Lunch for Preschool

If your child is just starting preschool, packing a lunch for him or her will be an eye-opening experience. It may seem pretty simple, but it isn't always easy to provide daily healthy portable meals that your child will actually eat and not get bored with. I was shocked at the sack lunches I saw when I went on a field trip with my son Robert's preschool class. Let's just say those parents must have run out of good ideas.

Here are the basic tools you'll need for packing lunches:

- An insulated lunch bag or box
- An ice pack to keep cold foods cold
- A Thermos to keep hot foods hot
- Plastic utensils
- Napkins

You'll want to put as many of the food groups in your child's lunch as possible. Following are some ideas for main courses.

- **Sandwiches**: There are lots of things you can put between bread slices besides peanut butter and jelly or bologna! And make those bread slices whole-grain ones if possible.
    - Cheese and tomato (or just cheese)
    - Shrimpy Spread (page 280)
    - Peanut butter mixed with mashed banana
    - Chicken Salad with Mango (page 315)
    - Ham and cheese
    - Cream cheese with fruit purée or jam
- **Cute sandwiches**: For this age group, looks do matter!
    - Cookie-cutter sandwiches: Cut sandwiches in the shape of your child's favorite animal or holiday shape. Cheese or lunch meat sandwiches work best for this.
    - Different breads: Use one slice of whole-wheat bread and one slice of Iron Kids white bread for a striped sandwich.
    - Finger sandwiches: Cut off the crusts and cut sandwiches into tiny triangles—perfect for small fingers!
- **Wraps**: Roll up these tasty fillings inside a round tortilla or a square sandwich wrap.
    - Refried beans and cheese
    - Cream cheese with carrot
    - Chicken salad with shredded cabbage
    - Tuna salad with shredded spinach
    - Chef salad wrap with ham, cheese, hard-boiled egg, tomato, and lettuce
    - Hummus Spread (page 280) with grated carrot

- Chicken Salad with Mango (page 315)
- Cheese and avocado
- Cheese and rice or other grain
- Salmon with spinach

- **Cracker sandwiches**: My son Robert sometimes wanted to take homemade "lunchables" to preschool. We'd go so far as to get a small empty box, put in the customary foods, and tape it shut! The nice thing about making your own version of this popular processed food is that you get to include all your child's favorites, as well as foods you want your child to eat.
  - Cheese squares with wheat crackers
  - Peanut butter on graham crackers
  - Tuna or chicken salad with crackers on the side
  - Tuna and cream cheese with crackers on the side
  - Hummus Spread (page 280) with cucumber and carrot

- **Thermos foods**: When my kids were smaller, they hardly ever used the cute matching Thermoses that came with their lunch kits. However, I was recently begged to buy a Thermos so my fifth-grader could bring baked beans, ravioli, or soup to school. Using a Thermos expands the number of foods you can pack for your child's school lunch.
  - Leftovers: pasta with sauce, casserole, soup, stew, chili
  - Canned meals: soup, canned pastas
  - Cold foods: fruit salad, yogurt-fruit parfait, homemade pudding, chef salad

- **Convenience foods**: There are convenience foods that are healthy enough to consider sending with your child to school. (Make sure to send them with an ice pack to keep them cool.) Some are better than others; following are a few I recommend.
  - Lunchables: In the past I've been opposed to sending Lunchables to school on a regular basis. However, this brand now has a healthier line called Sensible Solutions that contains less fat and sodium. Some include 100 percent fruit juice. If you send Lunchables with your child, it's also a good idea to send a fresh fruit to round out the meal.
  - Gerber Lil' Entrees are kid-friendly meals that have much less sodium than adult entrées.
  - Ian's Natural Foods makes mini chicken sandwiches and mini cheeseburgers. They're hormone- and antibiotic-free.

Beyond the main course, you should also send:

- Fruit or veggie
- Something to drink if your child's school doesn't provide milk: You might send a small juice box *plus* a water bottle. (Buy 100 percent fruit juice, Vruit juice, or veggie juice.) Single-serving soymilk and rice milk drink boxes are a good

option, too. They're shelf-stable, just like juice boxes, so they don't have to be kept cold. Don't send soda.

- A healthy treat or occasional splurge: A healthy treat might be a yogurt or some animal crackers. Don't send dessert every day, and when you do, make it something small like one or two low-sugar cookies. Do not send candy!

> **Peanut Butter Reminder**
>
> Peanut butter can be a choking hazard, so always spread it thinly or mix it with fruit. If your child is at high risk for allergy, avoid peanut products until he or she is at least three years old.

Here are some fruits that pack well:

- Packaged cut fruits: These make it easy to send fresh fruit to school with your little one.
- Grapes, cut in half
- Apple slices (sprinkled with lemon or orange juice)
- Orange sections (in a zipper bag to prevent leaks)
- Kiwi fruit slices (or halves sent with a plastic spoon)
- Cantaloupe or seedless watermelon chunks
- Fresh blueberries
- Fresh strawberries
- Fresh nectarine
- Any fresh or canned fruit packed in a plastic container

And here are some veggies that pack well:

- Baby carrot sticks (steam them for two- and three-year-olds)
- Bell pepper strips
- Grape tomatoes, cut in half
- Grated carrot and raisin salad in a plastic container

Keeping Fit as a Family

Your toddler may not be ready to run a marathon, but he or she is ready to be involved in family fitness. Today's children are at high risk of overweight and all the health problems that go with it—high blood pressure, diabetes, heart disease, stroke, cancer, and more.

Family fitness is your best chance at lowering these risks for your child. Regular physical activity also helps build brain connections and forms habits that are hard to shake. If you make fitness a priority now, with luck it will stick with your child even when other activities start crowding the calendar.

Do some kind of exercise together every day, even if it's just tossing a ball, stretching, or touching toes together. Here are some fun physical activities everyone can enjoy:

- Take a walk with your child, alternately walking and riding in the stroller.
  - To hold your child's interest, find an interesting place to walk, such as near a river or along a beach.
  - Turn your walk into a treasure hunt. Ask your child to try to spot five different birds or to count the number of different animals you see. Or search for interesting rocks.
- Enroll your child in a swim class.
- Attach a bike trailer to your bike so the whole family can go bike riding. Choose a destination where your child can get out and run, jump, hike, or climb—such as a playground on the other side of town or a local nature preserve.
- While you walk on a walking path, let your child ride alongside you on a tricycle.
- Play catch. Kick a ball around. Play baseball—with a toddler-size bat and tee, of course. Rig up a small, low basketball hoop.
- Play croquet.
- Play bocce ball.
- Take your child to a neighborhood park. If you push your child in a stroller or carry your child in a back carrier, you'll get your exercise en route. Once you get there, your child will get lots of exercise climbing, swinging, and running around.

> ### Tales from the Trenches: Christine and Tony Cut a Rug
>
> Christine, who lives in Minnesota, sees plenty of snowy days. For active fun in the wintertime, she and her three-year-old, Tony, grab some drums, shakers, and tambourines, put on some music, and march around the rooms of the house. It's great exercise and teaches rhythm and melody, too!

- Yard work can be a great family activity. Give your child small jobs like pulling weeds, emptying the bucket of weeds, and watering the flowers. (However, don't expect your child to be a huge help.) If your yard isn't enormous, consider using a reel (manual) lawnmower instead of a gas-powered or electric one. It's a great workout, with no noxious fumes and no fuel costs. And because it's so much safer, your child can "mow" right alongside you with a toy lawnmower—he or she will put on a lot of miles darting back and forth across the yard.

- If you have a fenced yard, install a swing set and slide (visible from your kitchen) to encourage independent active play when your child is three years and older.
- For birthday and holiday gifts, choose active toys for your child: balls, hula hoops, pool toys, jump ropes, Frisbees—anything that adds fun to physical activity.
- A sandbox will keep your toddler entertained for hours on end with creative, active play.

Being cooped up with an energetic toddler is no fun. Here are some active activities especially for rainy, snowy, windy, or cold days:

- If you have a basement, make your own mini-gym. Pad the floor with puzzle mats. Stock some baskets with all kinds of soft balls. Put up an indoor basketball hoop. Hang a baby/toddler swing from the ceiling. Set up a small playhouse, play tent, or baby/toddler-size play structure. Park a few push toys or trikes in the corner.

- Take your child to Gymboree or another kid-friendly program or a local recreation center.

- Go to the mall—not to shop, but to walk.

- Go to the play area of your local fast-food restaurant. If you choose to eat there, make healthy choices.

Chapter 18

Preventing Childhood Obesity

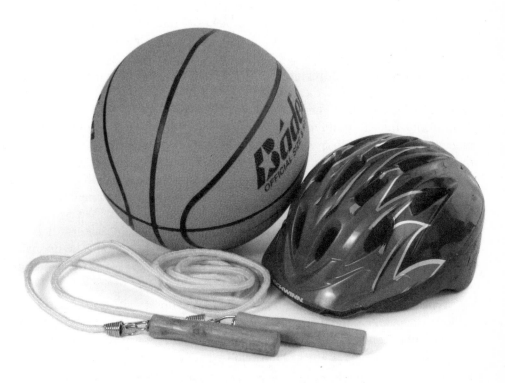

Life expectancy would grow by leaps and bounds
if green vegetables smelled as good as bacon.

–Doug Larson

Throughout this book, I've discussed the importance of good infant and toddler nutrition and how it can help your child form healthy eating habits that last a lifetime. In this final chapter, I'd like to discuss how instilling good eating habits in your child today can prevent childhood obesity later in life. I hope to enlighten and motivate you and your family so you can prevent your child from being another statistic in what's become a worldwide pandemic.

What Is Childhood Obesity?

Childhood obesity is the new buzzword in nutrition, and with good reason. (See sidebar for definition of terms.) In the last two decades, the obesity rate in the United States has nearly tripled from 5 percent to 14 percent for children two to five years old and from 5 percent to 17 percent in children twelve to nineteen years old. For children six to eleven years old, the obesity rate has quadrupled from 4 percent to 19 percent[1]. Approximately one in six U.S. children is now overweight; if the current trend continues, one in five children will be obese by 2010.

Beyond the United States, childhood obesity is a global problem. Approximately 22 million children under five are estimated to be overweight worldwide.[2] According to the World Health Organization (WHO), obesity rates have risen three times or greater since 1980 in some areas of North America, the United Kingdom, Eastern Europe, the Middle East, the Pacific Islands, Australia, and China. In the European Union, 24 percent of children are estimated to be overweight or obese.[3] Twenty-six percent of children in Canada are either overweight or obese, and the rates are similar in preschool children.[4, 5] The problem may be even greater in the Native Canadian community: one study showed 28 percent of boys and 34 percent of girls two to nineteen years old were overweight.[6] However, the obesity pandemic is not restricted to developed countries; obesity rates are also rising in developing countries.

So why are health professionals as well as politicians paying attention to childhood obesity? For one thing, we know obesity in childhood often persists throughout life—four out of five obese teenagers remain obese as adults.[7] We also know obesity can increase the risk of coronary heart disease, certain cancers, diabetes, hypertension, digestive disorders, joint problems, and depression. The financial and social cost of these diseases is tremendous. We already see the following problems in overweight and obese kids:

- Type 2 diabetes, which used to be called "adult-onset diabetes" because it previously appeared only in adults, is now being diagnosed in overweight children and adolescents at an alarming rate. The rate of type 2 diabetes in children and youth has doubled in the last ten years.[8]

- Many overweight children have high cholesterol and high blood pressure.

- Sleep apnea, which is interrupted breathing while sleeping, is one of the most severe problems overweight children face.

- Obese children have a high incidence of orthopedic problems, liver disease, and asthma.

Childhood Obesity and Overweight Defined

In this chapter, *overweight* and *obesity* will be used in general to describe excess body fat. The exact definitions of the terms change over time and from source to source. The term *childhood obesity* is most often used to describe the rising problem of childhood overweight.

At the center of understanding these terms is another term: *body mass index* (BMI). BMI is an indirect estimate of body fat using height and weight to determine a score. For adults over twenty years old, having a BMI between 25 and 29.9 is considered "overweight," and having a BMI over 30 is considered "obese." (Check out a BMI calculator at http://www.cdc.gov/nccdphp/dnpa/bmi/adult_BMI/english_bmi_calculator/bmi_calculator.htm.)

BMI for children two to nineteen years old is interpreted by comparing an individual score to a reference BMI for age and sex. This evaluation shows how your child's height and weight compares to other children of the same age and sex. According to the U.S. Centers for Disease Control (CDC), children in the eighty-fifth to ninety-fifth percentile range are considered "at risk of overweight." Children above the ninety-fifth percentile are considered "overweight." (To see a BMI-for-age growth chart for girls, visit http://www.cdc.gov/nchs/data/nhanes/growthcharts/set2/chart%2016.pdf. For a boys' chart, visit http://www.cdc.gov/nchs/data/nhanes/growthcharts/set2/chart%2015.pdf.)

Keep in mind that a BMI is just an *estimate* of body fatness. It's normal for children to have some body fat. Also, each child's body type is unique; BMI is often overestimated for children who are muscular. BMIs for children must be evaluated in light of current growth, puberty status, and so on. Some children gain weight before they grow taller—this can cause a temporary increase in BMI.

I consult at a public health clinic where I see high-risk clients. Sometimes I can tell at first glance when a child is way above the ninety-fifth percentile. Other children don't look overweight, but the BMI chart says they are. For those children, I look for visual signs of fatness, especially in the tummy area. One of my clients, Rosa, plotted above the ninety-fifth percentile, but the fat I could see around her waist was normal for a growing child. Her mother confirmed that Rosa was a very active little girl, ate a healthy diet, and watched little TV. Because her body was more muscular, her estimated body fatness was overestimated.

If you're concerned about your child's BMI, let your caregiver help you evaluate what it means.

- Children with early onset morbid obesity (achieving 150 percent of ideal body weight by age four) may have cognitive delay and lower IQ scores. This suggests obesity causes metabolic disturbances that can take a toll on young, developing brains.[9]
- The social discrimination obese kids face can be worse than the health-related problems, and it often leads to discouragement, low self-esteem, and depression.

What Causes Childhood Obesity?

That's the billion dollar question. The simple answer: childhood obesity is caused by an energy-balance problem. Obese children eat more calories than they need (too much energy in) and don't burn the calories through activity (not enough energy out). That simple answer gets complicated, however, once you consider the many factors that add to the risk of childhood obesity.

Genetics

Obesity does have a genetic component. Over 250 obesity-related genes have been discovered. Overall, there's a 25 to 50 percent chance children will be overweight if one parent is obese and a 75 percent chance if both parents are obese. However, genetic factors don't directly cause obesity in most cases—they only increase the chances of weight gain in children exposed to a "toxic" environment. (See next section.) So, children who have a genetic predisposition to obesity *plus* a sedentary lifestyle and a high calorie intake are more likely to become obese. In contrast, children who live in families that acknowledge their tendency to be overweight can keep the problem at bay with an active lifestyle and healthy eating habits.

"Toxic" Environment

As I mentioned above, environment is an even more significant cause of childhood obesity than genetics. Here are some factors that create a "toxic" eating environment for children and society in general:

- **Food everywhere.** Almost everywhere we go, there's always a vending machine or some other access to food.

- **Portion distortion.** Oversize portions have made us lose sight of what an appropriate serving size is for a healthy diet.

- **Energy-sparing conveniences.** Why walk when you can drive? Why get up to change the channel or turn on the fan when you can use the remote? Why take the stairs when you can ride the elevator? Why park far away and walk into the pharmacy when you can use the drive-thru? Because our lives are fast paced, we continuously look for ways to save time—and energy. Energy-sparing conveniences like elevators may add extra time to our days, but they also add extra pounds to our bodies.

- **Increased calorie intake.** We eat about two hundred more calories per day than we did twenty to thirty years ago. Doesn't sound like much, right? That's roughly the difference of a twenty-ounce soda per day. But two hundred extra calories a day can add up to *twenty pounds a year*!

- **Eating out more often.** We continue to eat out—a lot. In the United States, close to 30 percent of meals are eaten out, which accounts for up to 50 percent of families' food budgets. More restaurant meals translate into more calories, less fiber, and fewer nutrients—unless healthy choices are made.

- **Drinking more sweetened beverages.** Some studies show that consumption of sweetened beverages, such as soda and sugary juices, is associated with obesity in children.[10] Kids are now drinking less milk and more sweetened beverages, leading to calcium deficits, cavities, and sugar overloads. The Feeding Infants and Toddlers Study (FITS) showed that beverages other than milk make up about 10 percent of a toddler's total calorie intake by the age of two.[11]

- **Eating more fat.** Much of the food the average child eats is high in fat: ice cream, cookies, chips, fried foods, fast foods. This presents a twofold problem: First, fat is more calorie dense than carbohydrates or protein. Second, our bodies are designed to store excess fat rather than burn it.

- **Eating a diet full of junk food.** In the FITS study, almost half of seven- to eight-month-olds had at least one serving of a dessert, sweetened beverage, or salty snack per day. At fifteen to eighteen months, French fries are the most commonly eaten vegetable. By nineteen to twenty-four months of age, 10 percent of toddlers consumed candy; 23 percent consumed sodas or other sweetened beverages; 27 percent consumed salty snacks such as chips, popcorn, or cheese puffs; and 27 percent consumed hot dogs, sausages, or cold cuts.[12]

Decreased Activity

For many reasons, we're less active than we used to be, and kids have followed this trend. One study showed an 83 percent decline in habitual activity and a 35 percent decline in daily activity levels in children over a ten-year period. ("Habitual activity" includes all activities of daily life, such as walking from the bus stop, walking up and down the stairs, or taking out the trash. "Daily activity level" also usually includes the specific amount and intensity of exercise per day, such a thirty-minute brisk walk.) The decreased activity coincided with obesity rates doubling for adolescents between nine and nineteen years old.[13] School-age kids may get less daily activity because many schools are reducing the amount of PE and recess time. Also, more kids are going to sedentary afterschool care or are spending hours doing homework instead of shooting baskets or riding bikes with neighborhood friends. Younger kids in daycare may have limited opportunity or space for physical activity, and daycare providers often find it easier to show movies.

More TV Time

Kids who watch the most TV have the highest incidence of obesity. Watching TV can lead to health problems in many ways:

- Its hypnotic effect makes children forget playing outside is more fun, and it makes it hard for parents to pry them away.

Other Screen Time

While much of the research for screen time has been devoted to TV, we can assume that any "screen time"—including time with video games, computers, and hand-held entertainment—has much the same effect. For example, time spent on the computer has been liked to increased BMI in teens, and time spent playing video games was related to obesity in a study of first, second, and third graders.[20]

- Some researchers find that kids are in such an inactive state while watching the tube, they actually burn fewer calories than if they were sitting and not watching TV.[14]

- The more TV kids watch, the more they're at risk of being overweight. One research study showed that the risk of overweight increases by 6 percent for *each hour* of TV kids watch daily.[15] This finding becomes even more significant when you couple it with the fact that almost half of kids age eight to sixteen watch three to four hours of TV a day.[16]

- TV time also influences kids' food preferences and eating habits:
  - Kids are more likely to eat while watching TV than while doing other activities such as reading.[17]
  - Food advertisements can shape kids' food preferences—high-sugar and high-fat foods are often advertised on children's shows. One study showed that a brief advertisement imbedded into a children's program caused preschoolers to choose that food more often than an unadvertised food. Studies with older children showed similar results.[18]
  - In households where TV is on during mealtime, children consume fewer fruits and vegetables and more red meat, pizza, snack foods, and soda.[19]

Family Eating Behavior

Once they begin eating solids, children transition to their families' diets—for better or worse. Since many adults have poor eating habits, it follows that their kids will, too. Today's family is super busy. Between parents' work schedules and kids' after-school sports and activities, there's hardly time for cooking, much less eating! Fast and convenient foods are often the norm. These foods are not only prepared fast but also eaten fast, and obese children are known to eat faster than those who aren't.

Parenting Style

The way you approach the rules of the table can influence your child's eating habits and your child's risk of obesity.

- **Authoritarian—rigid and controlling.** Parents with this style are inflexible and don't include children in decisions about food. This is an ineffective style. For example, being overly strict about certain foods or using them only as rewards can lead children to overeat the food.[21] Also, many parents believe children will eat more fruits and vegetables with authoritarian parenting. In fact, it may achieve the opposite effect because kids can be uncooperative when they don't have control over what they eat.

- **Permissive—indulgent and lenient.** Parents with this style try to avoid food conflicts and tend to give in to children's demands, letting them eat what they like—sometimes becoming the "doting parent" or short-order cook. This style doesn't teach self-control, so it can lead to less than ideal eating habits as well as a tendency for overweight in some kids. Children need limits and structure in all areas to feel secure.

- **Authoritative—flexible yet firm.** Parents with this responsive style set appropriate limits with flexibility when needed, which allows children some input in meal planning and food selection. This is the preferred style of parenting. Because kids are not forced to eat any particular foods, they are less likely to develop aversions to the healthy foods their parents offer.

What Can You Do about Childhood Obesity?

When you think about the complex problem of childhood obesity, it can be overwhelming. However, you can do simple things from the very beginning as a parent to help prevent it.

Birth to Six Months

- Breastfeed exclusively—it reduces your child's risk for being overweight. One review study found that the longer babies are breastfed, the less chance they have of becoming overweight.[27] (See chart below.) Several theories suggest why breastfeeding may decrease the risk of obesity compared to formula-feeding:[28]

  - Breast milk contains hormones and other substances that help program a child's health and reduce the risk of obesity. One example is leptin, an appetite-regulating hormone.

  - Breastfed babies have greater control over their calorie intake and thus learn to trust their appetite. Parents are more likely to encourage formula-fed babies to have a "few more sips" or finish the bottle, which overrides the baby's own hunger cues.

  - Breastfed babies gain weight more slowly than formula-fed babies. Formula-fed babies have higher calorie and protein intake. This may lead to higher insulin levels, which play a role in the depositing of fat.

How Pregnancy Affects Childhood Obesity

Did you know that even before a baby is born, several factors during pregnancy can increase a child's risk of obesity and other health problems down the road?

- Being overweight before pregnancy may affect a mother's insulin and blood glucose levels, which can increase her baby's birth weight. Studies have shown that increased birth weight is, in turn, related to increased BMI later in life.[22]
- Children born to obese mothers are twice as likely to become obese by the age of two.[23]
- Excess weight gain during pregnancy can increase the likelihood of gestational diabetes, which can affect a baby's insulin production and sensitivity. This can lead to overweight and type 2 diabetes as the child grows.[24]
- Inadequate weight gain during pregnancy can create metabolic programming in the baby that encourages overweight in middle age as well as high blood pressure and reduced insulin sensitivity.[25]
- Studies have shown that smoking during pregnancy can increase a child's risk of obesity later in life, even though it's also related to lower birth weight.[26]

Breastfeeding Reduces Risk for Being Overweight

Breastfeeding Duration	Baby's Reduced Risk for Being Overweight
1 month	4%
1–3 months	19%
4–6 months	24%
7+ months	33%

- If you breastfeed, eat a wide variety of fruits, vegetables, and foods common to your culture. Flavors pass through the breast milk and help shape your baby's food preferences when he or she begins eating solids.[29]
- Always respect your baby's appetite, even if it's different than usual.
- If you formula-feed, follow your baby's cues. Don't encourage your baby to finish the bottle once he or she shows signs of being full.
- Whether you breastfeed or formula-feed, don't set a feeding schedule for your baby—let your baby be the boss!
- Don't introduce solid foods too early. (See Chapter 8.) Starting solids too early can cause allergies and intolerances. If babies eat gluten-containing foods (such as items made from wheat, rye, barley, and most oats) before they're four months old, they have a higher risk of developing allergies as well as higher levels of autoantibodies, which could lead to increased risk of type 1 diabetes in susceptible children.[30]

Six to Twelve Months

- It may take many tries—up to fifteen—for a baby to accept a new food, so when introducing solids, don't give up too easily. By the same token, don't keep forcing a food if your baby doesn't seem to like it. Wait a week or two and give it another try.
- Honor your child's appetite. Don't restrict your baby's food, but also don't push it when he or she shows signs of being full.
- Learn your child's cues. When babies turn their heads, it usually means they don't want more to eat, but they may want to drink. Or they may be saying, "Slow down!"

A Word of Caution

Children under the age of two need fat and should be eating as recommended elsewhere in this book. There are sad stories of babies who are diagnosed with "failure to thrive" because their parents took the obesity-prevention message too literally and put them on strict diets. In the process, they endangered their babies' health. Later in life, children and teens should never be put on a weight reduction diet without consulting your caregiver or preferably a health professional who specializes in childhood obesity.

- Try to follow your child's own eating pace. Some babies get frustrated because the food doesn't come fast enough; others savor each spoonful. Some babies prefer tiny bites; others like spoonfuls.
- Let your baby play with food. For babies, this exploration is an important step to self-feeding and having control over what they eat.
- Limit juice to four to six ounces a day and dilute it; remember that babies don't really *need* juice. It should be a treat.
- Don't introduce junk food to your baby.
- Ask your child if he or she is hungry at mealtimes. This helps your child connect the feeling of hunger with eating.

Twelve to Eighteen Months

- Keep following your toddler's cues. At this age, children can now communicate—verbally or otherwise—whether they are hungry or full.

- Trust your child's appetite. It slows down a lot during this stage, and your child may seem more interested in playing with food than eating it. That's okay. Your child will eat what he or she needs, so don't interfere.

- Keep offering new foods. Research shows that giving a taste of a previously disliked veggie fourteen days in a row increases the chance of the child's liking it.[31]

- Never use food as a reward.

- Be a model for healthy eating.

- Put off exposing your toddler to junk food and candy.

- Involve your child in shopping, cooking, or just deciding what goes on his or her plate. Give simple choices like "Peas or carrots?"

- Eliminate or limit TV time. The American Academy of Pediatrics (AAP) discourages any TV watching for kids under two.

- Provide opportunities for your child to be active in a safe environment. Share in the joy of being active and playing. Get down on the floor and have fun!

Eighteen Months to Two Years

- Continue encouraging water as the beverage of choice to quench thirst.

- Make sure your eating habits are ones you want your child to adopt.

- Don't force or bribe your child to eat. Continue honoring your child's appetite, which will continue to vary.

- Make a habit of family activity—walking to the park, playing at the park, playing chase, splashing in the baby pool, and going to indoor play areas in the winter.

- Avoid fast food for as long as possible. When you do indulge, make healthy choices—and talk about them.

- Accept that picky eating behaviors are temporary.

- Remember that you as a parent are responsible for serving appealing, appropriate meals and snacks; your child is responsible for deciding how much, if any, he will eat.

Two to Three Years

- During the "no" age, expect your child to say no when you ask if he or she is hungry. Respect that.

- Be ready for food jags (when your child eats nothing but one food item for every meal) and other seemingly strange food habits. They are completely normal.

- Let your child be a big helper in shopping and food preparation.

- Limit sweetened drinks.

- Continue offering fruits, vegetables, and whole grains at every meal, even if your child doesn't partake. Kids quickly learn to prefer high-fat and calorie-dense foods, so they need the opportunity to learn to like healthy foods, too.

- Limit TV time to one to two hours per day, per the AAP recommendation.[32] If you do let your child watch TV, watch PBS or educational videos and mute commercials for food. Also keep the TV out of your child's bedroom. One study showed that having a TV in a preschooler's bedroom increased the amount of viewing to four and a half hours per week and also increased the risk of being overweight by 31 percent.[33]

- Delay buying a video game console for your child. If you must, buy a system that allows for "exergaming" or exercise-based games. Here are some items to look for:
    - A dance mat so you can play interactive games like Dance Dance Revolution or interactive Ping-Pong. Chose appropriate games for your child's individual development.
    - A virtual reality attachment like EyeToy that allows the player to physically get into the game.

- A console like the Nintendo Wii system specially designed to be interactive.

- Provide daily opportunities for active play. The American Heart Association recommends that all children over two participate in thirty minutes of moderate activity per day and thirty minutes of vigorous activity three to four days a week. If thirty minutes at a time is not possible, break it up into two or three short activity breaks.[34] And don't be a couch potato yourself!

Three to Five Years

- Make family mealtime a priority.

- Watch out for the beginning of peer influences. Research shows that children are more likely to eat a food if they see family members or other children eating it. This can be both a positive or negative influence.

- Keep in mind that kids are starting to be influenced less by internal appetite cues and more by external stimuli such as amount of food served, taste of food, and availability of food. One result of this is that you need to watch your child's portion sizes; kids will begin eating more if more is on their plate.

- Continue to make water the drink of choice for thirst. Sweetened drinks should be an occasional treat.

- Continue to encourage exercise through sports and other family activities:
    - Do active chores as a family—raking leaves, flattening the recycling, getting the newspaper, or taking the dog for a walk. Make it fun.
    - Plan family vacations around activities such as skiing, swimming, or snorkeling.
    - Make a habit of enjoying family activities such as bowling, croquet, or Ping-Pong.

Five Years and Beyond: The School Years

- Continue to carve time out of your busy schedule for meals together.
- Continue watching your own eating habits; your child will continue to copy you.
- Teach your child about how nutrition affects his or her body.
- Peer influence becomes more prominent in the lunchroom. Let your child help pack his or her own lunch and discuss food options in the school cafeteria.
- Join your school's PTA or your district's advisory board made up of parents and community members to develop a wellness policy for area schools to make a difference in students' health. Advocate for a healthy school environment by asking for these things:
  - No sweetened drinks or high-fat snacks in vending machines
  - Availability of fresh fruits and vegetables
  - Adequate time for eating
  - Daily physical education that encourages lifelong fitness
  - Health curriculum that includes nutrition education
- Continue to provide fun opportunities for family activity as well as individual activity for your child. Most children are not developmentally ready for organized team sports at this age, so this is a good time for your child to master individual sports like swimming. If your child is interested in team sports, look for a noncompetitive and purely fun program. To encourage a lifetime of physical activity, encourage "lifestyle activities" such as walking, swimming, hiking, shooting baskets, and riding bikes.

References

Chapter 1

1. Schack-Nielsen L and Michaelse KF. Breastfeeding and Future Health. *Current Opinions in Clinical Nutrition and Metabolic Care.* 2006 May; 9(3)289–96.
2. Wilson AC et al. Relation of infant diet to childhood health: seven year follow up of cohort of children in Dundee infant feeding study. BMJ. 1998; 316(7124)6.
3. Burdette HL et al. Maternal infant-feeding style and children's adiposity at 5 years. *Archives of Pediatric and Adolescent Medicine.* 2006 May; 160(5)513–520.
4. Spruijt-Metz D et al. Relation between mothers' child-feeding practices and children's adiposity. *American Journal of Clinical Nutrition.* 2002 March; 75(3)581–586
5. Huotari, C. Breastfeeding statistics. La Leche League International Center for Breastfeeding Information. 2003. Available at http://www.lalecheleague.org/cbi/bfstats03.html. Accessed 1-20-06.
6. Ibid.
7. The National Board of Health and Welfare Center for Epidemiology. Official Statistics of Sweden. Breastfeeding, children born 2000. Available at http://www.sos.se/FULLTEXT/42/2002-42-7/2002-42-7.pdf. Accessed 10-14-06.
8. American Academy of Pediatrics Section on Breastfeeding. Policy Statement: Breastfeeding and the use of human milk. *Pediatrics.* 2005; 115(2)496–506.
9. Lawlor DA et al. Infant feeding and components of the metabolic syndrome: findings from the European Youth Heart Study. *Archives of Disease in Childhood.* 2005;90(6):582–8.
10. Ibid.
11. American Academy of Pediatrics Section on Breastfeeding. Policy Statement: Breastfeeding and the use of human milk. *Pediatrics.* 2005; 115(2)496–506.
12. Breastfeeding may prevent rheumatoid arthritis. November 4, 2004. *The National Women's Health Information Network.* Available at http://www.4women.gov/news/english/522140.htm Accessed 4-18-05
13 Groer MW. Differences between exclusive breastfeeders, formula feeders and controls: a study of stress, mood and endocrine variables. *Biological Research for Nursing.* 2005; 7(2):106-117.
14. Weimer J. The Economic benefits of breastfeeding; a review and analysis. *Food Assistance and Nutrition Research Report.* (FANRR13) March 2001.
15. Furman L, Minich N and Hack M. Correlates of lactation in mothers of very low birth weight infants. *Pediatrics.* 2002; 109(4):e57.
16. American Academy of Pediatrics Section on Breastfeeding. Policy Statement: Breastfeeding and the use of human milk. *Pediatrics.* 2005; 115(2)496–506.
17. Ibid.

Chapter 2

1. Lawrence RA and Lawrence RM, editors. *Breastfeeding: A Guide for the Medical Profession.* St. Louis: Mosby Inc. 1999. p 121-123.
2. American Academy of Pediatrics Section on Breastfeeding; Breastfeeding and the use of human milk. *Pediatrics.* 2005; 115(2) 496-506.
3. Ibid.
4. Taylor JS et al. A systematic review of the literature associating breastfeeding with type 2 diabetes and gestational diabetes. Journal of the American college of nutrition. 2005; 24(5)320-326
5. Qureshi IA. Et al. Hyperlidaemia during normal pregnancy, parturition and lactation. Annals of the academy of medicine Singapore. 1999;28(2)217-221.
6. Cohen A et al. Number of children and risk of metabolic syndrome in women. Journal of women's health. 2006; 15(6)763-773.
7. United States Breastfeeding Committee. Economic benefits of breastfeeding. Found at http://www.usbreastfeeding.org/Issue-Papers/Economics.pdf. Accessed 10-14-06.
8. Ibid.
9. The National Coalition on Health Care. Health Insurance Cost. Available at http://www.nchc.org/facts/cost.shtml. Accessed 10-15-06
10. Michels DL. A quick look at breastfeeding's most revolutionary year yet. From *Leaven.* August-September 1998; 34(6):115-118. Available at http://www.lalecheleague.org/llleaderweb/LV/LVDec98Jan99p115.html. Accessed 11-22-05
11. International Lactation Consultant Association. Evidence Based Guidelines for Breastfeeding Management during the First Fourteen Days, 1999.
12. Arnold LDW. The cost effectiveness of using banked donor milk in the neonatal intensive care unit: preven-

tion of necrotizing enterocolitis. Journal of human lactation. 2002; 18(2)172.

13. Schanler RJ, Shulman RJ, and Lau C. Feeding Strategies for Premature Infants: Beneficial Outcomes of Feeding Fortified Human Milk Versus Preterm Formula. *Pediatrics*. 1999; 103(6):1150-1157.

14. Hale TW et al. Transfer of metformin into human milk. *Diabetologia*. 2002. 45;1509-1514.

15. Loma Linda University Sweet Success Program. Women with diabetes can breastfeed. Available at http://www.llu.edu/llumc/sweetsuccess/special/. Accessed 10-18-06.

16. American Diabetes Association. Position statement: Nutrition recommendations and interventions for diabetes-2006. Diabetes care 2006. 29 (9): 2140-2157.

17. Jones NA. The protective effects of breastfeeding for infants of depressed mothers. *Breastfeeding abstracts*. 2005: 24(3) 19-20.

18. Gjerdingern D. The effectiveness of various postpartum depression treatments and the impact of antidepressant drugs on nursing infants. *Journal of the American Board of Family Practice*. 2003:16;372-382.

19. Hale, T. Using antidepressants in breastfeeding mothers. Keynote address at La Leche League of Illinois. October 26,2002. Available at http://www.kellymom.com/health/meds/antidepressants-hale10-02.html#Zoloft. Accessed 10-19-06.

20. American Academy of Pediatrics. Committee on drugs. The transfer of drugs and other chemicals into human milk. Pediatrics. 2001;108(3) page 776-789.

21. Ibid.

22. Judd K et al. Safety of bilaminar silicone nursing pads; randomized prospective single-blinded comparison of silicone versus traditional nursing pads. Unpublished research. Available at http://www.ardo.ch/downloads/stillhilfen/LilyPadz_Studie-E.pdf. Accessed 10-19/06

23. Fewtrell M et al. Randomized study comparing the efficacy of a novel manual pump with a mini-electric breast pump in mothers of term infants. *Journal of Human Lactation*. 2001;17(2)126-131

24. Fewtrell MS et al. Randomized trail comparing the efficacy of a novel manual breast pump with a standard electric breast pump in mothers who delivered preterm infants. *Pediatrics* 2001;107:1291-1297.

25. The Baby Friendly Hospital Initiative, Available at: www.babyfriendlyusa.org, Accessed 9-20-06.

26. International Lactation Consultant Association. Evidence based guidelines for breastfeeding management during the first fourteen days. April 1999. Available at: http://www.ilca.org/pubs/ebg.pdf Accessed 9-04.

27. Rasmussen KM, Kjolhede CL Pre-pregnant, overweight and obesity diminish the prolactin response to suckling in the first week postpartum. *Pediatrics*. 2004; 113 (5) e465-471.

28. Lawrence RA and Lawrence RM, editors. *Breastfeeding: A Guide for the Medical Profession*. St. Louis: Mosby Inc. 1999. p 259.

29. Bonyata K. I have thrush. Can I give my baby expressed milk? Available at http://www.kellymom.com/bf/concerns/thrush/thrush-expressed-milk.html. Accessed 1-20-06.

30. Lawrence RA and Lawrence RM, editors. *Breastfeeding: A Guide for the Medical Profession*. St. Louis: Mosby Inc., 1999. pp 610-611

31. Vaginal yeast infection. *Medline Plus Medical Encyclopedia*. Available at http://www.nlm.nih.gov/medlineplus/ency/article/001511.htm. accessed 1-20-06.

32. Meek, JM, with Tippins S. ed, American Academy of Pediatrics. *New Mother's Guide to Breastfeeding*. 2002. New York, Bantam Books. P 117-120.

Chapter 3

1. Butte NF and Hopkinson JM. Body Composition Changes during Lactation Are Highly Variable among Women. *The Journal of Nutrition*. 1988; 128(2)381S-385S.

2. Taheri S. et al. Short sleep duration is associated with reduced leptin, elevated ghrelin, and increased body mass index. *Public Library of Science Medicine*. 2004;1(3):e62. Epub.

3. Gangwisch JE et al. Inadequate sleep as a risk factor for obesity: analyses of the NHANES I. *Sleep*. 2005; 28(10)1289-1296.

4. Avas NT et al. A prospective study of self-reported sleep duration and incident diabetes in women. *Diabetes Care*. 2003; 26(2) 380-384.

5. Gangwisch JE et al. Short sleep duration as a risk factor for hypertension: analyses of the first national health and nutrition examination survey. *Hypertension*. 2006; 47(5)833-839.

6. From: Breastfeeding, Guide for the Medical Profession by Ruth Lawrence M.D. and Robert Lawrency M.D.

7. Polatti F et al. Bone mineral changes during and after lactation. *Obstetrics and Gynecology*. 1999; 94(1) 52-56.

8. McCrory MA et al. Randomized trial of the short-term effects of dieting compared with dieting plus aerobic exercise on lactation performance.. *American Journal of Clinical Nutrition*. 1999; 69(5):959-967.

9. AP, Leaf A and Salem N. Workshop on the Essentiality of and Recommended Dietary Intakes for Omega-6 and Omega-3 Fatty Acids. National Institutes of Health. Bethesda, MD. *Journal of the American College of Nutrition*. 1999; 18(5):487-489

10. Laurberg P, Nohr SB, Pederson KM and Fuglsang E. Iodine nutrition in breast-fed infants is impaired with

maternal smoking. *The Journal of Clinical Endocrinology and Metabolism.* 2004;89(1) 181-187

11. CSPI's Guide to Food Additives. Available at http://www.cspinet.org/reports/chemcuisine.htm. Accessed 12-13-05.
12. Conti, A. Identification of the human beta-casein C-terminal fragments that specifically bind to purified antibodies to bovine beta-lactoglobulin. *Journal of Nutritional Biochemistry.* 2000 Jun;11(6):332-7.
13. Chandra RK. Five-year follow-up of high-risk infants with family history of allergy who were exclusively breast-fed or fed partial whey hydrolysate, soy, and conventional cow's milk formulas. Journal of Pediatric Gastroenterology and Nutrition 1997; 24:380-8.
14. Businco L, Marchetti F, Pellegrini G, Cantani A, Perlini R. Prevention of atopic disease in "at-risk newborns" by prolonged breast-feeding. Annals of Allergy 1983; 51:296-9.
15. Chandra RK, Puri S, Suraiya C, Cheema PS. Influence of maternal food antigen avoidance during pregnancy and lactation on incidence of atopic eczema in infants. Clinical Allergy 1986; 16:563-9.
16. American Academy of Allergy, Asthma and Immunology. Tips to remember: prevention of allergies asthma in children. 2006. Available at www.aaaai.org. Accessed 11-11-06
17. Prescott SL and Tang ML Australasian Society of Clinical Immunology and Allergy position statement: Summary of allergy prevention in children. Medical Journal of Australia 2005; 182(9)464-467
18. American Academy of Pediatrics Committee on Drugs. Policy Statement: The transfer of drugs and other chemicals into human milk. Pediatrics. 2001;108(3)776-778.
19. Meek, JY ed. with Tippins S. *American Academy of Pediatrics New Mother's Guide to Breastfeeding.* New York, Bantam Books, 2002. p 136
20. Mennella JA. Pepino MY, Teff KL, Acute Alcohol Consumption Disrupts the Hormonal Milieu of Lactating Women. *The Journal of Clinical Endocrinology & Metabolism.* 2004; 90(4):1979-1985

Chapter 4

1. National Academy of Sciences. *Infant Formula: Evaluating the Safety of New Ingredients.* Washington DC. National Academy Press; 2004.
2. Koo WW at al. Reduced bone mineralization in infants fed palm olein-containing formula: a randomized, double-blinded, prospective trial. *Pediatrics.* 2003;111(5 Pt 1):1017-23.
3. Nelson SE, Frantz JA, Ziegler EE: Absorption of fat and calcium by infants fed a milk based formula containing palm olein *Journal of the American College of Nutrition.* 1998;17:327-332.
4. Lawrence RA and Lawrence RM, editors. *Breastfeeding: A Guide for the Medical Profession.* St. Louis: Mosby Inc. 1999. p 121-123.
5. Smith W, Erenbert A and Nowak A. Imaging evaluation of the human nipple during breast-feeding. American Journal of Diseases of Children. 1988. 142 (1):76-78
6. Recommended nipples for bottle supplementation. Available at http://www.bfar.org/nipples.shtml. Accessed 11-29-05.
7. Shelov SP. American Academy of Pediatrics Your Baby's First Year. Second Edition. New York. Bantam Books. 2005. p 144.
8. Greer FR, Shannon M. and the Committee on Nutrition and the Committee on Environmental Health, American Academy of Pediatrics. *Pediatrics.* 2005;116(3):784-786.
9. US Department of Agriculture A Guide for Use in Child Nutrition Programs. Food and Nutrition Service. Available at http://www.fns.usda.gov/tn/Resources/ch4.pdf Accessed 2-5-05.
10. Environmental Protection Agency. Bottled Water Basics. September 2005. Available at http://www.epa.gov/safewater/faq/pdfs/fs_healthseries_bottlewater.pdf. Accessed 12-10-05.
11. World Health Organization Questions and Answers on *Enterobacter sakazakii* in powdered infant formula. Version 4. February 2004. Available at http://www.who.int/foodsafety/publications/micro/en/qa2.pdf. Accessed 11-16-06
12. Ibid.
13. Bowen AB and Braden CR. Invasive *Enterobacter sakazakii* disease in infants. *Emerging Infectious Diseases.* 2006 Aug. Available from http://www.cdc.gov/ncidod/EID/vol12no08/05-1509.htm. Accessed 11-16-06.
14. Pediatric Nutrition Practice Group of the American Dietetic Association. Guidelines for preparation of formula and breastmilk in health care facilities. As adapted from Infant feedings: guidelines for preparation of formula and breast milk in health care facilities. 2003. Available at http://www.eatright.org/cps/rde/xchg/ada/hs.xsl/nutrition_5441_ENU_HTML.htm. Accessed 11-16-06.
15. Baker RD. Commentary: Infant Formula Safety. *Pediatrics.* 2002 110(4) 833-835.
16. Shelov SP. Ed. *Your Baby's First Year.* Elk Grove, IL: American Academy of Pediatrics. 2005.

Chapter 5

1. Breastfeeding on a worldwide scale; how the United States lags behind its international counterparts. Available at: http://www.house.gov/maloney/issues/breastfeeding/worldwide.htm. Accessed 1-14-06.
2. Bonoan R. Breastfeeding Support at the Workplace; Best Practices to Promote Health and Productivity. March 2000 (2) Washington Business Group on Health. . Available at http://www.businessgrouphealth.org/

pdfs/wbgh_breastfeeding_brief.pdf Accessed 1-26-05

3. Susan Kobara CLE, Breastfeeding Update, San Diego Breastfeeding Coalition, May 2001. Available at: http://www.breastfeeding.org/newsletter/v1i2/page1.html Accessed 1-27-05.

4. Cohen R, Mrtek MB, Mrtek RG. Comparison of maternal absenteeism and infant illness rates among breast-feeding and formula-feeding women in two corporations. *American Journal of Health Promotion.* 1995;10(2):148-53.

5. Recommended nipples for bottle supplementation. Available at http://www.bfar.org/nipples.shtml. Accessed 11-29-05.

6. Hanna N et al. Effect of storage on breast milk antioxidant activity. *Archives of Disease in Children. Fetal and Neonatal Edition.* 2004;89(6):F518-20.

7. National Women's Health Information Center. Breastfeeding made easier at home and work. Updated June 2004. Available at http://www.4women.gov/breastfeeding/index.cfm?page=237. Accessed 11-22-05.

8. Duke CS. Common Concerns When Storing Human Milk. . La Leche League International. *New Beginnings*; 1998; 15 (4):109.

Chapter 6

1. Shelov SP, editor. *American Academy of Pediatrics Caring for Your Baby and Young Child.* New York NY: Bantam, 2004: p. 505-509.

2. Kleinman RE, ed, *Pediatric Nutrition Handbook*, 5th edition, Elk Grove Village, Illinois: American Academy of Pediatrics 2004: p. 471-479.

3. Turck D et al. *Journal of Pediatric Gastroenterology and Nutrition.* 2003; 37(1):22-6. Incidence and risk factors of oral antibiotic-associated diarrhea in an outpatient pediatric population.

4. National Center for Complimentary and Alternative Medicine. Project concept review: Probiotics and infectious diarrhea. Available at: http://nccam.nci.nih.gov/research/concepts/consider/probiotics.htm. Accessed 8-04.

5. Weizman Z. Asli G and Alsheikh A. Effects of a probiotics infant formula on infections in child care centers: comparison of two probiotics agents. *Pediatrics* 2005 115(1):5-9. Available at http://www.pediatrics.org/cgi/content/full/115/1/5. Accessed 11-22-05.

6. Saavedra JM, Abi-Hanna A, Moore N. Long term consumption of infant formulas containing live probiotics bacteria: tolerance and safety. *American Journal Clinical Nutrition.* 2004; 79(2):261-7. Available at http://www.ajcn.org/cgi/reprint/79/2/261. Accessed 11-22-05.

7. Burks AW et al. Randomized clinical trial of soy formula with and without added fiber in antibiotic induced diarrhea. *Journal of Pediatrics.* 2001; 139(4)578-582.

8. Shelov SP, editor. *American Academy of Pediatrics Caring for Your Baby and Young Child.* New York NY: Bantam, 2004:p. 505-509.

9. American Academy of Pediatrics. Guide to treating diarrhea and dehydration. 2000. Available at: http://www.medem.com/MedLB/article_detaillb.cfm?article_ID=ZZZAHYUYQ7C&sub_cat=107 Accessed June 15, 2004.

10. Lloyd B, Halter RJ, Kuchan, MJ et al. Formula tolerance in post breastfed and exclusively formula-fed infants. Pediatrics. January 1999;103(1):E7 Available at: http://www.ncbi.nlm.nih.gov/entrez/query.fcgi?cmd=Retrieve&db=pubmed&dopt=Abstract&list_uids=9917487 Accessed 6-20-04.

11. Children's Digestive Health and Nutrition Foundation. Parents' Take Home Guide to GERD. May 2004. Available at: http://www.cdhnf.org/openbinfile.php?app=pdf&subfold=pdf&name=GERDParents_Handout.pdf Accessed July 2004

12. Rudolph CD et al. Guidelines for evaluation and treatment of gastroesophageal reflux in infants and children: recommendations of the North American Society for Pediatric Gastroenterology and Nutrition. Journal of Pediatric Gastroenterology and Nutrition. 2001; 32(Suppl 2): S1-S31.

13. Ostrom KM etal. Decreased regurgitation with a soy formula containing added soy fiber. *Clinical Pediatrics.* 2006; 45(1)29-36.

14. Children's Digestive Health and Nutrition Foundation. Parents' Take Home Guide to GERD. May 2004. Available at: http://www.cdhnf.org/openbinfile.php?app=pdf&subfold=pdf&name=GERDParents_Handout.pdf Accessed July 2004

15. Kleinman, RE. editor. American Academy of Pediatrics. Pediatric Nutrition Handbook, 5th Edition. 2004. pp251-252

16. Ibid.

17. Zeiger RS. Food Allergen Avoidance in the Prevention of Food Allergy in Infants and Children. *Pediatrics.* 2003:111(6Pt3):1662–1671

18. Salam MT, Li,YF, Langholz B, Gilliland FD. Early-Life Environmental Risk Factors for Asthma: Findings from the Children's Health Study. *Environmental Health Perspectives.* 2004; (112(6):760-765.

19. Food Allergy and Anaphylaxis Network. Do you have a food allergy? Available at: http://foodallergy.org/downloads/DoyouhaveFA.pdf. Accessed 6-15-04

20. Food Allergy and Anaphylaxis Network. Do you have a food allergy? Available at: http://foodallergy.org/

downloads/DoyouhaveFA.pdf Accessed 6-15-04

21. Prescott SL and Tang MLK. The Australasian society of clinical immunology and allergy position statement: summary of allergy prevention in children. *Medical Journal of Australia*. 2005; 182(9):464-67 Available at http://www.mja.com.au/public/issues/182_09_020505/pre10874_fm.html#i1085929. Accessed 11-22-05.

22. Lawrence RA and Lawrence RM, editors. *Breastfeeding: A Guide for the Medical Profession*. St. Louis: Mosby Inc. 1999. p 620

23. Rautava S, Kalliomaki M, Isolauri E. Probiotics during pregnancy and breast-feeding might confer immunomodulatory protection against atopic disease in the infant. *Journal of Allergy and Clinical Immunology*. 2002;109(1):119-21.

24. Zeiger RS. Food Allergen Avoidance in the Prevention of Food Allergy in Infants and Children. *Pediatrics*. 2003;111(6Pt3):1662–1671

25. Brostoff J and Gamlin L. *Food Allergies and Food Intolerances; The Complete Guide to Their Identification and Treatment*. Rochester, Vermont: Healing Arts Press. 2000. p. 277.

26. American Academy of Allergy, Asthma and Immunology. Tips to remember: prevention of allergies asthma in children. 2006. Available at www.aaaai.org. Accessed 11-11-06

27. Prescott SL and Tang ML Australasian Society of Clinical Immunology and Allergy position statement: Summary of allergy prevention in children. Medical Journal of Australia 2005; 182(9)464-467

28. Palmer DJ and Makrides M. Diet of lactating women and allergic reactions in their infants. Current Opinion in Nutrition and Metabolic Care. 2006; 9(3)284-288.

29. Committee on Nutrition, American Academy of Pediatrics. *Hypoallergenic infant formulas. Pediatrics*. 2000; 106(2):346-349. Available at: http://aappolicy.aappublications.org/cgi/reprint/pediatrics; 106/2/346.pdf Accessed 6-20-04

30. Zeiger RS. Food Allergen Avoidance in the Prevention of Food Allergy in Infants and Children. *Pediatrics*; 2003;111(6Pt3):1662–1671

31. Gray L, Watt LM Blass EM. Skin-to-skin contact is analgesic in healthy newborns. *Pediatrics*. 2000;105(1): e14. Available at http://pediatrics.aappublications.org/cgi/content/full/105/1/e14. Accessed 11-22-05.

32. Hill DJ et al. Effect of a low-allergen diet on colic among breastfed infants: a randomized, controlled trial. *Pediatrics*. 2005; 116(5):e809-e715.

33. Savino F et al. Bacterial counts of intestinal Lactobacillus species in infants with colic. *Pediatric Allergy and Immunology*. 2005; 16(1):72-75. Available at http://www.ncbi.nlm.nih.gov/entrez/query.fcgi?cmd=Retrieve&db=pubmed&dopt=Abstract&list_uids=15693915&query_hl=37. Accessed 11-29-05.

34. Duro D, Rising R, Cedillo M, Lifshitz F. Association Between Infantile Colic and Carbohydrate Malabsorption From Fruit Juices in Infancy. *Pediatrics*. 2002;109(5): 797-805

35. Committee on Nutrition American Academy of Pediatrics. The Use and Misuse of Fruit Juice in Pediatrics. *Pediatrics*. 2001;107(5) 1210-1213. Available at: http://aappolicy.aappublications.org/cgi/reprint/pediatrics;107/5/1210.pdf Accessed 6-17-04.

36. Committee on Child Abuse and Neglect. American Academy of Pediatrics. Shaken Baby Syndrome: Rotational Cranial Injuries. Technical Report *Pediatrics*. 2001;108(1):206-210

Chapter 7

1. WHO Working Group on Infant Growth, Nutrition Unit, World Health Organization. An evaluation of infant growth. 1994. Available at http://www.breastfeedingbasics.org/cgi-bin/deliver.cgi/content/Growth/gro05_research_who_workgroup.html. Accessed 11-24-06.

2. Shelov SP and Hannemann RE, ed. The American Academy of Pediatrics. *Caring for Your Baby and Young Child. Birth to Age Five*. 4th edition; Bantam. New York; 2004. p. 144

3. Ibid. 178

4. Kelly Bonyata BS, IBCLC. *Growth Spurts*. Available at: www. kellymom.com. Accessed 2-26-05.

5. U.S. Department of Agriculture. Dietary Guidelines for Americans 2005. Available at http://www.healthierus.gov/dietaryguidelines/. Accessed 11-24-06

6. Gartner LM, Greer FR, Section on Breastfeeding and Committee on Nutrition. Prevention of rickets and vitamin D deficiency. *Pediatrics*. 2003 111(4) 908-910.

7. Food and Nutrition Board, Institute of Medicine, National Academies. *Dietary Reference Intakes (DRIs): Recommended Intakes for Individuals*, Tolerable Upper Intake Levels, Vitamins. Washington DC: National Academies Press; 2004.

8. Kleinman R, ed. Pediatric Nutrition Handbook. Fifth edition. Elk Grove, IL: American Academy of Pediatrics; 2004. p. 793.

9. Dewey KG et al. Iron Supplementation Affects Growth and Morbidity of Breast-Fed Infants: Results of a Randomized Trial in Sweden and Honduras. *Journal of Nutrition*. 2002; 132: 3249-3255.
10. Bakerink, J.A et al. Multiple organ failure after ingestion of pennyroyal oil from herbal tea in two infants. *Pediatrics*. 1996; 98 (5):944-947.
11. Woolf AD. Herbal Remedies and Children: Do They Work? Are They Harmful? *Pediatrics*. 2003; 112 (1):240-246.
12. Fox et al. Feeding Infants and Toddlers Study: What foods are infants and toddlers eating? Journal of the American Dietetic Association. 2004; 104: S22-S30.
13. Briefel R et al. Feeding infants and toddlers study; do vitamin and mineral supplements contribute to nutrient adequacy or excess among US infants and toddlers. Journal of the American Dietetic Association 2006:106(1S) S52-S65.
14. Mangels R. *Feeding Vegan Kids*. The Vegetarian Resource Group. Updated April 2004. Available at: www.vrg.org/nutshell/kids.htm. Accessed 3-6-05.
15. Simopoulos AP, Leaf A and Salem N. Workshop on the Essentiality of and Recommended Dietary Intakes for Omega-6 and Omega-3 Fatty Acids. National Institutes of Health. Bethesda, MD. *Journal of the American College of Nutrition*. 1999; 18(5):487-489 :, 1999.
16. Davis BC and Kris-Etherton PM. Achieving optimal essential fatty acid status in vegetarians: current knowledge and practical implications. *American Journal of Clinical Nutrition*. 2002; 78(3):640S-646S.
17. Ibid.
18. Food and Agricultural Organization of the United Nations. Carbohydrates in Human Nutrition. Report of a Joint FAO/WHO Consultation. 1997. Available at http://www.fao.org/docrep/W8079E/w8079e00.HTM. Accessed 11-26-06.
19. Swan IL Teething complications: a persisting misconception. *Postgraduate Medical Journal*. 1979; 55:24.
20. Coreil J et al. Recognition and management of teething diarrhea among Florida pediatricians. *Clinical Pediatrics* (Phila).1995;34(11):591-8.
21. Macknin ML et al. Symptoms Associated With Infant Teething: A Prospective Study *Pediatrics*. 2000;105(4):747-752.
22. Academy of General Dentistry. Medications and cough syrup may cause cavities. Available at http://www.agd.org/media/2005/Dec/cavities.asp. Accessed 1-17-06.
23. Kashket S, Zhang J and Van Houte J. Accumulation of fermentable sugars and metabolic acids in food particles that become entrapped on dentition. *Journal of Dental Research*. 1996. 75(11):1885-1891.
24. Von Fraunhofer A and Rogers MM. Effects of sports drinks and other beverages on dental enamel *General Dentistry*. 2005; 53 (1):28-31.
25. Li Y. and Caufield PW. The fidelity of initial acquisition of mutans streptococci by infants from their mothers. *Journal of Dental Research*. 1995; 74:681-685.
26. American Academy of General Dentistry. See a baby tooth? See a dentist. Available at: http://www.agd.org/consumer/topics/baby/tooth.asp. Accessed 3-6-05.

Chapter 8

1. Meek JY. *American Academy of Pediatrics New Mother's Guide to Breastfeeding*. New York, NY. Bantam Books; 2002: p. 180
2. Shelov SP and Hannemann RE, ed. The American Academy of Pediatrics. *Caring for Your Baby and Young Child. Birth to Age Five*. 4th edition; Bantam. New York; 2004:p. 21
3. Kleinman R, ed. *Pediatric Nutrition Handbook*. Fifth edition. Elk Grove, IL: American Academy of Pediatrics; 2004: p. 110.
4. Krebs NF et al. Meat as a first complementary food for breastfed infants: feasibility and impact on zinc intake and status. *Journal of Pediatric Gastroenterology and Nutrition*. 2006; 42(2)207-214.
5. Regan FM et al. The impact of early nutrition in premature infants on later childhood insulin sensitivity and growth. *Pediatrics*. 2006; 118(5)1943-1949.

Chapter 9

1. Food and Nutrition Service, USDA. Home prepared baby food. A guide for use in the child nutrition programs. http://www.fns.usda.gov/tn/Resources/ch12.pdf. Accessed 4-21-05

Chapter 10

1. National Institute of Allergy & Infectious Disease, National Institutes of Health. Health Matters: Foodborne Diseases. April 2002, Updated November 2003. Available at http://www.niaid.nih.gov/factsheets/foodbornedis.htm Accessed 8-04.
2. Canadian Food Inspection Agency. Causes of food borne illness. 8-2-06. Available at http://www.inspection.gc.ca/english/fssa/concen/causee.shtml. Accessed 11-29-06

3. Food Standards Australia New Zealand. Incidence of foodborne illness. Available at www.foodstandards.gov.au. Accessed 11-29-06
4. Modified from U.S. Department of Health and Human Services, U.S. Food and Drug Administration. (October 1995, revised July 2002.) Can Your Kitchen Pass the Food Safety Test? [Electronic version] FDA Consumer.
5. Clemson University Cooperative Extension Service. Safe Handling of Fish. HGIC 3508. 1999. Available at http://hgic.clemson.edu/factsheets/HGIC3508.htm. Accessed 11-28-06.
6. Center for Disease Control and Prevention. Salmonellosis. October 31, 2006. Available at http://www.cdc.gov/ncidod/dbmd/diseaseinfo/salmonellosis_g.htm. Accessed 11-29-06.
7. Ibid.
8. Partnership for Food Safety Education. Modified from Fight Bac® Six steps to safer fruits and vegetables, 2004. Retrieved March 8, 2005 from http://portal.fightbac.org/pfse/toolsyoucanuse/phec/Produce%20factSheet.pdf
9. U.S. Environmental Protection Agency. Mid Atlantic Lead Paint. Frequently asked questions about lead. Updated June 2004. Available at http://www.epa.gov/reg3wcmd/lp-faqhealth.htm. Accessed November 19,2005.
10. Center for Disease Control. Second National Report on Human Exposure to Environmental Chemicals: Metals. March 2003. Available at: http://www.cdc.gov/exposurereport/2nd/pdf/lead.pdf Accessed 9-04
11. USDA and USDHHS. What you need to know about mercury in fish and shellfish. 2004 EPA and FDA advice for women who might become pregnant, women who are pregnant, nursing mothers, and young children. March 2004. Available at http://www.cfsan.fda.gov/~dms/admehg3.html. Accessed 11-24-05
12. Modified from: Santerre, CR. Fish for your health™. Advice for pregnant or nursing women, women that will become pregnant and children under 6 years of age. version 2.1. 2006. Available at http://fn.cfs.purdue.edu/anglingindiana/FishAdvisory04.PDF. Accessed 11-29-06
13. Ibid.
14. Ibid.
15. Environmental Working Group. Shopper's Guide to Pesticides in Produce. October 2006. Available at http://www.foodnews.org/pdf/EWG_pesticide.pdf Accessed 11-28-06
16. Groth III. E, Benbrook CM, Lutz K. Update: Pesticides in Children's Food; An analysis of 1998 USDA PDP data on pesticide residues. Consumers Union of U.S., Inc. May 2000 Available at http://www.ecologic-ipm.com/PDP/UpdateChildrensFoods.pdf accessed 1-20-05
17. Meadows M. Plastics and the microwave. U.S. FDA. FDA Consumer November-December 2002.
18. American Academy of Pediatrics Medical Library. Choking Prevention. 2001. Available at: http://www.medem.com/search/article_display.cfm?path=n:&mstr=/ZZZSEN9YA7C.html&soc=AAP&srch_typ=NAV_SERCH Accessed 1-20-05

Chapter 11

1. Allen LH. Multiple micronutrients in pregnancy and lactation: an overview. *American Journal of Clinical Nutrition*. 2005; 81(5)1206S-1212S.
2. Norris JM et al. Risk of celiac disease autoimmunity and timing of gluten introduction in the diet of infants at increased risk of disease. *Journal of the American Medical Association*. 2005; 293(2):343-51.
3. Norris JM et al. Timing of initial cereal exposure in infancy and risk of islet autoimmunity. *Journal of the American Medical Association*. 2003; 290(13):1713-1720.
4. Poole JA. Et al. Timing of initial exposure to cereal grains and the risk of wheat allergy. *Pediatrics*. 2006; 117(6)2175-2182.
5. Ivarsson A, Hernell O, Stenlund H and Persson LA. Breast-feeding protects against celiac disease. *American Journal of Clinical Nutrition*. 2002; 75(5)914-921,
6. Dietz W.H. & Stern L (Eds). *American Academy of Pediatrics Guide to your Child's Nutrition*. New York: Villard; 1999
7. Ibid.

Chapter 12

1. Greer FR, Shannon M. and the Committee on Nutrition and the Committee on Environmental Health, American Academy of Pediatrics. *Pediatrics*. 2005; 116(3):784-786. Accessed 1-19-06.
2. University of Wisconsin Cooperative Extension. Food facts for you: June 2004 Newsletter. Available at http://www.wisc.edu/foodsafety/assets/foodfacts_2004/wffjune2004.htm. Accessed 12-3-06
3. Food and Agriculture Organization of the United Nations. Food safety and quality as affected by organic farming. July 2000. Available at http://www.fao.org/docrep/meeting/X4983e.htm#b2. Accessed 1-18-06.
4. Greer FR and Shannon M. and the American Academy of Pediatrics Committee on Nutrition and the Committee on Environmental Health. *Pediatrics*. 2005; 116(3)784-786.
5. University of Wisconsin Cooperative Extension. Food facts for you: June 2004 Newsletter. Available at

http://www.wisc.edu/foodsafety/assets/foodfacts_2004/wffjune2004.htm. Accessed 12-3-06

6. American Egg Board. *Basic Egg Facts*. Available at: http://www.aeb.org/facts/facts.htmilliliters#21. Accessed 4-2-05.

7. American Frozen Food Institute. *FDA Rules Frozen Fruits and Vegetables Have Equivalent, If Not Better, Nutrient Profile than Fresh Product*. 1999. Available at www.healthyfood.org/sub/news_03.25.98.htmilliliters. Accessed 3-10-05.

Chapter 13

1. Butte, N., Cobb K., Dwyer, J., Graney, L., Heird W., & Rickard, K. The start healthy feeding guidelines for infants and toddlers. *Journal of the American Dietetic Association*. 2004; 104(3):442-454.

2. University of Minnesota. *The Whole Grain*. 1-26-05. Available at: http://www.wholegrain.umn.edu/health/index.cfm. Accessed 3-15-05

Chapter 14

1. US Department of Agriculture. US Department of Health and Human Services. Finding your way to a healthier you: based on the dietary guidelines for Americans. Available at http://www.health.gov/dietaryguidelines/dga2005/document/html/brochure.htm#b1. Accesed 6-15-05.

Chapter 15

1. Benton D. Role of parents in the determination of the food preferences of children and the development of obesity. *International Journal of Obesity and Related Metabolic Disorders*. 2004. 28(7):858-869.

2. Ibid.

3. Parents Action for Children. *Marketing Bad Habits to Children*. Available at: http://www.iamyourchild.org/learn/features/marketingeating/ Accessed 3-20-05.

4. Nemours Foundation. Kids Health for Parents *How TV Affects Your Child*. 2-05. Available at: http://kidshealth.org/parent/positive/family/tv_affects_child.html. Accessed 3-30-05.

5. National Academy of Sciences. Board on Children, Youth and Families, Food and Nutrition Board, Food Marketing to Children: Threat or Opportunity. 2006. National Academies Press. Washington DC. P. ES 1-ES7. Available at http://www.nap.edu/books/0309097134/html/4.html. Accessed 12-3-06.

6. Ibid. Accessed 1-21-06

7. American Academy of General Dentistry. *Soft Drink Logos On Baby Bottles Encourage Soda Drinking*. Available at www. www.agd.org/consumer Accessed 3-10-05.

8. Committee on Public Education. American Academy of Pediatrics Policy Statement. Children, Adolescents and Television. *Pediatrics*. 2001; 107(2):423-426.

9. The New Family Dinner: Different Ways to Come Together, *Parents Magazine*, May 1999. Available at http://www.parents.com/articles/family_time/4001.jsp?page=2 Accessed 3-30-05.

10. Building Blocks for School Success: Four HGSE Alumni Making a Difference in Early Childhood Education. *HGSE News; The News Source of the Harvard Graduate School of Education*. April 1, 2005. Available at: http://www.gse.harvard.edu/news/features/blocks04012005.html. Accessed April , 2005.

11. On Monday, Invite the Whole Family to Dinner. *Salt Lake Tribune*. Sept. 19, 2001.

12. Neumark-Sztainer D, Wall M, Story M, Fulkerson JA. *Are family meal patterns associated with disordered eating behaviors among adolescents? Journal of Adolescent Health*. 2004; 35(5):350-9.

13. Eisenberg, M.E., et al., Correlations between family meals and psychosocial well-being among adolescents. *Archives of Pediatrics and Adolescent Medicine*. 2004; 158(8):792-796.

Chapter 17

1. Lee KW, Kim YJ, Lee HJ, Lee CY. Cocoa has more phenolic phytochemicals and a higher antioxidant capacity than teas and red wine. Journal of Agricultural and Food Chemistry. 2003; 51(25):7292-5.

Chapter 18

1. Institute of Medicine. National Academy of Sciences. Progress in Preventing Childhood Obesity: How do we measure up. September 2006.

2. World Health Organization. Obesity and Overweight. 2005 http://www.who.int/dietphysicalactivity/publications/facts/obesity/en/. Accessed April 13, 2005.

3. International Obesity Task Force. EU childhood obesity out of control. Childhood Obesity Report. May 2004.

4. Statistics Canada. Health reports: regional difference in obesity. The Daily. August 22, 2006. Available at http://www.statcan.ca/Daily/English/060822/d060822b.htm. Accessed 11-21-06

5. Canning PM, Courage ML and Frizzell LM. Canadian Medical Association Journal. 2004(171)3:240-242.

6. Hanley AJ et al. Overweight among children and adolescents in a Native Canadian community: prevalence

and associated factors. American Journal of Clinical Nutrition. 2000;71(3)893-700.

7. Whitaker RC, Wright JA, Pepe MS, Seidel KD, Dietz WH. Predicting obesity in young adulthood from childhood and parental obesity. N Engl J Med 1997; 337: 869–873.

8. National Academy of Sciences. Board on Children, Youth and Families, Food and Nutrition Board, Food Marketing to Children: Threat or Opportunity. 2006. National Academies Press. Washington DC. P. ES 1-ES7. Available at http://www.nap.edu/books/0309097134/html/4.html. Accessed 1-21-06.

9. Miller J. et al. Neurocognitive findings in Prader-Willi syndrome and early onset morbid obesity. Journal of Pediatrics. 2006;149(2)192-198.

10. Ebbeling CB, Pawlak DB, Ludwig DS. Childhood obesity: public-health crisis, common sense cure. The Lancet. 2002;360(9331):473-482.+

11. Fox, MK, Pac S, Devaney B, Jankowski MS. Feeding infants and toddlers study: What foods are infants and toddlers eating? Journal of the American Dietetic Association. 2004; (104 (Suppl 1):s22-30. Lederman SA et al. Summary of the Presentations at the Conference on Preventing Childhood Obesity, December 8, 2003. Pediatrics. 2004; 114(4):1146-1173.

12. Ibid.

13. Kimm SYS, Barton BA, Obarzanek E, et al. Obesity development during adolescence in a biracial cohort: the NHLBI Growth and Health Study. Pediatrics. 2002;110(5):E54-E58.

14. Robinson TN. Television viewing and childhood obesity. Pediatric Clinics of North America. 2001; 48(4):1017-1025.

15. Dennison BA, Erb TA and Jenkins PL. Television viewing and television in bedroom associated with overweight risk among low-income preschool children. Pediatrics. 2002; 109(6):1028-1035.

16. Torgan, C. Childhood obesity on the rise. Word on Health; Consumer health information based on research from the National Institutes of Health. July 2002. Available at http://www.nih.gov/news/WordonHealth/jun2002/childhoodobesity.htm. Accessed 4-14-05

17. Mateson DM et al. Children's Food Consumption during television viewing. American Journal of Clinical Nutrition. 2004;79(6)1088-1094.

18. Goldberg ME, Gorn GJ, Gibson W. TV messages for snack and breakfast foods: do they influence children's preferences? Journal of Consumer Research. 1978; 5:73-81.

19. Coon K, Goldberg J, Rogers B, Tucker K. Relationships between use of television during meals and children's food consumption patterns. Pediatrics [serial online] 2001;107:e7. Available at http://pediatrics.aappublications.org/cgi/content/abstract/107/1/e7. Accessed 11-21-06

20. Stettler N., Signer TM, Suter PM. Electronic games and environmental factors associated with childhood obesity in Switzerland. Obesity Research. 2004;12: 896-903

21. Skelton JA. Child Obesity Overview. Pediatric Perspectives Newsletter Volume 3, series 3. Mead Johnson Nutritionals. Evansville, Indiana, 2004.

22. Lederman SA et al. Summary of the Presentations at the Conference on Preventing Childhood Obesity, December 8, 2003. Pediatrics. 2004; 114 (4):1146-1173.

23. Whitaker RC. Prediction preschooler obesity at birth: the role of maternal obesity in early pregnancy. Pediatrics. 2004;114(1):e29-e36.

24. Ibid.

25. Salsberry PJ and Reagan PB. Dynamics of early childhood overweight. Pediatrics. 2005; 116(6):1329-1338.

26. Lederman SA et al. Summary of the Presentations at the Conference on Preventing Childhood Obesity, December 8, 2003. Pediatrics. 2004; 114 (4):1146-1173.

27. Harder T, Bergmann R, Kallischnigg and Plagemann A. Duration of breastfeeding and risk of overweight: a meta-analysis. American Journal of Epidemiology. 2005; 162(5):397-403. Available at http://aje.oxfordjournals.org/cgi/content/abstract/162/5/397. Accessed 1-24-06.

28. Okie S. Fed up! Winning the war against childhood obesity. 2005. Washington DC. Joseph Henry Press. Pp 170-172.

29. Mennella JA, Jagnow CJ, Beauchamp GK. Prenatal and postnatal flavor learning by human infants. Pediatrics. 2001;107(6):e88 . Available at: www.pediatrics.org/cgi/content/full/107/6/e88. Accessed 3-05.

30. Ziegler AG, Schmid S, Huber D, Hummel M, Bonifacio E. Early infant feeding and risk of developing type 1 diabetes-associated autoantibodies. Journal of the American Medical Association. 2003; 290(13):1721 –1728

31. Wardle J et al. Increasing children's acceptance of vegetables; a randomized trial of parent-led exposure. Appetite. 2003; April 40(2):155-62

32. American Academy of Pediatrics Committee on Public Education. Children, Adolescents and television. Pediatrics. 2001; 107(2):423-426.

33. Dennison BA, Erb TA and Jenkins PL. Television viewing and television in bedroom associated with overweight risk among low-income preschool children. Pediatrics. 2002; 109(6):1028-1035.

34. Exercise (Physical Activity) and Children. AHA Scientific Position http://www.americanheart.org/presenter.jhtml?identifier=4596. Accessed 4-14-05.

Index

Baby's Only Organic Soy Toddler Formula, 295

Bacteria
    causing food-borne illnesses, 202–203
    cavity formation and, 170
    powdered formula and, 91
    in sprouts, 204

Bacterial meningitis, 20

Baked Oatmeal, 299

Bananas, 211

Barber, Marianne, 166

Barley cereal, 219

Basic Bean Puree, 265–266

Basic Cream Veggie Soup, 267

Basic Fish Recipe, 264

Basic Meat Recipe, 264

Beans
    canned, 262
    cooking, 265–267
    recipes using, 265–266, 267, 269, 303

Bed sharing, 38

Beechnut, 185

Beer, 74

Beet Puree, 244

Behan, Eileen, 36

Bell peppers, 211, 228

Bell-shaped bottle nipples, 84

Berens, Pamela, 69

Berkeley Parents Network, 111

Berry n'Ice, 281

Beta carotene. *See* Vitamin A

Beverages
    dental health and, 169
    introducing a cup and, 222
    maternal weight loss and, 59
    packed in lunches, 328–329
    smoothie recipes, 281, 303, 304, 314, 326
    sweetened, and childhood obesity, 336
    vegetables in, 325

Bibs, 177

Bioavailability, 19

Bird food personality, 307

Birth experience, 25–26, 37–38

Birth injury, 24

Birth site, as part of breastfeeding team, 34–35

Birth to six months, preventing childhood obesity
    during, 339–340

Black Bean Soup, 303

Blankets, 11

Blenders
    cleaning, 192
    grinding brown rice with, 238
    for homemade whole-grain cereal, 224

Blood glucose, 27

Blueberry Sauce, 282

B lymphocytes, 18

Bobo Baby, 185

Body mass index (BMI), 144, 335

Body mass index for age, 145

Body weight. *See* Weight gain (baby); Weight
    loss (baby); Weight loss (mother)

Bone density, 63

Bone growth, 148

Bonyata, Kelly, 74

Books. *See* Resources

Boppy (pillow), 31

Bottle
    cereal in a, 181
    for formula-feeding, 82–83
    introducing breastfed baby to, 108–111
    stopping use of, 222
    switching to a cup from, 292–293

Bottle brushes, 84

Bottle drying rack, 84

Bottle warmer, 84

Botulism, 20

Bowel movements. *See* Poop

Bowel obstruction, 122

Brassica Protection Products, 204

Braun blender, 238

Breast abnormalities, 29

Breast cancer, 6

Breast engorgement, 45–46

Breastfeeding. *see also* Breast milk
    after cesarean section, 25–26
    alcohol intake and, 74
    allergies and, 138
    artificial sweeteners used during, 70–71
    basic guidelines for, 41
    with breast conditions, 28–29
    caffeine intake and, 73
    calcium intake for, 63
    challenges affecting, 7–8, 24–29
    checklist for early, 39
    childhood obesity and, 339–340
    chosen over formula feeding, 4–5
    common questions on, 42–44, 63–66
    continued after going back to work, 98–99
    convenience of, 7
    cost benefits of, 6, 22–23
    determining if baby is drinking during, 44
    with diabetes, 27
    diet for, 66–68
    drugs and, 68
    engorgement and, 45–46
    exposure to chemicals and, 71–72
    expressing wishes on, at birth site, 37
    first feeding and, 38–39
    formula-feeding combined with, 94
    frequency of, 42–43, 45
    gathering information on, 36–37
    gearing up for, 29–33
    GERD in baby and, 132
    global impact of, 22–24
    growth patterns and, 145–146
    health benefits of, 4, 5–6, 21
    how long to breastfeed and, 34
    iron and, 216
    knowing if baby is eating enough and, 43–44
    latching and, 44–45
    length of feedings and, 43
    letdown problems and, 47–48
    mastitis and, 51

Cow's milk
    allergy to, 138
    comparison of alternatives to, 294–295
    cow's milk formula *vs.*, 95
    protein in, 79
    switching to, 293–294
Cow's milk formula, 77, 95, 122
Crackers, 185
Cracker sandwiches, 328
Cradle hold, 39
Cream Carrot-Cauliflower Soup, 301
Cream cheese, 303
Creamy Spinach, 280
Crock-Pot, 189
Cross cradle hold, 39
Crunchy Cream Cheese Spread, 303
Crying, 41. *see also* Colic
Cubed foods, 182
Cup
    introducing a, 221–222
    switching from bottle to, 292–293
Custard recipes, 272
Cutting boards, 196, 198
Cytomegalovirus (CMV), 8

D

Dairy products. *see also* Milk
    allergies to, 73
    choosing low-fat, 321
    introducing, 255–256, 262–263
    snacks with, 311
    storing, 206
Daycare centers, 115–116
*Defining Your Own Success: Breastfeeding after Breast
    Reduction Surgery* (West), 36
Dehydration, 42, 127
Deli meats, 203
Dental health
    candy and, 324
    cavity formation and, 169–170
    drinking from a cup and, 292
    plaque and, 260
    teeth brushing and, 170–171
    teething and, 167–169
    of toddlers, 323–324
    visiting a dentist and, 170
Dentists, 170
Deoxyribonucleic acid (DNA), 19
Depression, 28
DHA. *See* Docosahexaenoic acid (DHA)
DHA supplements, 64
Diabetes, 8, 20, 27
Diapering
    changing cloth diapers and, 121
    place for, 11
Diapering supplies, 11
Diarrhea, 20
    causes of, 123–124
    dehydration and, 127
    diagnosis of, 123
    formula-feeding and, 129

prevention of, 128
    treatment for, 124–126
Diary, food, 59
Diced family fare, 194
Diet
    baby's sensitivity to mother's, 52–53, 123, 129
    balancing physical activity with, 275
    best breastfeeding, 66–68
    breast milk affected by mother's, 61–63
    choosing from every food group for, 275
    colic and, 140
    for eleven-month-old, 277–278
    fad, 152–153
    with food allergies, 163–166
    gas and, 130
    getting most nutrition from calories and, 275–276
    of nine-month-olds, 258
    of one-year-old, 284
    of six-to-eight-month olds, 231–233
    of a ten-month-old, 258
    of two-year-old, 321–323
    of vegan ten-month-old, 259
    vegetarian. *See* Vegan/vegetarian diet
Dietary fiber, in formula, 81
Dietary reference intake (DRI), 156, 295
Dietary supplements. *See* Supplements, dietary
Digestive symptoms, 219
Digestive system, 52–53. *see also* Poop
Dinnertime
    de-stressing, 308–309
    importance of family, 296–297
Dioxins, 210
Dips
    Spinach Dip, 300
    Strawberry Crème Dip, 302
    vegetables in, 325
    veggie, 313
Dishwashing, 197, 200
Disposable pads, 30, 82
Distillation water treatment, 87
Distilled water, 87, 88
Docosahexaenoic acid (DHA)
    in breast milk, 5, 17
    commercial baby foods with, 185
    in eggs, 229
    in infant formula, 79, 81
    mother's diet and, 62
    vegan diet and, 159
Doctor (baby's), 33–34
Down syndrome, 7, 24
DRI. *See* Dietary reference intake (DRI)
Dried fruit, 245
Drinker food personality, 307
Drinking water, 87
Drinks. *See* Beverages
Drugs and Lactation (LactMed) Database, 69
Drugs, breastfeeding and, 8, 69. *see also* Medication
Drugs in Pregnancy and Lactation
    (Briggs/Freeman/Yaffee), 69
Drug Therapy and Breastfeeding (Ilett/Hale), 69
D-Tagatose, 71

Also from Meadowbrook Press

Eating Expectantly, by dietitian Bridget Swinney, offers a practical and tasty approach to prenatal nutrition, combining nutrition guidelines for each trimester with 200 complete menus, 85 tasty recipes, plus cooking and shopping tips. Cited by *Child* magazine as one of the "10 best parenting books of 1993," *Eating Expectantly* is newly revised with the most current nutrition information.

Healthy Food for Healthy Kids, by dietitian Bridget Swinney, offers a practical guide to selecting and preparing healthy meals for kids and teaching healthy attitudes toward food. More than just a cookbook, this is a user-friendly book with real-world advice for parents who want their children to eat better.

Breastfeeding with Confidence is a practical guide to breastfeeding that's designed to provide new mothers with the practical skills and confidence they need to have a positive breastfeeding experience. Internationally known lactation expert Sue Cox explains both the art and the method of breastfeeding, and addresses the fact that making milk comes naturally but breastfeeding is a learned skill. She provides invaluable information, advice, resources, and encouragement for new mothers.

100,000+ Baby Names is the #1 baby name book and is the most complete guide for helping you name your baby. It contains over 100,000 popular and unusual names from around the world, complete with origins, meanings, variations, and famous namesakes. It also includes the most recently available top 100 names for girls and boys, as well as over 300 helpful lists of names to consider and avoid.

Feed Me! I'm Yours is an easy-to-use, economical guide to making baby food at home. More than 200 recipes cover everything a parent needs to know about teething foods, nutritious snacks, and quick, pleasing lunches. Now recently revised.

First-Year Baby Care is one of the leading baby-care books to guide you through your baby's first year. It contains complete information on the basics of baby care, including bathing, diapering, medical facts, and feeding your baby. Now recently revised.

The Toddler's Busy Book, ***The Preschooler's Busy Book***, ***The Arts and Crafts Busy Book***, and ***The Wiggle & Giggle Busy Book*** each contain 365 activities (one for each day of the year) for your children, using items found around the home. The books offer parents and child-care providers fun reading, math, and science activities that will stimulate a child's natural curiosity. They also provide great activities for indoor play during even the longest stretches of bad weather!

Baby Play and Learn, by child-development expert Penny Warner, offers ideas for games and activities that will provide hours of developmental learning opportunities and fun for babies. The book contains step-by-step instructions, illustrations, and bulleted lists of skills your baby will learn through play activities.

**We offer many more titles written to delight, inform, and entertain.
To order books with a credit card or browse our full
selection of titles, visit our website at:**

www.meadowbrookpress.com

or call toll free to place an order, request a free catalog, or ask a question:

1-800-338-2232

Meadowbrook Press • 5451 Smetana Drive • Minnetonka, MN • 55343